EXERCISE THERAPY

Prevention and treatment of disease

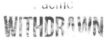

EXERCISE THERAPY

Prevention and treatment of disease

Edited by

John Gormley and Juliette Hussey

School of Physiotherapy, Trinity Centre for Health Sciences,
University of Dublin, Trinity College

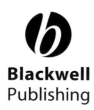

Blackwell
Publishing

© 2005 by Blackwell Publishing Ltd

Editorial offices:
Blackwell Publishing Ltd, 9600 Garsington Road, Oxford OX4 2DQ, UK
 Tel: +44 (0)1865 776868
Blackwell Publishing Inc., 350 Main Street, Malden, MA 02148-5020, USA
 Tel: +1 781 388 8250
Blackwell Publishing Asia Pty Ltd, 550 Swanston Street, Carlton, Victoria 3053, Australia
 Tel: +61 (0)3 8359 1011

First published 2005 by Blackwell Publishing Ltd

Library of Congress Cataloging-in-Publication Data
Exercise therapy: prevention and treatment of disease/edited by John Gormley and
Juliette Hussey.
  p. ; cm.
Includes bibliographical references and index.
ISBN 1-4051-0527-5 (pbk. : alk. paper)
1. Exercise therapy. I. Gormley, John. II. Hussey, Juliette.
[DNLM: 1. Exercise Therapy. 2. Preventive Medicine. WB 541 E96 2004]
RM725.E95 2004
615.8′2–dc22
2004015072

ISBN-10: 1-4051-0527-5
ISBN-13: 978-1-4051-0527-9

A catalogue record for this title is available from the British Library

Set in 10/12.5 pt Sabon
by Graphicraft Limited, Hong Kong
Printed and bound in India
by Replika Press Pvt Ltd

The publisher's policy is to use permanent paper from mills that operate a sustainable
forestry policy, and which has been manufactured from pulp processed using acid-free
and elementary chlorine-free practices. Furthermore, the publisher ensures that the text
paper and cover board used have met acceptable environmental accreditation standards.

For further information on Blackwell Publishing, visit our website:
www.blackwellpublishing.com

CONTENTS

PREFACE

Exercise has always been one of the key skills of physiotherapy. The use of exercise in the treatment of musculoskeletal disorders and acquired cardiorespiratory diseases is a theme of most undergraduate physiotherapy courses. Today, healthcare faces new challenges with the increased prevalence of other acquired disorders such as obesity, diabetes and osteoporosis. Physiotherapists therefore need the knowledge and skills to effectively deal with these conditions. Furthermore, in the area of neurological rehabilitation, where treatment was previously aimed at the restoration of movement, there is now a new focus on the promotion of physical activity and exercise training.

This book explores the use of exercise in the treatment of the above conditions. The use of exercise in the prevention of many of these conditions is also documented. This emphasis on prevention as well as treatment is essential. Physical inactivity is an independent risk factor for coronary heart disease, while physical activity can positively effect risk factors such as hypertension, hyperlipidaemia and obesity. As health professionals, it is our responsibility to advise when necessary on the positive health benefits of exercise and prescribe an appropriate programme. To recommend a programme of exercise, knowledge of the assessment of physical activity is required. It is also important to be aware of factors that influence participation in exercise. This text examines these issues so as to optimise the physiotherapist's exercise prescription.

During the assessment of patients the physiotherapist may discover that lack of physical activity may be a contributory factor to the presenting complaint. Patients who have been prescribed exercise may present with comorbities such as pain in weight bearing joints which require consideration in the prescription of exercise. With their clinical background, physiotherapists are uniquely placed to manage such scenarios. This text aims to enable the physiotherapist to manage conditions through the use of exercise as a preventative measure and as a treatment modality.

In editing this book we hope we have provided the reader with a useful text that informs both the undergraduate student and the clinician. It will also provide a reference text for students in the areas of health promotion, sports science, physical activity and exercise rehabilitation.

John Gormley
Juliette Hussey

ACKNOWLEDGEMENTS

The editors wish to thank everyone associated with this book. Thanks to all the contributors, whose expertise is evident throughout the chapters. Thank you to Mr Peter Yung and our colleagues at Trinity College and associated hospitals for creating an environment that is conducive to a venture of this nature. To all at Blackwell Publishing: Amy Brown, Lisa Whittington and our editorial project manager, Shahzia Chaudhri. We must express our gratitude to Caroline Connelly, the commissioning editor, for her help and patience over the last two years.

The support of our families has been immense. Thank you to our sisters and brothers. A special word of thanks to our parents for their help and encouragement, both during this project and throughout the years. One regret is that John Gormley (Snr) did not live to see the book in print. Finally, thanks to Berna and Garry, Robert and Gavin for their love, understanding and patience, without which this book would never have been completed.

CONTRIBUTORS

Editors

John Gormley BSc(Hons), MA, DPhil, Lecturer, School of Physiotherapy, Faculty of Health Sciences, Trinity College, Dublin, Ireland

Juliette Hussey MSc, MA, MISCP, Head of Department, School of Physiotherapy, Faculty of Health Sciences, Trinity College, Dublin, Ireland

Contributing authors

Tony Ashton BSc(Hons), PhD, SRD, Head of Department of Sport Science, Bedford Faculty, De Montfort University, Bedford, UK

Christopher Bell PhD, DSc, FTCD, Professor of Physiology, Faculty of Health Sciences, Trinity College, Dublin, Ireland

Judy M. Bradley PhD, MCSP, Lecturer/Practitioner in Cardiopulmonary Physiotherapy, School of Rehabilitation Sciences, University of Ulster, Jordanstown Campus, Newtownabbey, and Belfast City Hospital, Northern Ireland

Margaret G. Brownlee BA, DipTP, MCSP, Lecturer, Division of Physiotherapy, School of Health and Social Care, Glasgow Caledonian University, Glasgow, UK

Gareth W. Davison BA(Hons), MSc, PhD, Lecturer in Exercise Physiology, School of Applied Medical Sciences and Sports Studies, University of Ulster, Jordanstown Campus, Newtownabbey, Northern Ireland

Lindsey Dugdill BA, MA, MPhil, PhD, Reader in Exercise and Health, School of Community, Health Sciences and Social Care, Faculty of Health and Social Care, University of Salford, UK

Brian Durward MSc, PhD, MCSP, Head of School of Health and Social Care, Glasgow Caledonian University, Glasgow, UK

Rebecca Graham BSc, Research Institute for Sport and Exercise Sciences, Liverpool John Moores University, Liverpool, UK

Richard J. Hawksworth BSc, Respiratory Scientist, Department of Respiratory Medicine, Adelaide & Meath Hospital, Dublin, Ireland

Ciara M. Hughes BMedsci, MMedsci, PhD, Lecturer in Clinical Physiology, School of Applied Medical Sciences and Sports Studies, University of Ulster, Jordanstown Campus, Newtownabbey, Northern Ireland

Stephen J. Lane MB, PhD, FRCP, MRCPI, Consultant Respiratory Physician, Department of Respiratory Medicine, Adelaide & Meath Hospital, Dublin, Ireland

Fidelma Moran BSc(Hons), MCSP, PGCUT, Lecturer in Physiotherapy, School of Rehabilitation Sciences, University of Ulster, Jordanstown Campus, Newtownabbey, Northern Ireland

John Nolan BSc, MB, FRCPI, Associate Professor, Metabolic Research Unit, Department of Clinical Medicine and Department of Biochemistry, Trinity College, Dublin, and Consultant Endocrinologist, St James's Hospital, Dublin, Ireland

Donal O'Gorman BSc, MSc, Lecturer, Centre for Sport Science and Health, Dublin City University, Ireland

Brenda O'Neill BSc(Hons), MCSP, Lecturer, School of Rehabilitation Sciences, University of Ulster, Jordanstown Campus, Newtownabbey, Northern Ireland

Saoirse E. O' Sullivan BA, PhD, Research Fellow in Cardiovascular Science, School of Biomedical Sciences, Queen's Medical Centre, Nottingham, UK

Alison Quinn BA, BSc, MISCP, Senior Physiotherapist, Weight Management Service, St. Columcille's Hospital, Loughlinstown, Ireland

Fiona Wilson-O'Toole BSc, MSc, MCSP, MISCP, Lecturer, School of Physiotherapy, Faculty of Health Sciences, Trinity College, Dublin, Ireland

SECTION 1

Chapter 1

INTRODUCTION

Juliette Hussey

Key words: physical activity, exercise, physical fitness.

Exercise as a part of physiotherapy

Physiotherapy originally developed from three key areas: massage, medical gymnastics and electrotherapy. The early examination system emphasised the diversity of the profession with separate qualifications in these three areas. Historically, the Chartered Society of Physiotherapy began in 1894 as the Society of Trained Masseuses and became the Incorporated Society of Trained Masseuses in 1900. In 1920 exercise was formally recognised as part of the profession and the Society became the Chartered Society of Massage and Medical Gymnastics. In 1944 this was renamed the Chartered Society of Physiotherapy. In 1985 the SRGRT (Society of Remedial Gymnasts and Recreational Therapists) voted and agreed on the merger with the CSP. Therefore, in 1986 the Remedial Gymnasts Board was formally disbanded by Parliament and remedial gymnasts became members of the CSP.

In 1994 the profession reached its centenary and this provided the Chartered Society of Physiotherapy with an opportunity to reflect on its origins and the changes that had occurred since its birth. New methods and theories have come in and out of vogue in the physiotherapy management of patients and sometimes . . . 'Fashion, prejudice and ignorance, rather than scientific reasoning, often dictate practice or dismiss new modalities that could be valuable assets' (Thornton, 1994). There is sufficient scientific reasoning and evidence to support the use of exercise therapy in the prevention and treatment of many chronic diseases.

If we now try to look forward and predict the role of physiotherapists in 100 years time it is possible that we will be more involved in the prevention of disease. Advising on how to maintain health may become a higher priority than the traditional curative role (Wise and Hemmings, 1994). Indeed, this is already occurring, particularly in the area of ergonomics. However, the prevention of many chronic diseases that are becoming ever more prevalent in Western societies should also become a focus for the profession.

Exercise recommendations for health

It is necessary to define the concepts of 'physical activity' and 'exercise'. Physical activity is defined as body movement produced by skeletal muscles and resulting in energy expenditure (Caspersen et al., 1985). Exercise is defined as a subclass of physical activity that includes planned, structured and repetitive bodily movement, which is done to improve or maintain one or more components of physical fitness (ACSM, 2000). Recommendations for exercise have moved from emphasising vigorous activity for cardiorespiratory fitness to the option of moderate levels of activity for health benefits. The ACSM recommend that people of all ages accumulate 30 minutes of moderate physical activity on most, if not all, days of the week. Brisk walking is an example of the type of activity recommended and can easily be incorporated into most people's lives. Examples of activities that can be included in this recommendation are stair climbing, gardening, household chores, as well as activities such as swimming, cycling and playing sports. The greatest health benefits from an increase in activity occur when those most sedentary begin a regular programme of moderate intensity activity. Adherence to a regular programme is essential as the health benefits are quickly lost on cessation of activity.

Physical activity and its health benefits

Today much is known about the beneficial effects of physical activity in the prevention of many acquired diseases, but it would appear that this knowledge has not influenced the behaviours of the vast majority of the population of the developed world. Indeed, unprecedented levels of inactivity are being seen. The prevalence of people who are overweight and obese worldwide is increasing at such a dramatic rate that it is now considered a global epidemic. The increased prevalence is seen both in developed and less developed countries, as the latter evolve towards westernisation (International Obesity Task Force (IOTF, 2003). It is estimated that there were 200 million adults worldwide with obesity in 1995. By 2000 this figure had increased to 300 million. In developing countries it is estimated that more than 115 million people suffer from problems related to obesity (IOTF, 2003). The incidence of obesity in Europe in the last decade has increased by about 10–40% in most European countries, with the most significant increase seen in the United Kingdom, where it has doubled since 1980 (IOTF, 2003). In the United States it is estimated that 19.8% of adults were obese in 2000, which represents an increase of 61% since 1991 (Mokdad et al., 2001). This figure continues to rise (Mokdad et al., 2003). In children, increasing levels of obesity and accompanying health consequences are of considerable concern. Obesity in children has been linked to sedentary behaviours. Current data suggest that 20% of children in the US are overweight (Goran, 2001). In England, between 1984 and 1994, there was an increase from 5% to 9% and 9% to 13% in obesity levels in boys and girls respectively (Chinn and Rona, 2001). Even in children as young as four years of age there had been a significant increase in weight and body mass index between 1989 and 1998

(Bundred et al., 2001). Booth et al. (2001) state that the prevalence of chronic diseases linked to physical inactivity is increasing so rapidly that the costs to US society will be greater than $1 trillion (one thousand million) in the next decade. In terms of human cost it has been estimated that there are 250 000 deaths in the US annually as a result of physical inactivity (Booth et al., 2001). In the European Union a study involving 15 239 adults found obesity and higher body weight were strongly associated with a sedentary lifestyle (Martinez-Gonzalez et al., 1999).

The cost of obesity to the individual, society, the health service and the economy is significant. Health problems associated with obesity include cardiovascular, respiratory, musculoskeletal, metabolic and psychological disorders. Mortality and morbidity rates also increase with increasing levels of obesity. It is estimated that 2–8% of total sick care costs in Western countries can be attributed to obesity (IOTF, 2003). One of the most common health problems associated with obesity is the development of diabetes mellitus. In the US, the prevalence of this disease has increased from 4.9% in 1990 to 7.3% in 2000 (Mokdad et al., 2001). In the European Union 42% of all deaths are attributed to cardiovascular disease. Lack of weight-bearing exercise is associated with osteoporosis, and the National Osteoporosis Society estimates that 3 million people in the UK suffer from osteoporosis, costing the NHS and Government over £1.7 billion each year.

There is, therefore, an onus on health professionals to utilise every opportunity to prescribe exercise when involved with individuals with chronic diseases or with risk factors for these conditions. Combating the global epidemic of type 2 diabetes may be one of the greatest health care challenges of this century.

How physical activity levels have decreased

Throughout history humans have been physically active, from the hunter gatherer way of life, to active farming, to the industrial revolution just over 100 years ago. Both hunting and farming also involved travelling great distances by foot. Nowadays few occupations demand physical work. Technological advances have decreased the need for physical labour and therefore there is a need to schedule exercise/physical activity into our lives. In the home, over the past 40 years, there has been an increase in labour-saving devices such as dishwashers, vacuum cleaners and even automatic lawnmowers.

Motorised transport is dominant and people often try to find the closest parking spot to the door (for example, at the supermarket). In some cases now we do not even have to push a trolley up and down the aisles of a supermarket, pack bags, and load them in and then out of our car, as we can shop online, only having to move the mouse around the virtual supermarket. In shopping centres and malls people are willing to queue for the escalators or lifts rather than walk up usually empty stairs. At work many sit at desks for prolonged periods, communicating documents by email, thereby removing the need to walk to the fax machine. Communication with colleagues at work is by email instead of walking along the corridor to another office.

There is increased concern for personal security, particularly of children, and therefore they are often driven short distances to school. Concerns about safety may result in discouraging spontaneous play outdoors unless in the garden or supervised by an adult. Many children have little free time as they are ferried from one after school activity to another. Any free time is often spent in front of the television, without even moving to change the channel. This should cause concern as more than two hours spent sedentary in front of the television has been correlated to increased body fat in children (Andersen et al., 1998).

We increasingly need to build in leisure time activity in a world with more choices and less time for leisure. Despite the frequent claim that there is little leisure time which can be devoted to exercise, many adults, nonetheless, engage many hours passively in front of the television.

The future

Epidemiological evidence supports the importance of regular physical activity in the prevention of many acquired chronic diseases and in the enhancement of overall health (Southern et al., 1999). Physical inactivity is an independent risk factor for coronary heart disease (Paffenbarger, 1993) and regular physical activity has been shown to reduce the risk of hypertension, type 2 diabetes and to maintain optimal bone mineral density. Type 2 diabetes, previously only seen in middle to old age is now being seen in teenagers (Pinhas-Hamiel et al., 1996), dramatically affecting quality of lives and set to place an enormous strain on health services. Regular physical activity can relieve symptoms of depression and in the elderly it may reduce the risk of falling. For patients with osteoarthritis regular physical activity is necessary for maintaining normal muscle strength, joint structure and joint function.

Exercise should be considered, for the vast majority, to prevent disease. It is an inexpensive intervention strategy which could help to prevent more costly treatments later on. This economic gain has been appreciated by many American companies who have established worksite exercise programmes to reduce health insurance premiums. It is not sufficient just to advise individuals to be more active. In many cases there is a need to measure activity levels and prescribe individualised programmes which are re-evaluated and progressed at regular intervals.

With the rise in obesity and type 2 diabetes physiotherapists are well suited to have a dramatic effect on the health of individuals and help in the prevention of many acquired diseases, through the promotion of activity. Physiotherapists are ideally positioned and educated for this. As physiotherapists have professional autonomy and are often the first point of contact for many patients then it could be argued that it is our professional responsibility to advise the patient on risk factors they present with and those that are discovered as part of the physiotherapy assessment. Even if we are not the first point of contact the GP may only see the patient for a short period of time and may not address the risk factors of inactivity. The health professional needs an understanding of what exercise is, its health benefits and how to prescribe appropriate exercise for the individual.

In children, the increasing levels of obesity and the accompanying health consequences are of considerable concern. Obesity in children has been linked to sedentary behaviours. The importance of daily physical activity cannot be overstressed and daily physical education in schools would go some way to providing this.

In this book the argument is presented for exercise as an essential component in both the prevention and treatment of many of the diseases that are common today. In Section One, the physiology of exercise is outlined in relation to the cardiovascular system, the pulmonary system and the musculoskeletal system, as is the theory behind exercise in diabetes and obesity. In Section Two, the application of exercise in conditions affecting these systems are described. Chapter 6 discusses the measurement of exercise capacity and activity, introduces the reader to the evaluation of the patient, and sets the scene for Chapter 7 on exercise prescription. Chapters 8–12 examine the role of exercise in various clinical conditions. The issues surrounding adherence to exercise and health promotion are described in the final chapters.

References

American College of Sports Medicine (2000). *Guidelines for Exercise Testing and Prescription*, 6th edn. Lippincott Williams and Wilkins, Baltimore.

Andersen, R.E., Crespo, C.J., Bartlett, S.J., Cheskin, L.J. and Pratt, M. (1998). Relationship of physical activity and television watching with body weight and level of fatness among children. *Journal of American Medical Association* 279, 938–42.

Booth, F.W., Gordon, S.E., Carlson, C.J. and Hamilton, M.T. (2001). Waging war on modern chronic diseases: primary prevention through exercise biology. *Journal of Applied Physiology* 88, 774–87.

Bundred, P., Kitchiner, S.D. and Buchan, I. (2001). Prevalence of overweight and obese children between 1989 and 1998: population based series of cross sectional studies. *British Medical Journal* 322, 313–4.

Caspersen, C.J., Powell, K.E. and Christenson, G.M. (1985). Physical activity, exercise, and physical fitness: Definitions and distinctions for health-related research. *Public Health Reports* 100, 126–31.

Chinn, S. and Rona, R.J. (2001). Prevalence and trends in overweight and obesity in three cross sectional studies of British children, 1974–94. *British Medical Journal* 322, 24–6.

Goran, M.I. (2001). Metabolic precursors and effects of obesity in children: a decade of progress, 1990–1999. *American Journal of Clinical Nutrition* 73, 158–71.

International Obesity Task Force (2003). www.iotf.org

Martinez-Gonzalez, M.A., Alfredo Martinez, J., Hu, F.B., Gibney, M.J. and Kearney, J. (1999). Physical inactivity, sedentary lifestyle and obesity in the European Union. *International Journal of Obesity and Related Metabolic Disorders*, 23, 1192–1201.

Mokdad, A.H., Bowman, B.A., Ford, E.S., Vinicor, F., Marks, J.S. and Koplan, J.P. (2001). The continuing epidemics of obesity and diabetes in the United States. *Journal of American Medical Association* 286, 1195–200.

Mokdad, A.H., Ford, E.S., Bowman, B.A., Dietz, W.H., Vinicor, F., Bales, V.S. and Marks, J.S. (2003). Prevalence of obesity, diabetes and obesity – related health factors, 2001. *Journal of American Medical Association* 289, 76–9.

Paffenbarger, R.S., Hyde, R.T., Wing, A.L., Lee, I.M., Jung, D.L. and Kampert, J.B. (1993). The association of changes in physical activity level and other lifestyle characteristics with mortality among men. *New England Journal of Medicine* **328**, 538–45.

Pinhas-Hamiel, O., Dolan, L.M., Daniels, S.R., Standiford, D., Khoury, P.R. and Zeitler, P. (1996). Increased incidence of non-insulin-dependent diabetes mellitus among adolescents. *The Journal of Pediatrics* **128**, 608–15.

Southern, M.S., Loftin, M., Suskind, R.M., Udall, J.N. and Blecher, U. (1999). The health benefits of physical activity in children and adolescents: implications for chronic disease prevention. *European Journal of Pediatrics* **158**(4), April, 271–4.

Thornton, E. (1994). 100 years of Physiotherapy Education. *Physiotherapy* **80**, 11A–19A.

Wise, J. and Hemmings, G. (1994). Physiotherapy to 2094. *Physiotherapy* **80**, 100A–101A.

Bibliography

Oxford Concise Medical Dictionary (1996). Oxford University Press, Oxford, New York.

Chapter 2

CARDIOVASCULAR RESPONSES TO EXERCISE

Christopher Bell and Saoirse E. O'Sullivan

Key words: cardiac output, central adaptations, peripheral adaptations.

Introduction

Undertaking physical exercise requires a number of cardiovascular adjustments. First, and most obviously, there must be increased regional blood flow in order to provide for the metabolic demands of the active muscles. Second, the effect of this regional hyperaemia on systemic distribution of cardiac output must be compensated for, so as to sustain adequate perfusion of other aerobic organ systems. Third, preventing hyperthermia due to metabolic heat produced by muscle activity requires elevation of skin blood flow. Finally, pulmonary ventilation/perfusion matching has to be optimised in order to ensure that gas exchange matches the elevated metabolic demands.

All of the above adjustments are seen most dramatically in response to dynamic exercise (for example, walking or running) and constitute an important part of the therapeutic approach to patient care. Resistive exercise (for example, weightlifting) initiates a similar pattern of underlying processes, but their final manifestation is distorted by the static nature of the exercise and may under some circumstances be deleterious to the patient.

In this chapter we will discuss the various cardiovascular responses to acute exercise and consider the influences of chronic activity (training), gender and age on cardiovascular variables. No attempt will be made to detail the basics of cardiovascular structure and function; it is presumed that the reader is familiar with these and, in the case of any doubt, information can readily be obtained from any one of the numerous textbooks of physiology for students of health sciences. For reference, two flow diagrams are included which summarise the interrelationships between the various acute and chronic cardiovascular responses to exercise (Figs 2.1, 2.2).

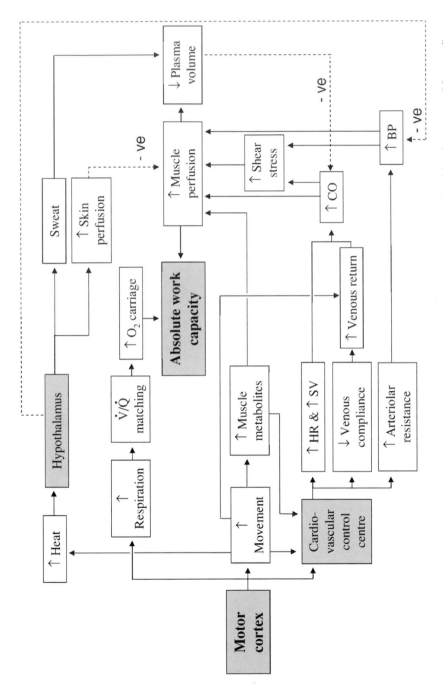

Figure 2.1 Interaction of the various factors in cardiovascular response to acute exercise. BP– blood pressure, CO – cardiac output, HR – heart rate, SV– stroke volume, $\dot{V}/\dot{Q}$ – ventilation:perfusion ratio.

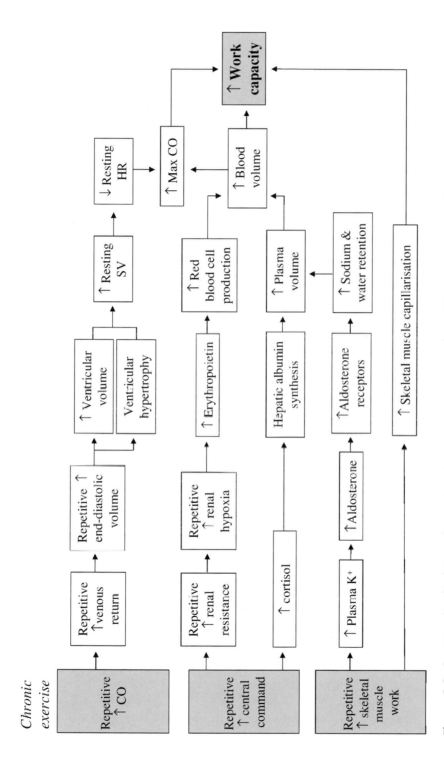

Figure 2.2 Processes involved in cardiovascular adaptations to chronic exercise. CO – cardiac output, HR – heart rate, SV – stroke volume.

Acute exercise

Muscle blood flow

At rest, blood flow through the skeletal musculature is only around 20% of cardiac output, despite the fact that muscle typically represents about 60% of body mass. This relatively low level perfusion is due primarily to the fact that the muscle bed is a major site of sympathetically mediated vascular resistance associated with baroreflex regulation of blood pressure. The ongoing sympathetic vasoconstrictor drive also overrides the critical closing pressure for many terminal arterioles, with the result that only a fraction of the capillary bed is perfused.

During aerobic muscle activity, regional blood flow increases proportionately to the elevation of metabolism to attain peak values of the order of 20 times that at rest (typically around 25–50 ml/min per 100 ml tissue). This hyperaemia represents both an overall decrease in arteriolar vascular resistance and perfusion of previously non-perfused capillaries. The dominant hyperaemic stimulus is a rise in interstitial concentration of metabolic by-products, which include potassium ions, adenine breakdown molecules, protons, lactate and phosphates. No single factor appears to be the primary dilator mediator and probably the end result is due as much to an overall dilator effect of elevated interstitial osmolarity as it is to the chemical actions of individual factors. There is also a dilator effect of reduced interstitial oxygen tension, mediated through specific hypoxia receptors on the vascular smooth muscle cells. In addition to these metabolically linked contributors to hyperaemia, the reduced vascular resistance in exercising muscle itself leads to further dilation, since the increased blood flow exerts shear stress on the precapillary endothelium, which releases local dilator factors such as nitric oxide (NO).

The traditional viewpoint has been that the dilator potency of these various factors overrides any vasoconstrictor effect of ongoing sympathetic discharge. Techniques of regional denervation, however, indicate convincingly that there is flow limitation by sympathetic activity at all workloads of whole-body exercise and that muscle perfusion is appreciably enhanced by removal of this sympathetic input (O'Sullivan and Bell, 2000). However, there does not appear to be sympathetic limitation of local flow when only small muscle groups are activated, suggesting that activation of sympathetic drive to muscle occurs only in compensation for large falls in peripheral resistance due to high levels of muscle hyperaemia. It is still uncertain whether this flow limitation has a concomitant limiting influence on whole-body aerobic work capacity.

Anticipation of exercise has been shown to provoke, at least in certain individuals, an increase in muscle blood flow that is not restricted to the muscles that will be activated. Additionally, some evidence has shown that the time course of hyperaemia at the onset of exercise is too rapid (1–2 sec) to be caused by the release of metabolic vasodilators (> 4 sec). The mechanisms underlying this response are a matter of some debate, with some studies supporting a role of active dilator processes (either neural or via circulating adrenaline) and others suggesting passive dilation by withdrawal of vasoconstrictor tone (Joyner and Halliwill, 2000; O'Sullivan and

Bell, 2000). It is possible that this response has some biological significance, but at present no evidence exists to suggest that it contributes functionally to the efficiency of subsequent exercise.

Because cardiac muscle relies entirely on aerobic metabolism, it is of utmost importance that coronary blood flow matches cardiac energy demands. As in working skeletal muscle, a number of local metabolites and dilators such as NO, adenosine and endothelial-derived hyperpolarising factor, are released and act locally to increase coronary conductance. Additionally, up to around 25% of cardiac hyperaemia arises from noradrenaline, released by sympathetic nerve endings in the cardiac muscle, acting on coronary beta-adrenoreceptors. Thus, the sympathetic activity that increases cardiac contractility also directly causes coronary vasodilation, in a feed-forward manner.

Systemic circulatory adjustments

During exercise, the motor cortex influences the cardiovascular control centre in the hindbrain to modulate cardiac function. There is withdrawal of vagal cardio-inhibitory drive and increased sympathetic cardio-excitatory drive to the sinoatrial node, increasing heart rate. As heart rate rises there is concomitant progressive shortening of the ventricular action potential plateau from its resting value of around 350 msec to around 200 msec at maximal heart rate. This decreased systolic period is essential for maintained ventricular filling in the face of a greatly reduced diastolic period.

Sympathetic activation also increases cardiac muscle cell contractility and speeds up Purkinje system conduction, leading to increased efficiency of cardiac emptying. In parallel, cardiac filling is enhanced by compression of lower limb veins through contraction of the surrounding muscles and by the increased pressure gradient for venous return generated by exaggerated inspiratory movements. Especially at low workloads, when filling time is not so constrained, the consequent increase in end-diastolic volume acts through the Frank-Starling relationship to further increase stroke volume. During swimming, the contributions of muscle pumping and thoracic suction to venous return are somewhat less than during upright terrestrial exercise, but instead there is mobilisation of blood from veins in the body wall due to external compression and absence of any tendency for gravitational pooling because of the horizontal posture. These increases in stroke volume and heart rate together increase cardiac output, with tachycardia contributing around 60–70% of the total increase in an untrained individual.

Descending inputs from the motor cortex to the cardiovascular control centre also activate sympathetic vasoconstrictor nerves to the peripheral vasculature, most dramatically in the abdominal viscera (the splanchnic circulation), with associated marked reduction of blood flow through these tissues. For example, the normal blood flow to the kidneys of around one litre per minute can be reduced to as little as 250 ml per minute during heavy exercise. Although the coronary and cerebral beds receive innervation from the sympathetic nervous system, these nerves appear to be exempted from the sympathetic activation initiated from the hindbrain centre. Sympathetic vasoconstriction in working skeletal muscles is largely counteracted by the simultaneous local dilator factors (see section on muscle blood flow, p. 12).

Sympathetic activation also affects function of segments of the vascular tree other than precapillary resistance vessels. In the proximal aorta there is reduced wall compliance, reinforcing the rise in peak systolic pressure that follows from increased stroke volume; in the veins there is reduced capacitance, increasing effective circulating blood volume. Collectively these changes, together with the elevated heart rate, provide for diastolic arterial blood pressure to be maintained despite the large absolute reduction in total peripheral resistance that is associated with skeletal muscle hyperaemia. Because of the increased systolic pressure, mean blood pressure also increases, so the pressure gradient for tissue perfusion is somewhat elevated; a useful safety factor under circumstances where the external compression of blood vessels by skeletal muscles means that muscle perfusion is phasic rather than continuous. This situation demands that the sympathetic discharge resulting from motor activation is accompanied by depression of arterial baroreflex drive. The baroreceptors normally respond to changes in arterial pressure only below a value of around 150 mmHg (Chapleau and Abboud, 2001). During exercise, by contrast, a combination of descending motor command and input from limb receptors resets the reflex so that it operates in a higher pressure range, the absolute level of which is proportional to exercise intensity. The resetting is probably irrelevant to blood pressure control during exercise, since the exercise-induced sympathetic activation and the impact of mechanical factors on venous return would override any other factors. It may, on the other hand, contribute to the rapidity of restoration of resting heart rate and blood pressure in the immediate post-exercise period.

The systemic sympathetic activation secondary to motor cortex activation is enhanced by other excitatory inputs to the hindbrain cardiovascular centre. During dynamic exercise, there is discharge of receptors in the moving limbs at a rate that reflects the acceleration and magnitude of joint movement. Also, the skeletal muscle interstitium contains chemoreceptive axons that are activated by accumulation of acidic metabolites. This combination of sensory modalities, each providing inputs with an intensity proportional to muscle activation, ensures that cardiovascular performance is matched to the demands of exercise.

In addition to the direct effects of sympathetic nerve fibres on heart and vasculature, the same process of descending sympathetic activation releases adrenaline into the circulation from the adrenal medulla. This reinforces sympathetic cardioexcitation. In the vasculature, the circulating adrenaline has dual effects. In most beds it augments the neurally induced vasoconstriction via alpha-adrenoreceptors but, in skeletal and cardiac muscle, where beta-adrenoreceptors exist in large numbers, it tends to induce vasodilation and so supplements the hyperaemic action of local factors.

Pulmonary circulatory adjustments

The same descending excitatory signals from the motor cortex that activate limb muscles and systemic cardiovascular responses also influence the respiratory centres, leading to increased depth of ventilation. This has several consequences for the pulmonary circulation. First, dilution of dead-space air during inspiration results in an increase in alveolar PO_2, causing vasodilation of the pulmonary arteriolar bed by withdrawal of activation of vascular hypoxia receptors. Second, the increased thoracic volume during inspiration expands areas of lung parenchyma that are partially collapsed at rest, with resultant reduction of arteriolar resistance in that section of the pulmonary vasculature. Third, there is increased right heart filling due to increased inspiratory suction. This, together with the other processes discussed above that elevate venous return, increases right ventricular ejection volume and pulmonary systolic pressure. This leads to more efficient perfusion of areas of the pulmonary bed that are gravitationally above the level of the heart. Collectively, these changes therefore result in more efficient ventilation:perfusion matching and a reduction in the right ventricular work that is needed to match right heart cardiac output to the systemic demands.

Cardiovascular limitations to acute exercise

Due to the existence of anaerobic metabolic pathways in many muscle fibres, whole-body exercise can be performed for a short period at an intensity that is far in excess of the capacity of the circulation to deliver oxygen and remove muscle waste products. Beyond that time, however, muscle performance is strictly determined by circulatory performance and so the maximal workload sustainable can be described in terms of the factors that limit elevation of cardiac output and maintenance of blood pressure, and hence the delivery of fresh blood to the working muscle.

Limits to heart rate

The maximal heart rate attainable is determined by the maximum discharge frequency of the sinoatrial pacemaker cells. This allows a rate of around 220–240 bpm at birth but the maximum decreases progressively with age. For normal adults, it can be approximated as being (220 bpm – age in years) for subjects of average build or (200 bpm – 0.5 age in years) for obese subjects (Plowman and Smith, 2003). Since the sympathetically mediated shortening of ventricular action potential plateau cannot produce a systolic period less than 200 msec in duration, progressive tachycardia impinges selectively on the time available for diastolic relaxation and ventricular refilling. This has the consequence that even with the improved central venous drainage achieved by respiratory suction and decreased venous pooling there is little change in ventricular filling at heart rates above those developed during moderate exercise. While progressive sympathetic inotropic activation causes progressive increases in the efficiency of cardiac ejection, this also has limits imposed by the structure of the ventricles. Together, these factors mean that stroke volume typically can rise only around 50% above its resting value. Thus, a 20-year-old with a resting heart rate of 70 bpm could typically increase cardiac output by 1.5-fold through increased stroke volume and by a little under 3-fold through tachycardia ((220 – 20)/70), giving an overall rise of around 4.3-fold, that is, a maximal output of 21–22 litres/min assuming an initial resting output of 5 litres/min. The muscular work intensity that can be achieved is therefore constrained by the nutrient and metabolite exchange that can be serviced by this flow rate.

Limits to effective blood volume

In reality, the above figures give an overestimation of the situation except with extremely short episodes of exertion. First, the fall in precapillary resistance in vasculature of active muscle necessarily elevates the capillary hydrostatic pressure, with resulting movement of plasma water outwards into the muscle interstitium. With whole-body exercise, the volume involved before pressures re-equilibrate is of the order of 15% of plasma volume, which leaves the vascular compartment over 10–15 min. Second, metabolic heat is generated by exercise of large muscle groups at a faster rate than it can be dissipated from the body by passive processes, so core temperature begins to rise. Detection of this by the hypothalamic thermoregulatory centre leads to inhibition of sympathetic discharge to the skin (cutaneous) circulation and to activation of eccrine sweating. The withdrawal of sympathetic vasoconstriction and the local metabolic hyperaemia that accompanies sweat secretion, together result in skin blood flow rising from what may be trivial levels to several litres/min, imposing a new limit on the proportion of cardiac output that is available for muscle perfusion. Third, the absolute amount of heat exchange needed to accommodate the metabolic output from whole-body exercise requires in excess of 1 litre/hr of sweat to be evaporated from the skin. Since the plasma is the immediate source of water and electrolytes necessary to produce this fluid, exercise that continues for longer than around 20 min is associated with a further progressive decline in circulating blood volume at a rate that depends on the effectiveness of the heat loss processes.

This sequence of depletion of effective blood volume (first by capillary extravasation, then by cutaneous dilation and finally by sweat production) is reflected in the fact that while a cardiac output may be maintained at a steady level during heavy, whole-body exercise for around an hour without fluid replacement, this is achieved by a progressive rise in heart rate after about 15–20 min have elapsed. The drive for this additional tachycardia probably originates from low-pressure atrial baroreceptors detecting cardiac filling, but it is possible that muscle metaboreceptors may also be involved. The decline in blood volume not only limits capacity to sustain cardiac output and peripheral perfusion, but since there is a progressive rise in haematocrit and hence blood viscosity, cardiac workload rises disproportionately.

By contrast with the situation during exercise modalities on land, depletion of effective blood volume is minimal during prolonged swimming. On the one hand, external compression by the medium increases extravascular hydrostatic pressures in the musculature and reduces outward fluid movement. More importantly, the high conductive index of water means that metabolic heat is lost effectively enough not to induce a rise in deep body temperature and so skin vasodilation does not occur to any significant extent.

Limits in women and children

The patterns of circulatory adjustments during exercise are similar in age-matched men and women and in children and adults. However, both women and children have smaller hearts than men, so that a greater increment in heart rate is required in order to provide a given elevation of cardiac output. In consequence, a lower absolute maximum level of work is achievable. For children, this limitation is somewhat less than for adult women, since the maximum heart rate that can be achieved is higher in children. Women also have two additional circulatory limitations to work capacity, relative to men. First, blood oxygen carriage is higher in men because of the higher haematocrit that results from erythropoietic stimulation by testosterone. Second, the greater proportional contribution of adipose tissue to body mass in women means that fractional muscle mass is reduced and that in consequence an additional increment of afterload and hence of cardiac work is imposed during exercise. With age, changes in cardiovascular structure and function occur that result in greater limits on exercise capacity in both men and women. This is discussed in a later section (Exercise in the ageing patient, p. 111).

Potentially adverse cardiovascular effects of exercise

Renal ischaemia

Although the intense vasoconstriction that occurs in the splanchnic vasculature throughout a bout of exercise causes relative ischaemia of the kidney and digestive organs, this is not usually associated with significant tissue damage. In the case of the digestive tract, the processes of nutrient digestion and absorption induce a high degree of local metabolic dilation and this, at least largely, counteracts the vasoconstrictive effects of sympathetic activation and so limits the proportion of cardiac output available for muscle perfusion. There is therefore a logical biological reason for advising people not to exercise soon after a meal. In the case of the kidney, sustained intense exercise can produce sufficient hypoxia to cause reversible damage to the nephron epithelium, with consequent appearance in the urine of protein and sometimes cellular debris. This normalises over several days after exercise, without residual deficits.

Haemolysis

Damage to both red and white blood cells has been reported in response to acute exhaustive exercise. The damage is thought to arise through increased oxidative stress, secondary to release of free radicals from activated mitochondria in the working muscles and other sites. In addition, prolonged running on hard surfaces can cause significant traumatic destruction of blood cells as they pass through vessels on the soles of the feet and this may lead to excretion of haem proteins in the urine. However, the extent of haemolysis is not sufficient to have any deleterious effects of haematocrit or to cause renal damage.

Hyperthermia

The amount of metabolic heat generated by dynamic whole-body exercise always elevates core body temperature, with values of 39–40°C being common in endurance athletes. The increased thermal gradient induced by this hyperthermia means that under optimal conditions the protective processes of cutaneous dilation and sweating are sufficient to prevent any further rise. Nonetheless, this ideal situation can easily be circumvented. The decline in blood volume during sustained exercise means that exercise periods of over around one hour are not possible without fluid and electrolyte replacement. In the absence of this, the cardiac output becomes insufficient to service either the metabolic demands of the central nervous system and musculature, or the need for delivery of heat to the skin. With upright exercise, activity usually terminates with fainting because of cerebral hypoxia (heat stress) before the thermal implications of hypovolaemia can develop. Nonetheless, after exercise ceases a substantial residual heat load remains in the body and care must be taken to ensure that thermal exchange is optimised during recovery.

If thermal exchange is sub-optimal either because of extremely hot, humid conditions or because the individual is wearing garments that prevent convective and evaporative heat loss from the skin (as occurs commonly, for instance, in members of the armed services, firefighters and players of American football), then core temperature may rise to values greater than 40°C in parallel with or even before cerebral perfusion begins to fall. Under these conditions, direct effects of hyperthermia on the central nervous system become evident, with disorientation and collapse (heat stroke). Since these neurological effects reflect potentially irreversible damage to neuronal proteins, the occurrence of heat stroke is an event of the utmost seriousness and rapid reduction of body temperature becomes urgent.

Foetoplacental insufficiency

Although exercise is beneficial during pregnancy, especially in order to maintain skeletal muscle tone and joint integrity, theoretically there are potential dangers that reduced plasma volume may compromise foetoplacental perfusion and that the foetal heat load coupled with the mother's reduced surface area-volume ratio might lead to an undesirable degree of hyperthermia. Under most conditions, these factors are probably unlikely to be sufficient to contraindicate moderate exercise. In cases of doubt, however, the implications for maintenance of effective circulating blood volume may make swimming preferable to terrestrial exercise.

Syncope

With resistive exercise, the external compression of body compartments by sustained muscle contraction imposes potentially dangerous effects on the circulation that are absent with dynamic exercise. One of these is the increase in intrathoracic pressure, which is usually well in excess of normal pulmonary arterial pressure and may reach values of 50–60 mmHg. This dramatically reduces venous return, cardiac output and consequently systemic blood pressure, with the result that cerebral perfusion is often compromised in the upright position and consciousness may be impaired. In some circumstances, such as competitive weightlifting, resistive exercise is characteristically preceded by hyperventilation. The resulting hypocapnia and consequent cerebral vasoconstriction further reduces delivery of blood to the cerebral cortex. In patients receiving medication with drugs that deplete fluid volume (for example, diuretics) or damp reflex cardiovascular control (for example, adrenoreceptor antagonists), the reduced capacity to compensate rapidly for a fall in cardiac ejection also enhances the potential for this to occur. The potential for sudden loss of consciousness and for fall-related injuries must therefore always be kept in mind when supervising resistive exercise. Chronic resistive training may also induce unfavorable changes in the left ventricular wall thickness:internal volume ratio (see Chronic exercise, below).

Hypertension

Paradoxically, when the intensity of resistive effort is insufficient to compromise venous return and induce hypotension, the potential danger is production of an excessively high arterial pressure. During isometric activation of large muscle groups, the occlusive compression of all intramuscular vessels causes a substantial rise in total peripheral resistance. In individuals whose vasculature is atherosclerotic or otherwise weakened, for example, by connective tissue deterioration, these hypertensive episodes may lead to infarcts or strokes. For this reason as well as for the greater adaptive benefits (see below), dynamic exercise has substantial advantages over resistive exercise in a rehabilitation setting.

Chronic exercise

Blood volume changes

The first detectable effect of sustained exercise is an increase in circulating blood volume of around 10–20% (500–1000 ml), which can be seen almost to its full extent after even a two-hour aerobic training bout and is sustained throughout a period of regular training (Fletcher, 1994). The initial response to a single training bout is renal retention of water and electrolytes, which is attenuated by blockade of aldosterone synthesis but is not associated with persistently elevated plasma aldosterone, suggesting upregulation of aldosterone-dependent sodium channels in the distal tubule. The trigger is not certain. However, since muscle activity releases potassium ions into the circulation and the resulting hyperkalaemia is known to increase aldosterone secretion, this is likely to be the sequence leading to the elevated channel expression.

Within 2–3 days of continued training, plasma protein content has returned to normal. The recurrent muscle and respiratory pumping will speed up lymphatic drainage and return of interstitial proteins, but such a large rise in total plasma protein must also involve stimulation of hepatic protein synthesis, probably as a result of exercise-induced cortisol secretion. At this stage, the expanded plasma volume dilutes the blood and causes a fall in haematocrit that might be erroneously interpreted as mild anaemia, although of course there is no real reduction in blood cell numbers. Over the succeeding several weeks haematocrit returns to normal, presumably because of increased erythropoietin release due to the recurrent renal hypoxia associated with each exercise bout. The increased circulating fluid volume itself has a substantial beneficial effect on exercise performance because a higher maximum cardiac output can be achieved and thermal demands for skin perfusion will cause less deprivation of muscle blood flow. The eventual restoration of normal haematocrit will be accompanied by an increase in oxygen carrying capacity that contributes further to the overall benefits of training.

Cardiac changes

Similarly to skeletal muscle, cardiac muscle has the adaptive capacity to respond to chronically increased workload by laying down additional contractile sarcomeres (hypertrophy). In a highly trained individual, this hypertrophy can amount to almost a doubling of normal cardiac mass, from around 300 g to up to 500 g (Huonker et al., 1996).

The hypertrophic response to increased work occurs both during work involving elevated preload (such as, increased stretch during filling seen during dynamic exercise) and that involving elevated afterload (such as, increased pressure during emptying seen during resistive exercise), but the implications for cardiac efficiency are quite different. With chronically increased diastolic stretching of the ventricles during aerobic training, new sarcomeres are laid down along an increased chamber diameter, resulting in larger volume ventricles surrounded by a wall that is similar in relative thickness to the pretraining situation (eccentric hypertrophy). As a consequence, end-diastolic volume is increased and stroke volume also increases for a given degree of end-diastolic filling pressure in accordance with the Frank-Starling relationship.

At rest, stroke volume in an endurance athlete may exceed 100 ml and this increased ejection capacity by itself confers the ability to increase cardiac output during exercise to a greater value than in an untrained person. Coupled with the increased stroke volume, is a reduced resting heart rate, so that cardiac output at rest remains constant but there is a greater heart rate reserve available. Typical resting heart rate in an elite athlete would be around 35–45 bpm. If we compare this with the untrained individual discussed on p. 15, whose ability to increase cardiac output during exercise allowed an increment of 4.3 times the resting value, an athlete of the same age (20 years of age), whose stroke volume also rose 50% during exercise might typically achieve an increment of $1.5 \times ((220 - 20)/40)$ or 7.5 times, to peak at around 35 litres/min (assuming a resting heart rate of 40 bpm).

Resistive exercise, by contrast, does not increase end-diastolic volume to the same extent as does dynamic exercise, mainly because of the mechanical obstruction to venous return. The hypertrophy induced by cardiac work against the elevated peripheral resistance that is induced by muscle contraction therefore takes place around a ventricular chamber that is unchanged in size from rest. This results in a thickened ventricular wall (concentric hypertrophy) without increased stroke volume at rest and so no appreciable resting bradycardia occurs. Thus, although structured resistance training may be beneficial in improving the work capacity of skeletal muscles and mobility, this is not coupled with enhancement of the maximum attainable cardiac output and aerobic work capacity.

Both eccentric and concentric hypertrophy are associated with increased coronary capillary density. This provides for nutrient and gas exchange in the myocardium to be matched relatively well to the increased work capacity of the muscle, although the match can never be perfect because of the longer diffusional pathway between interstitium and sarcoplasm that results from the increased myocardial cell diameter. Further details of the mechanisms underlying angiogenesis appear in the section 'Structural and functional adaptations of the vasculature', p. 22. With eccentric hypertrophy, the capillary sprouting enhances absolute trans-capillary exchange at rest because the hypertrophy is not associated with any elevation in cardiac work, due to the coexisting bradycardia. This improvement in myocardial nutrition is probably one of the major benefits of aerobic exercise programmes. With concentric hypertrophy, on the other hand, cardiac work is increased even at rest, so there is less benefit of increased vascularisation.

Thickening of the myocardium results, during contraction, in an increased pressure in the endocardial layer, which causes relative impairment of endocardial coronary perfusion. In the presence of dramatic concentric left ventricular hypertrophy, as occurs in response to severe hypertension or aortic stenosis, this impairment appears to be of clinical significance, since most infarcts are localised to the inner layers of the ventricular wall. Resistance training, where afterload is only elevated for brief periods, produces far less pronounced hypertrophic changes than occur in response to continual pathologically increased afterload, and there is no convincing evidence that in healthy individuals resistive training can lead to coronary insufficiency. Notwithstanding, the implications of endocardial pressures for coronary efficiency should be borne in mind in relation to possible abuse of anabolic steroids, since these agents themselves elevate blood pressure and afterload.

The bradycardia that accompanies training is likely to be predominantly due to a resetting of autonomic control of the sinoatrial node, secondary to the increased stroke volume. This involves an increase in parasympathetic activity and/or a decrease in sympathetic activity. However, it appears more rapidly than the structural ventricular changes (over the order of weeks rather than months), and so is likely to reflect the effect of increased blood volume on cardiac filling (Huonker et al., 1996; O'Sullivan and Bell, 2000). For example, an 8% increase in blood volume would be sufficient to cause continually elevated discharge from low-pressure baroreceptors in the right atrium, which are capable of causing reflex enhancements of vagal tone. Similarly, strong ventricular distension excites ventricular receptors located at the apex of the heart, which also brings about vagally-mediated bradycardia.

Blood pressure control

Regular exercise leads to a reduction in blood pressure by several mmHg, most notably in systolic pressure. This response occurs after only a few weeks of exercise and is more pronounced in people where blood pressure is already raised above normal levels (see Chapter 8). Exercise is therefore being increasingly favoured as a therapeutic aid for patients with hypertension and associated cardiovascular diseases. The bradycardia resulting from training will predispose to a fall in blood pressure, but the major cause of the depressor effect appears to be a reduction in resting peripheral resistance. This is due in large part to attenuation of central sympathetic drive, although increased resting skeletal muscle conductance and increased basal production of vasodilator substances also contribute (see 'Structural and functional adaptations of the vasculature' below).

The mechanisms underlying the reduced sympathetic vasoconstrictor drive are still unclear. As with the concomitant bradycardia, one potential contributor is stimulation of low-pressure baroreceptors in the atria as a result of training-induced blood volume expansion. Additionally, central down-regulation of sympathetic output from the medullary cardiovascular centre may result from chronic input from joint mechanoreceptors, muscle chemoreceptors and descending motor pathways. A further contributing factor is chronic elevation in concentration of the endorphins that are known to be liberated during exercise, and have a sympatho-inhibitory effect.

Changes in sympathetic activity are not only seen at rest, but also during acute episodes of cardiovascular activation. Sympathetically mediated cardiovascular responses mediated by descending cortico-medullary pathways in response to dynamic or to isometric exercise, and also in response to exercise-unrelated situations such as cold exposure or mental arousal, appear to be blunted post-training. These changes suggest that training may help to protect against cardiovascular morbidity not only by the effect on resting circulatory status but in addition by reducing the surges in cardiac workload that accompany a variety of stressors in everyday life.

Structural and functional adaptations of the vasculature

With training, structural and functional changes in the vasculature are observed which enhance oxygen delivery and uptake during exercise. Repetitive enhancements of intraluminal shear stresses during exercise induce cellular reorganisation and endothelial-mediated alterations in gene expression of a number of substances (Huonker et al., 1996). One effect of this is upregulation of endothelial paracrine dilator processes. Additional structural adaptations include angiogenesis and arterial and venous remodelling.

In the peripheral circulation, basal production of a number of dilator substances, including nitric oxide (NO), prostacyclin and adenosine, is enhanced after as little as four weeks training. The vasculature also shows increased sensitivity to endothelium-dependent, but not endothelium-independent vasodilator stimuli. Conversely, there is diminished sensitivity to vasoconstrictors such as noradrenaline.

Enhancement of endothelium-dependent dilator function may occur preferentially in vessels of the trained muscle groups. However, improved dilator function in forearm vasculature has also been observed in athletes who do not participate in substantial upper body activity (O'Sullivan, 2003). Nonetheless, at least for NO, which is the most well studied of the endothelium-derived dilators, it is doubtful that an increase in these responses affects maximal work capacity since NO does not appear to contribute substantially to skeletal muscle hyperaemia during exercise. As in the peripheral vasculature, NO synthesis is increased in coronary endothelium with training and the sensitivity of coronary vascular smooth muscle to vasoactive agents is also altered, but it remains uncertain whether these changes contribute significantly to coronary perfusion in the trained heart.

The stimulation of training-induced angiogenesis in skeletal and cardiac muscles arises from increases in growth factors such as vascular endothelial growth factor (VEGF) and basic fibroblast growth factor. An increase in gene expression of VEGF has been identified in human skeletal muscle after a single bout of exercise, as well as post-training. Some potential triggers for growth factor activation and release include locally increased muscle blood flow, muscle contraction, local release of paracrine molecules such as NO, changes in the biochemical milieu such as acidosis and hypoxia and, in the case of the coronary circulation, the passive distension caused by increased preload.

As well as exhibiting increased capillary density in working muscles, trained individuals also have larger luminal diameters of their large conducting arteries, including the major coronary arteries, than do sedentary controls (Plowman and Wright, 2003). This remodelling is probably a response to chronically elevated flow and, although the conducting arteries do not constitute the main site of peripheral resistance, an increased diameter will lead to some attenuation of cardiac work during ejection, as well as to better coronary perfusion.

With the prolonged, intensive training characteristic of highly trained individuals, there is elevated compliance in both large arteries and large veins. In the venous compartment, the increased compliance tends to result in poor orthostatic tolerance, with sub-optimal reflex ability to maintain arterial pressure in the upright stationary position. The fact that compliance changes are seen only after months of training at relatively high intensity contrasts with the reductions in sympathetic vasomotor tone that are seen after several weeks training at even moderate workloads. The effect on compliance cannot therefore be ascribed to reduced sympathetic vasoconstriction but must reflect structural changes, probably an altered balance between vascular elastin and collagen. Nonetheless, it is possible that the long-term alteration of sympathetic discharge may contribute to these changes through altering the trophic environment of the vessel wall.

Cardiovascular detraining

After a high level of fitness has been established, cardiovascular adaptations and work capacity may be maintained for at least up to one month, after training is reduced in intensity by up to 70–80%. If, however, exercise ceases completely, then the functional adaptations decline rapidly over the first month, although structural adaptations persist for somewhat longer.

Blood volume is the most rapidly reversed parameter, with protein and plasma volume falling to values only slightly above pretraining values within about seven days. This is correlated with reductions in resting and exercise-induced stroke volume and thus maximum cardiac output, with an associated fall in work capacity. At this stage, if plasma volume is restored to the trained value with dextran solution, maximum stroke volume and work capacity can be returned nearly to the levels seen during training. Resting plasma levels of NO have fallen significantly within one month's cessation of exercise and have returned to untrained values after two months detraining. Predictably, structural adaptations to training are reversed over a longer timespan. For recreational athletes, left ventricular hypertrophy is reversed within 1–2 months. However, substantial chamber dilatation may persist in elite athletes after several months, and even after several years, detraining. The persistence of elevated left ventricular volume accounts for the fact that maximum cardiac output and stroke volume do not reach pretraining values until after several months detraining. Similarly, skeletal muscle capillarisation is still elevated above untrained values for several months. The cardiovascular correlates of detraining are similar in males and females.

Exercise in the ageing patient

Ageing is accompanied by a variety of cardiovascular changes, which include, in Western populations, increases in resting sympathetic drive, peripheral resistance and blood pressure, reduced resting stroke volume, maximal heart rate and cardiac adrenoreceptor responsiveness, decreased peripheral vasodilator capacity and decreased blood volume. All of these factors could potentially limit exercise capacity with progressive ageing. However, the most dramatic factor is the reduction in maximum cardiac output that follows from the reduced stroke volume, which may be only around 60–70% of that in young individuals and from the lower maximum heart rate. Given that resting heart rate does not change with age, it can be seen that resting cardiac output must fall proportionately to stroke volume and so at the age of 60 years may be of the order of 3.0–3.5 litres/min rather than the 5 litres/min typical of youth. Hence, using the same calculations that were employed earlier (on p. 15) to estimate the potential increment in cardiac output during exercise, we can assume that a 60-year-old might be able to increase his output by $1.5 \times ((220 - 60)/70)$ or 3.4-fold, attaining a maximal output of around only 12 litres/min. Limits to circulatory performance are therefore a substantial consideration in absolute exercise capacity in older populations.

A further set of limiting factors associated with ageing is centred on the fact that many autonomically mediated reflex responses, including those involved in baroreflex regulation and thermoregulation, tend to show lower gain with age. In the aged population, therefore, syncope during resistive exercise and the potential for hyperthermia during endurance events are both enhanced.

The cardiovascular benefits of regular exercise in a young population have been described earlier, so it is relevant to ask how chronic exercise affects the cardiovascular correlates of ageing. As in younger subjects, one of the quickest and most pronounced effects of training in an older population is an increase in blood volume, which correlates well with the training-induced increase in exercise capacity. Associated with this is an increase in end-diastolic left ventricular function and an increase in both resting and exercise stroke volumes, consequently increasing maximum cardiac output. Cardiac contractility is also improved by enhanced β-adrenoreceptor responsiveness. Thus, the increase in fitness with training in older athletes is due mainly to these responses reversing the age-related decline in cardiac performance.

With age, there is faster regression of ventricular muscle mass and ventricular volume during detraining than is seen in young subjects. It is, however, uncertain to what extent ageing affects the rapidity of cardiovascular detraining responses after different durations of physical conditioning.

References

Chapleau, M.W. and Abboud, F. (2001). Neuro-cardiovascular regulation: from molecules to man. *Annals of The New York Academy of Science*, 940.

Fletcher, G.A. (ed.) (1994). *Cardiovascular Response to Exercise* (American Heart Association Monograph). Futura Publishing Company, Mount Kisco, New York.

Huonker, M., Halle, M. and Keul, J. (1996). Structural and functional adaptations of the cardiovascular system by training. *International Journal of Sports Medicine* 17, S164–172.

Joyner, M.J. and Halliwill, J.R. (2000). Sympathetic vasodilation in human limbs. *Journal of Physiology* (London) 526, 471–80.

O'Sullivan, S.E. (2003). The effects of exercise training on markers of endothelial function in young healthy men. *International Journal of Sports Medicine* 24, 404–9.

O'Sullivan, S.E. and Bell, C. (2000). The effects of exercise and training on human cardiovascular reflex control. *Journal of the Autonomic Nervous System* 81, 16–24.

Plowman, S.A. and Smith, D.L. (2003). *Exercise Physiology for Health, Fitness and Performance*, 2nd edn. Benjamin Cummings, San Francisco.

Rowell, L.B. and Shepherd, J.T. (eds) (1996). Exercise: Regulation and Integration of Multiple Systems (*Handbook of Physiology* Section 12). Oxford University Press, Oxford.

Bibliography

Several of the standard textbooks of exercise physiology have extensive citations to primary sources in this area. Among the more comprehensive of these are:

Robergs, R.A. and Roberts, S.O. (2000). *Fundamental Principles of Exercise Physiology for Fitness, Performance and Health*. McGraw-Hill, Boston.

Additional materials that provide introductions to the literature on particular themes are:

Balady, G.J. (ed.) (2000). Exercise in the modification of cardiovascular disease risk: biological mechanisms. *Coronary Artery Disease* **11**, 97–135.

Lakatta, E.G. (1993). Cardiovascular mechanisms in advanced age. *Physiological Reviews* **73**, 413–67.

McAllister, R.M. (ed.) (1995). Endothelial-mediated control of coronary and skeletal blood flow during exercise. *Medicine and Science in Sports and Exercise* **27**, 1122–57.

Scheuer, J. and Tipton, C.M. (1977). Cardiovascular adaptations to physical training. *Annual Review of Physiology* **39**, 221–51.

Seals, D.R. and Esler, M.D. (2000). Human ageing and the sympathoadrenal system. *Journal of Physiology* (London) **528**, 407–17.

Chapter 3

EXERCISE AND THE PULMONARY SYSTEM

Stephen J. Lane and Richard J. Hawksworth

Key words: ventilation, maximum oxygen uptake, maximal ventilation at peak exercise.

Introduction

This chapter will concentrate on the pulmonary system and how it changes throughout life. Furthermore, the adaptations that occur during exercise in healthy subjects and in patients with lung disease are discussed.

The external environment and the lung

At sea level an atmospheric pressure of 760 mmHg or 100 kPa is exerted on the surface of the earth. This is called 1 atmosphere or 1 bar (1000 millibars). This total pressure is equal to the sum of the partial pressures of its constituent gases, which essentially are 20% oxygen (O_2) and 80% nitrogen (N_2). Dalton's Law informs us that atmospheric pressure decreases as one ascends, although the relative proportions of the gases remain the same as per Table 3.1.

Therefore, at sea level we have a fractional inspired oxygen concentration (FiO_2) of 20–21% available for respiration. The primary purpose of the lung is to

Table 3.1 Total pressure and oxygen and nitrogen partial pressures under varying conditions.

Ambient condition	Total pressure in mmHg (kPa)	Partial pressure O_2 in mmHg (kPa)	Partial pressure N_2 in mmHg (kPa)
Sea level, 1 atmosphere; 1 bar	760 (100)	160 (20)	600 (80)
16 000 feet altitude	380 (50)	80 (10)	300 (40)
30 foot sea dive	1520 (200)	320 (40)	1200 (160)

transfer this oxygen from the atmosphere to the arterial blood and to correspondingly remove carbon dioxide CO_2. The lung achieves this through the processes of ventilation and gas exchange.

Structure and function of the lung

The lung in biology resembles a tree in both structure and function. The trachea can be likened to the trunk of the tree, the bronchi to the branches and the alveoli to the leaves. At rest, when one inhales a breath of approximately 500 ml, air flows under negative pressure through the trachea, down through the bronchial branches until it arrives at the alveoli, where gas exchange occurs. The branching of the tracheobronchial tree is mirrored by similar branching of the pulmonary arterial, venous and connective tissue systems. Thus there are two functional zones of the lung, i.e. the conducting zone from the trachea to the terminal bronchioles and the gas exchange zone at the alveoli. There are 23 divisions of the tracheobronchial tree from the trachea to alveolus, comprising a volume of 150 ml, which is the anatomical dead space. The corresponding cumulative cross-sectional area of the tree is constant to approximately the 7th airway division and increases dramatically thereafter toward the alveoli. Just as a tree is mainly made up of leaves, the lung is mainly made up of alveoli, and this makes sense as the primary function of the lung is gas exchange. The surface area of the gas exchange zone has been estimated at a dramatic 100 m², the size of a football pitch, with a thickness of just 1 μm.

Air flow in and out of the normal lung at rest depends predominantly upon a pressure gradient between the alveolus and atmosphere. This pressure gradient results from changes in volume of the thoracic cavity between inspiration and expiration, generated by the rhythmic contraction of the muscles of respiration as per Boyle's Law. Inspiration occurs when the intra-alveolar pressure is less than atmospheric and expiration occurs when intra-alveolar pressure is greater than atmospheric (Table 3.2).

The contraction of the respiratory muscles is under central midbrain neural control, mediated predominantly by the phrenic nerve. In disease states such as asthma, airflow becomes more dependent on the resistance to flow, which is determined by the cumulative cross-sectional area of the structures through which the flow is occurring, in this case the bronchial tubes or branches. In the tracheobronchial

Table 3.2 Volume and flow changes during respiration.

	Atmospheric pressure in mmHg	Intra-alveolar pressure in mmHg	Thoracic cage volume	Movement of air
Before inspiration	760	760	Minimum	No flow
During inspiration	760	759 (−1)	Increasing	Inspiratory flow
During expiration	760	761 (+1)	Decreasing	Expiratory flow

tree there are two sites of resistance to airflow, namely a site of high resistance, low cross-sectional area from trachea to the the 7th branching of the tree (90% total resistance), and a site of low resistance, high cross-sectional area from the the 8th to the 23rd branches (10% total resistance).

Control of ventilation

Like the heartbeat, breathing occurs in a continuous cyclical pattern. Inspiratory muscles must rhythmically contract and relax to alternately fill the lungs with air and empty them. Neural control of respiration involves two main components:

(1) Factors responsible for generating the pacemaker rhythm of inspiration and expiration.
(2) Factors regulating the rate and depth of ventilation.

There are also factors that modify respiratory activity to serve other purposes, such as speech, breath holding and singing.

The inherent pacemaker rhythm is generated from interrelated complex groups of neurones within the medulla of the midbrain. These groups are finely tuned by centres from within the pons. The resultant activity is an inspiratory discharge approximately every 3–4 seconds that results in the 'firing' of the efferent inspiratory nerves, which serve the muscles of inspiration. The main inspiratory muscle is the diaphragm, which is innervated by the phrenic nerve. Thus, unlike the sinoatrial node within the heart muscle, the midbrain respiratory centres are geographically displaced from the muscles of inspiration and are interconnected by efferent nerves such as the phrenic.

The rate and depth of ventilation is controlled by the partial pressure of carbon dioxide (pCO_2), partial pressure of oxygen (pO_2) and the pH. The dominant factor in the minute-to-minute control of ventilation is the pCO_2. An increase in the pCO_2 is the most potent stimulus for increasing ventilation via the central medullary chemoreceptors. These receptors do not respond to the CO_2 itself but rather to the hydrogen ions (H^+) generated within the cerebrospinal fluid (CSF) by the law of mass action as it applies to the reaction: $CO_2 + H_2O = H_2CO_3 = H^+ + HCO_3^-$. This local increase in the CSF H^+ concentration directly stimulates the chemoreceptors, leading to an increase in ventilation which blows off more CO_2. Remember that this is a local effect as plasma H^+ are unable to cross the blood brain barrier. In contrast to normal reflex control of ventilation, very high levels of pCO_2, such as 9–10 kPa, actually suppress respiration. In addition, prolonged hypoventilation, as seen in some patients with chronic lung diseases such as COPD, leads to blunting of the CO_2 effect on ventilation as more HCO_3^- crosses the blood brain barrier to buffer the H^+ ions. Thus the central chemoreceptors are no longer aware of the elevated pCO_2 as the CSF H^+ is normal. These patients' ventilation is driven by their hypoxaemia and administering oxygen to these patients paradoxically worsens their condition.

Arterial O_2 concentration is monitored by the peripheral chemoreceptors in the carotid and aortic bodies. In contrast to CO_2, these receptors are relatively insensitive to small changes in O_2 and indeed the pO_2 must fall below 600 mmHg (8 kPa) before ventilation in activated. This only happens in severe disease states and so is not very relevant in normal reflex regulation of ventilation. The reason for this relative insensitivity is because of the margin of safety afforded by the unique relation of O_2 to its carrier molecule haemoglobin. Because of the shape of the O_2-Hb curve, Hb is still 90% saturated at 8 kPa O_2, but falls precipitously thereafter.

Changes in the arterial H^+ concentration also affect ventilation. An increase in H^+ generated secondarily to high CO_2 states, such as in type 2 respiratory failure, increases ventilation predominantly via CO_2 generated CSF H^+, but also by a direct action of plasma H^+ on the peripheral chemoreceptors. Indeed, the peripheral chemoreceptors are more sensitive to changes in H^+ concentration than to changes in CO_2 or in O_2. In acidotic states not related to CO_2 levels, such as in diabetic ketoacidosis or renal failure, H^+ are added to the plasma and directly stimulate ventilation via the peripheral chemoreceptors. Indeed, changes in ventilation induced by a falling pH are one of the most important regulatory mechanisms of body acid-base balance. Hyperventilation blows off CO_2 and so buffers H^+ increases. Conversely, low levels of H^+ result in hypoventilation and CO_2 retention in order to keep the pH steady.

The usual volume of an inhalation at rest is approximately 500 ml of air, the tidal volume (TV). The typical inspiratory phase lasts one second and the expiratory phase lasts three seconds. Thus the respiratory cycle lasts four seconds, yielding 15 breaths per minute (bpm) or respiratory rate (RR). The minute ventilation (MV), or the product of respiratory rate and tidal volume per breath is thus 15 bpm × 500 mls air = c.7.5 litres/minute at rest. The volume of the conducting airways is approximately 150 ml, the anatomic dead space, so that only 350 ml reaches the alveolar compartment to participate in gas exchange. Thus alveolar ventilation, as opposed to minute ventilation, is 350 ml × 15 bpm = 5 litres/min. Of this 5 litres of air entering the alveoli, only 300 ml of oxygen moves across into the blood each minute, to be replaced by 250 ml of CO_2. Thus, less than 5% of the inhaled gas volume is exchanged with gas in the blood. During exercise the oxygen uptake may increase to as high as 6 litres/min, giving an increase of 20-fold as shown in Table 3.3.

Table 3.3　Effect of exercise on ventilatory parameters.

Ventilatory parameter	Litres per minute
Minute ventilation	7–8
Alveolar ventilation	5.25–5.5
Oxygen uptake per min at rest	0.30
CO_2 exhaled per min at rest	0.25
Potential oxygen uptake during exercise	6

Respiratory failure

Respiratory failure is defined on arterial blood gas analysis as a PaO_2 of < 8 kPa breathing room air of FiO_2 21% at sea level at rest. When one analyses the arterial blood gas abnormalities in respiratory failure two patterns consistently emerge. The first blood gas pattern is a PaO_2 < 8 kPa associated with a low $PaCO_2$, a high pH. This is called type 1 respiratory failure with respiratory alkalosis. The second blood gas pattern is a PaO_2 < 8 kPa associated with a high $PaCO_2$ and a low pH. This is type 2 respiratory failure with respiratory acidosis. These two obviously different patterns predict two different mechanisms of respiratory failure.

The key to understanding the pathogenesis of respiratory failure is to understand the factors governing CO_2 levels in the blood (see above). Volatile carbon dioxide, equivalent to carbonic acid, is the principle acid product of metabolism. Its arterial concentration is fixed by the lungs to 5 kPa by minute ventilation stimulated by the action of CO_2 on the medullary chemoreceptors. At this concentration pulmonary excretion equals metabolic production. Minute ventilation increases in response to increased production in order to keep this level constant. Conversely, changes in alveolar ventilation will alter CO_2 levels. A decrease in minute ventilation, as occurs when one holds one's breath, will increase arterial CO_2. Indeed, in the resting non exercising subject, there is an inverse linear relationship between minute ventilation and arterial CO_2 such that doubling minute ventilation from 7 to 14 litres/min will halve the arterial CO_2. Thus, type 1 respiratory failure is associated with minute (alveolar) hyperventilation, whereas type 2 respiratory failure is associated with alveolar hypoventilation.

Exercise and the pulmonary system

Multiparameter exercise testing is being increasingly used for exercise assessments within the hospital setting. The commonest indications are for determining the aetiology of dyspnoea, evaluating pulmonary disability, assessing the risk for cardiothoracic or major upper abdominal surgery and for the determination of the relative contributions of heart and lung disease to activity limitation. Measuring aerobic tolerance using the ventilatory threshold enables the clinician to determine the level of sustainable exercise. In addition, exercise testing can help unmask latent exercise-induced asthma and help in the assessment of portable oxygen requirements in patients with diffuse lung disease or patients after lung resection surgery. Laboratories may utilise both a cycle ergometer and a treadmill, and measure breath-by-breath % O_2, % CO_2 and airflow via a gas analyser attached to a non-rebreathing bag. By digitally integrating these values over time O_2 uptake, CO_2 output and minute exhaled ventilation ($\dot{V}E$) can be computed.

Intense exercise can elicit a rapid 15-fold increase in whole body oxygen uptake. This is accomplished by a 10-fold increase in minute ventilation, a 5-fold increase in cardiac output and a 3-fold increase in systemic oxygen extraction. In normal subjects cardiac output is the normal limiting factor for $\dot{V}O_2$max although elite athletes may exhaust their breathing reserves before attaining maximum cardiac output. PO_2 and PCO_2 remain within very narrow ranges, despite the huge alterations in metabolism induced by exercise. This occurs due to sophisticated matching of ventilation to blood flow and tissue metabolism. Exercise is usually limited by maximal cardiac output in normal subjects with residual unused ventilatory and skeletal muscle function.

Maximum oxygen uptake ($\dot{V}O_2$) is the most accurate and commonly used overall assessment of exercise capacity and can be measured absolutely in litres/minute or relative to body mass. $\dot{V}O_2$ is the product of cardiac output by the difference in oxygen content between arterial and venous blood. $\dot{V}O_2$ increases linearly with work rate and maximal $\dot{V}O_2$ in any particular individual is said to occur with symptom limitation, or $\dot{V}O_2max$. The maximally predicted $\dot{V}O_2$ for a particular individual is that maximal value predicted from age, gender, height and lean body weight. This true maximal predicted $\dot{V}O_2max$ is identified by a plateau of the $\dot{V}O_2$/work curve. It is rarely achievable except in very elite athletes who can achieve values of greater than 80 ml/kg/min. The normal $\dot{V}O_2max$ is greater than 20 ml/kg/min and a normal $\dot{V}O_2max$ usually rules out serious disease of the cardiac, pulmonary or neuromuscular systems. It increases with training and decreases with age.

Minute ventilation ($\dot{V}E$ in this context, or exhaled ventilation) can increase from approximately 7 litres/min at rest to up to 100 litres/min on exercise. This is achieved by a linear increase in respiratory rate up to 50 breaths per minute and a hyperbolic increase in tidal volume from a baseline of approximately 500 ml to up to 50% of the resting vital capacity, or up to 2 litres when elastic resistive forces come into play. The $\dot{V}O_2:\dot{V}E$ relationship is linear until the patient approaches the lactic or anaerobic threshold (LT) and metabolic acidaemia ensues. At this point the $\dot{V}E$ increases out of proportion to the $\dot{V}O_2$, a point called the ventilatory threshold. The ventilatory threshold can be used as a non-invasive marker of LT as they normally occur simultaneously. Thus, for practical purposes the LT, anaerobic and ventilatory thresholds are synonymous. The LT occurs at 40–60% $\dot{V}O_2max$ in normal individuals but is less in cardiovascular disease and higher in fit normal subjects. For normal individuals PCO_2 levels remain isocapnic until compensation for metabolic acidosis occurs at LT when CO_2 levels fall in late exercise. The pH can actually fall to 7.15 or less. Likewise PO_2 levels remain near resting levels despite the marked reduction in venous oxygen content.

Changes in the respiratory system with ageing

Throughout life indices of lung function are steadily changing and reflect the function of the body as a whole. Stature is positively correlated with lung size more than any other anthropometric index and consequently height is the reference variable of choice for most purposes. The correlation is almost linear in adults but in adolescents the relationship is in part exponential. The age of the individual has little bearing on lung size up to the age of about 25, after which the lung size declines in a linear fashion. This decline is greater in absolute terms in males than females due to the fact that the size and performance of the lung in males is superior to that in females. Specifically, vital capacity (VC), residual volume (RV) and total lung capacity (TLC) are positively correlated to body height up to the age of 25, after which age and height determine the lung size. Throughout adult life the function of the lung deteriorates, a change that is the result of a number of factors, including the composition of the lung tissue, a reduction in the respiratory muscle strength, an increase in the stiffness of the thoracic cage and fibrosis of the pulmonary arteries and venules. These intrapulmonary changes can partly be explained by the decreasing efficiency of the bronchial arteries to provide the nutrients to the cell, the loss of permeability of the cell membrane, thus affecting nutrient uptake, and the alteration in the molecular structure of collagen and other tissues. This collective effect on the lung will be manifested in the increasing rigidity and decreasing tensile strength of the tissue (Mittman et al., 1965). As the lung ages its recuperative powers from injury diminish.

The loss of elastic recoil as one ages has the effect of weakening the forces that prevent the closure of the respiratory bronchioles on expiration. This has the effect that with increasing age the closure of these small airways occurs at larger lung volumes. Thus the RV increases from an average of 1.5 litres at the age of 20 to about 2.2 litres at the age of 60. Interestingly TLC does not increase significantly as the respiratory muscle strength and thoracic compliance offset the decrease in the elastic recoil. In both males and females the RV as a percentage of the TLC increases from 25% at 20 years to approximately 37% at age 60.

With regard to the effect of ageing on the ventilatory capacity, all indices show a consistent decline. In healthy males of Western European descent the decline in FEV_1 is about 30 ml per year. This, however, is accelerated in smokers or chronic bronchitics to approximately 90 ml per year. The reasons are unequivocal: the ventilatory capacity is a reflection of the strength of the respiratory muscles and the resistance offered by the airways and the movement of the chest wall.

Respiratory responses to exercise

When an individual commences exercise the pulmonary system responds in a fashion to ensure that the oxygen requirements of the working muscles are met. This is achieved by the adaptation of the various components of the breathing cycle.

Dead space

Only part of the inhaled volume of air participates in gaseous exchange, known as the effective alveolar volume (VA); the part of the inspired volume that occupies the conducting airways is known as the dead-space volume (VD). During expiration the dead space is exhaled first and has a composition similar to moist inspired air. This is followed by the alveolar volume that contains high levels of CO_2 and low levels of O_2. The total expired air therefore contains a mixture of dead space and alveolar air or VT = VA + VD. At rest the tidal volume is typically 500 ml and of this approximately 150 ml is dead space. Not all the dead space can be attributed to the anatomical features of the respiratory tract; there are functional anomalies that can alter the dead space. These are more significant in lung disease than in normal subjects. Here we see a perfusion/ventilation inequality which can cause an increase in the physiological dead space.

The ratio of dead space to tidal volume is normally between 0.2 and 0.35 at rest. During exercise this ratio falls as tidal volume increases with increasing exercise intensity. The dead space has been shown to increase with exercise more markedly than at moderate increases in tidal volume (Asmussen and Nielsen, 1956; Bargeton, 1967).

Pulmonary ventilation

Pulmonary ventilation is calculated by multiplying the tidal volume by the number of breaths, or $\dot{V}_E = f\dot{V}_T$. Normally the respiratory frequency is between 10 and 20 at rest. With low increases in exercise the increase in pulmonary ventilation is attributed to the effective increase in tidal volume but when the rate of exercise is moderate to heavy then the respiratory frequency also increases. The maximal values for respiratory frequency decline with age, with children aged about 5 attaining a respiratory frequency of about 70, 12-year-olds attaining a respiratory frequency of about 55, and 25-year-old individuals attaining 40–45 (Astrand, 1952).

During exercise the increase in tidal volume is achieved by the use of the inspiratory and expiratory reserve volumes. The subject's vital capacity will ultimately limit the tidal volume but in normal subjects the proportion of vital capacity utilised rarely exceeds 60%. In pulmonary disease, however, where the vital capacity may be compromised, this ratio may well prove limiting in the level of exercise achievable in these patients.

Respiratory work

During breathing the role of the respiratory muscles is to overcome the elastic resistances and flow resistive forces. At rest the respiratory muscles require approximately 0.5–1.0 ml O_2 per litre of ventilation. This demand increases as exercise intensifies and ventilation rises. It has been reported that up to 10% of the oxygen uptake during maximal exercise is being used to service the respiratory muscles (Otis, 1964).

Even in athletes the maximal oxygen uptake is reached before the maximum ventilation. During extremely strenuous exercise the pulmonary ventilation increases without an increase in oxygen uptake, possibly indicating the extra oxygen production is being entirely utilised by the respiratory muscles, with no extra benefit to the rest of the exercising muscles in the body (Bye et al., 1983).

Minute ventilation

Minute ventilation ($\dot{V}E$) increases during increasing levels of exercise up to a maximal level. At rest the $\dot{V}E$ is about 6.0 litres/min and increases to 100, 150 and sometimes in top athletes to 200 litres/min. The relationship between $\dot{V}E$ and oxygen uptake by the cells ($\dot{V}O_2$) is semi-linear, with a greater increase in ventilation than oxygen uptake at maximal work intensities. Thus it is difficult to predict maximal oxygen uptake from maximal ventilation. If pulmonary ventilation is expressed in relation to oxygen uptake then resting levels in adults of 20 to 25 litres/litre O_2 are seen and this remains through moderate exercise, but increases to 30 to 40 litres/litre O_2 during maximal exercise. Maximal ventilation was shown by Astrand et al. (1973) to decline by only about 5% over a 33-year-period in adult females and males originally 22 and 26 years of age respectively.

Each subject will have a maximal ventilation rate that they can achieve during exercise; this value can be obtained either by performing a maximal voluntary ventilation test or by using formulae that use the subject's FEV_1. In normal healthy subjects this maximal ventilation is never reached, indicating that pulmonary ventilation is not an exercise limiting factor in normal subjects. This is not the case in pulmonary disease where ventilation can be a limiting factor.

Effects of physical activity and training on lung function parameters

The pulmonary characteristics of an individual are unique. However, in the laboratory we compare the different lung function indices against a predicted value. These predicted or normal values have been calculated by statisticians using lots of lung function data from a wide range of normal subjects. From this data they have formulated equations that by entering the patient's age, gender and height one can estimate the value that could be expected. These population studies are used as reference values to distinguish subjects with or without lung disease. It goes without saying that to have most lung function parameters greater than the norm is of benefit to the individual. It is also true to say that everybody is different, and the environment that one is brought up in can boost the development of the pulmonary system.

Habitual physical activity varies depending on access to transport, occupation (sedentary or manual) and leisure time activity. This level of activity can be analysed to differentiate those that have always had this level of activity or have developed it during adolescence or in adult life. There appears to be an association with increased lung size and its capabilities with regard to gas transfer particularly if a high level of habitual activity has been mandatory from an early age.

The following is a list of the main pulmonary parameters and how training can affect their development.

- *Lung volumes (ITGV, RV, TLC)* are not affected by training in adults. However, there is some evidence that training has a positive effect during adolescence (Astrand, 1956; Hamilton and Andrew, 1976).
- *Pulmonary ventilation (VE)* is not affected at rest. There is a decrease or no change at sub-maximal exercise and an increase at maximal exercise, secondary to the increase in maximal oxygen uptake (Ekblon et al., 1968).
- *Tidal air (TV)* is sometimes increased at rest, sub-maximal exercise and maximal exercise.
- *Respiratory rate (RR)* is sometimes decreased at rest and sub-maximal exercise and increased at maximal exercise secondary to the increase in maximal oxygen uptake.

- *Diffusion capacity (TLCO)* is not affected at rest or at sub-maximal exercise but is increased at maximal exercise secondary to the increase in maximal oxygen uptake (Anderson et al., 1968; Hamilton and Andrew, 1976; Saltin et al., 1967).
- *Vital capacity* can be increased, particularly by training the muscles of the shoulder girdle, which in turn increases the strength of the inspiratory accessory muscles. This can be seen in rowers, weightlifters and archers. However, interestingly, this does not increase the FEV_1 and consequently the FEV_1/FVC ratio is relatively low, but does not allow for the observation of airways obstruction without other clinical features.

References

Anderson, T.W. and Shephard, R.J. (1968). Physical training and exercise diffusion capacity. *Internationale Zeitschrift fur Angewandle Physiologic, Einschliesslich Arbeitsphysiologie* 25, 198.

Asmussen, E. and Nielsen, M. (1956). Physiological dead space and alveolar gas pressures at rest and during muscular exercise. *Acta Physiologica Scandinavica* 38, 1.

Astrand, P.O. (1952). *Experimental Studies of Physical Working Capacity in Relation to Sex and Age*. Munksgaard, Copenhagen.

Astrand, P.O. (1956). Human physical fitness with special reference to sex and age. *Physiology Review* 36, 307.

Astrand, I., Astrand, P.O., Hallback, I. and Kilbom, Å. (1973). Reduction in maximal oxygen uptake with age. *Journal of Applied Physiology* 35, 659.

Bargeton, D. (1967). Analysis of capnigram and oxygram in man. *Bull de Physio-Pathologie Respiratoire* 3, 503.

Bye, P.T.P., Farkas, G.A. and Roussos, C.H. (1983). Respiratory factors limiting exercise. *Annual Review of Physiology* 45, 465.

Ekblom, B., Astrand, P.O., Saltin, B., Stenberg, J. and Wallstrom, B. (1968). Effect of training on circulatory response to exercise. *Journal of Applied Physiology* 24, 518.

Hamilton, P. and Andrew, G.M. (1976). Influence of growth and athletic training on heart and lung functions. *European Journal of Applied Physiology* 36, 27.

Mittman, C., Edelman, N.H., Norris, A.H. and Shock, N.W. (1965). Relationship between chest wall and pulmonary compliance and age. *Journal of Applied Physiology* 20, 1211.

Otis, A.B. (1964). *The Work of Breathing, Handbook of Physiology*, Sec 3. Respiration 1, p. 463, American Physiological Society, Washington DC.

Saltin, B. and Astrand, P.O. (1967). Maximal oxygen uptake in athletes. *Journal of Applied Physiology* 23, 353.

Bibliography

Astrand, P.O. and Rodahl, K. (1986). *Textbook of Work Physiology*, 3rd edn. McGraw-Hill Book Company, New York.

Cotes, J.E. (1993). *Lung Function Assessment and Application in Medicine*, 5th edn. Blackwell Science, Oxford.

Sherwood, L. (2004). *Human Physiology From Cells to Systems*, 5th edn. Brook/Cole, California.

Chapter 4

EXERCISE AND THE MUSCULOSKELETAL SYSTEM

Gareth W. Davison, Tony Ashton and Ciara M. Hughes

Key words: muscle structure and function, muscle fibre, bone and joint structure.

Introduction

The musculoskeletal system is central to movement and the ability to perform daily tasks such as eating, walking and exercise. This chapter will focus initially on the structure and function of skeletal muscle, prior to reviewing the structure of bone and joint. The chapter also details muscle strength and endurance and adaptations to exercise. A final objective is to introduce and present current understanding of an emerging field of oxidative stress and antioxidant function and its relationship with skeletal muscle and exercise.

SKELETAL MUSCLE

Muscle structure and function

A fundamental principle of physiology is that the structure of a tissue reflects its function. Nowhere is this more appropriate than in the case of muscle, whose function is to generate force, and hence produce movement. In order to achieve this the muscle fibre must be able to move and this is reflected in its structure. Thus a muscle fibre is composed of contractile elements which 'slide' and allow the muscle to contract and produce movement. This is the means by which a muscle transforms chemical energy into kinetic energy, or movement.

However, a muscle must first receive a stimulus or signal to contract and this is provided by nervous innervation. A muscle must therefore be able to communicate with a nerve in order to send and receive these 'motor' signals and become 'excited'. However, there is a small gap between the muscle fibre and motoneuron called the neuromuscular junction, across which any communication signals must first pass. Here again structure reflects function, since in order to facilitate this the presence of transverse tubules allows the action potential to simultaneously reach all parts of the muscle fibre. Thus structure or 'form' reflects function in muscle and will be explained in further detail.

The muscle fibre

Three types of muscle fibre can be identified on the basis of their structure, contractile properties and control mechanisms. They are:

- Skeletal muscle
- Cardiac muscle
- Smooth muscle

This section will describe only skeletal muscle.

Human skeletal muscle

Structure

A single skeletal muscle cell is known as a muscle fibre. During the development of the foetus in the womb, these fibres are formed via the fusion of a number of undifferentiated, mononucleated cells called myoblasts, into a single, cylindrical, multinucleated muscle fibre. Muscle fibres have diameters between 10 and 100 μm with lengths of up to 20 cm. The term 'muscle' refers to a number of muscle fibres bound together by connective tissue and anchored to bone by bundles of collagen fibres known as tendons. This scaffolding is referred to as the muscle 'architecture'. In some muscles, individual fibres extend the entire length of the muscle, although more often the fibres are shorter and are frequently oriented at an angle to the longitudinal axis of the muscle.

Arguably, the most striking feature of a skeletal muscle is its alternating light and dark appearance when seen under a light microscope. This 'banding' is created by the presence of thick and thin filaments organised into roughly cylindrical bundles, 1–2 μm in diameter, and known as myofibrils. The thick filaments are primarily composed of the contractile protein myosin while the thin filaments are primarily composed of the contractile protein actin. Troponin and tropomyosin are other proteins that are important in the regulation of muscle contraction and will be considered later.

Each myofibril is composed of thick and thin filaments in a repeating pattern along the length of the myofibril. One unit of this repeating pattern is known as a sarcomere (*sarco* = muscle, *mere* = small). The thick filaments are located in the centre of the sarcomere where their organisation into parallel filaments produces a dark band called the A band (Figure 4.1). Additionally, each sarcomere contains

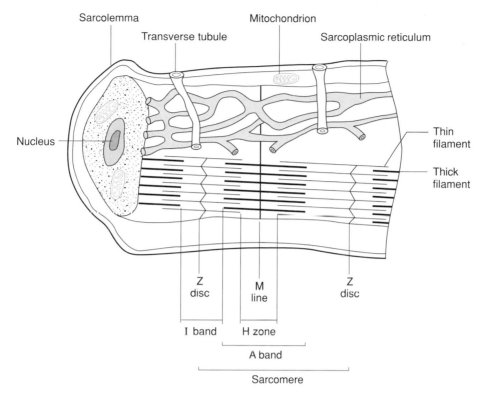

Figure 4.1 Organisation of a skeletal muscle fibre.

a set of thin filaments located at each end, with one end being anchored to the Z line with the other end overlapping the thick filaments. The Z line is essentially a network of interconnecting proteins with two successive Z lines encompassing one sarcomere. The Z line also bisects those parts of the thin filaments that are not overlapped by the thick filaments. Thus a light band, the I band, is seen between the ends of the A band of two adjacent sarcomeres.

The main function of the proteins troponin and tropomyosin is to regulate the making and breaking of contacts between thick and thin filaments during muscular contraction. Tropomyosins are long polypeptide molecules, which attach end to end with minimal overlap, forming two very thin continuous strands running along the length of the actin filament. Tropomyosins are rod-shaped in appearance, approximately 40 nm in length, and are positioned alongside each of the two grooves in the actin double helix. This structure allows each tropomyosin molecule to be in close proximity to seven actin monomers. Troponin is a more complex protein. The molecule contains three sub-units: a calcium binding protein (TN-C); an inhibitory protein (TN-1); a tropomyosin binding protein (TN-T). It is globular in shape, and is attached at regular intervals to both the actin and tropomyosin proteins. Tropomyosin and troponin work simultaneously with calcium ions to either maintain relaxation or initiate action of the myofibril. This interaction between molecules will be discussed later.

Skeletal muscle fibre types

Skeletal muscles are composed of various types of muscle fibres and based on metabolic and contractile characteristics are classified into two groups:

Type 1

Type 1 or slow-twitch fibres contain a large number of mitochondria and myoglobin and a high concentration of mitochondrial enzymes. This type of fibre has low myosin ATPase activity and slow calcium handling ability and shortening speed and hence generates comparatively less force. Type 1 fibres generate energy for ATP resynthesis mainly via oxidative phosphorylation. Thus, this type of fibre is predominately utilised during prolonged aerobic exercise since it is relatively fatigue resistant because of lower force generation, and also has an abundant supply of energy via oxidative phosphorylation.

Type 2

In contrast to type 1, type 2 or fast-twitch fibres possess a high capability for electrochemical transmission of action potentials and increased activity of myosin ATPase, and hence larger force generation. Calcium is also rapidly released by the sarcoplasmic reticulum, which contributes to this fibre's rapid ATP turnover for short, intense periods of muscular contraction. Type 2 fibres rely heavily on the glycolytic system for energy production; thus this fibre type is particularly suited to exercise of an anaerobic nature and correspondingly these fibre types also tend to fatigue more rapidly than type 1 fibres.

There are several subdivisions of type 2 fibres. The intermediate type 2a fibre (also termed fast-oxidative-glycolytic (FOG) fibre) has a moderate calcium capacity with a medium to high oxidative capacity. This fibre has the ability to generate a moderate force output. Thus this fibre type is best suited for exercise that involves the transfer of energy from both aerobic and anaerobic sources (McArdle et al., 2001). Type 2b fibres, in contrast, have a high glycolytic and low oxidative capacity. They have the ability to generate a large power output, and are therefore best suited to exercise of an anaerobic type.

Buller and colleagues provided the first important stimulus for studies on exercise-induced changes in muscle fibre type in 1960, when they showed the occurrence of fibre changes during the cross-innervation of slow muscles by fast nerves and vice versa. In past decades, research has shown that both endurance and strength training can cause the fibre type to change from type 2 to type 1 (Hamilton and Booth, 2000). The characteristics of fibre type that influence muscle fatigue and power output may also provide useful information on the risk of developing disease. Hamilton and Booth (2000) report that there exists an association between a high percentage of type 2 fibres and the 'metabolic syndrome' (the metabolic clustering of atherosclerosis, type 2 diabetes mellitus and hypertension). A cause-and-effect relationship between muscle fibre type and pathology has not been proven directly, rather it is the metabolic properties per se that are associated with different fibre types that appear to influence predisposition to disease.

Skeletal muscle connective tissue

Muscle connective tissue is essential, since it provides structure to the muscle belly and allows the force generated in the muscle to be transmitted to the tendon eliciting movement and/or force. There are three levels of organisation of muscle connective tissue, with each embedded in an amorphous protein based ground substance.

Epimysium
This is the outer muscle membrane covering the entire surface of the muscle belly, separating it from other muscles. It is composed of tight bundles of collagen fibres approximately 600 to 1800 nm in diameter.

Perimysium
This is the middle connective tissue membrane, which separates the muscle fibres into bundles called fascicles. The perimysium also provides a route for blood vessels and nerves to pass through the muscle belly. Thus, arguably, it is a type of conductance system.

Endomysium
The endomysium is a sheath of connective tissue covering each muscle fibre, and allows individual muscle fibres to be separated from adjacent fibres. The various sheaths of connective tissue blend with the tendon in a way that is determined by function and space.

Muscle innervation by the nervous system

Muscle fibres are innervated by motor neurons, which have responsibility for transmitting the electrochemical signal from the spinal cord to the muscle. The majority of motor neurons contain dendrites – the neuron receivers. The impulses coming into the nerve enter the neuron via these dendrites. These processes carry the impulses towards the cell body. The axon, in contrast, carries the impulse away from the cell body. Motor neurons have only one axon, which is myelinated and is the largest diameter axon in the human body. The latter point in particular allows for rapid transmitting of signals from the central nervous system to skeletal muscle fibres. Within skeletal muscle, the axon splits into numerous branches called the axon terminals. Each branch forms a single junction with a muscle fibre. Thus, a single motor neuron innervates many muscle fibres.

> Note: *myelin is a fatty substance that insulates the nerve, allowing faster nerve impulse transmission than in an unmyelinated nerve. In a myelinated nerve, impulses leap from node of Ranvier to node of Ranvier. This is a physical conduction rather than a chemical one and is known as saltatory conduction. See section on action potential conduction and synaptic transmission, p. 42.*

The plasma membrane contains channel proteins that allow the principal cellular ions, sodium (Na^+), potassium (K^+), calcium (Ca^{2+}) and chloride (Cl^-) to move through it at different rates down their concentration gradients. Ion concentration gradients and selective movement of ions through channels create a difference in electric potential between the inside and outside of the cell. This is known as the membrane potential and is measured in millivolts (mV). At rest the neuron contains a high concentration of K^+ ions inside the cell, and a high concentration of Na^+ ions on the outside. The resting membrane potential reflects a compromise between the equilibrium potentials for K^+ and Na^+ (that is, the movement of these ions into and out of the cell). At rest, the cell membrane of a neuron has a negative electrical potential of between -60 and -70 mV. When the charges across the membrane differ, the membrane is polarised.

The action potential is the signal that conveys information over distances in the nervous system. Each action potential usually lasts approximately 1 msec. The action potential arises due to a rapid reversal of the resting membrane potential where the intracellular environment becomes positively charged with respect to the outside. This change in potential is termed depolarisation and is due to a change in the permeability of the cell membrane to Na^+ ions brought about by an opening of the Na^+ ion channels. Thus there is an influx of sodium down its concentration gradient into the cell. This causes the number of positive ions within the cell to increase. The potential at this stage increases to approximately +30 mV. Action potentials follow the all or nothing principle, that is, if depolarisation reaches a certain level (approximately -55 mV) then the voltage-gated ion channels open, producing an action potential which is always the same size.

This depolarisation stimulates voltage sensitive K^+ channels to open causing K^+ ions to exit the cell. The loss of large quantities of K^+ brings the intracellular environment back to a negative value of approximately -90 mV. The membrane potential remains hyperpolarised until the voltage-gated K^+ channels close. During this phase, when a particular segment of an axon is generating an action potential and its sodium gates are deactivated, it does not have the ability to respond to other stimulus. This inability is referred to as the absolute refractory period. However, when the potassium gates are open, and repolarisation is occurring, the segment of the axon can then respond to a new stimulus as long as the stimulus is of a greater magnitude to evoke an action potential. This is termed the relative refractory period.

Because of the huge differences in concentration gradients across the membrane some sodium ions slowly leak into the cell while some potassium ions slowly leak out. The sodium/potassium pump corrects this 'leak current'. The pump is therefore responsible for the long-term maintenance of concentration gradients and is of central importance in metabolic physiology.

Action potential conduction and synaptic transmission

In order to communicate information to muscle, nerve impulses must travel from where they originate (axon hillock) to the axon terminals. The special mode of impulse travel is termed propagation or conduction. As Na^+ ions flow into the axon hillock of the nerve cells, the depolarisation subsequently stimulates the opening of voltage-gated Na^+ channels in adjacent portions of the membrane. Due to the membrane being refractory, the stimulus can move in one direction only. This type of *continuous conduction* is chemical in nature and occurs in muscle fibres and unmyelinated axons. In myelinated axons, wherever a myelin sheath covers the axolemma, such as those conducting impulses to skeletal muscle, there are few voltage-gated ion channels. At the nodes of Ranvier, the myelin sheath is interrupted and the axolemma has a high density of voltage-gated ion channels. Membrane depolarisation occurs only at these nodes; therefore the impulse appears to leap from node to node. This type of impulse conduction, characteristic of myelinated axons, is called saltatory conduction.

At the site of an axon terminal, an impulse transmission can travel from one neuron to another across a synapse. At a synapse the neuron sending the signal is called the pre-synaptic neuron. Similarly, the neuron receiving the signal is called the post-synaptic neuron, possessing post-synaptic receptors. There are two types of synapses that differ electrically and functionally: electrical synapses and chemical synapses. At an electrical synapse, ionic current spreads directly between adjacent cells through gap junctions. Each gap junction contains a hundred or so tubular proteins called connexons that form tunnels connecting the two cells. Both ions and molecules are able to flow back and forth through the connexons. Gap junctions are common in visceral smooth muscle and cardiac muscle and are also present in the central nervous system (CNS).

At a chemical synapse, the plasma membrane of the pre- and post-synaptic neurons do not touch each other. The axon terminals and the post-synaptic receptors are separated by a narrow gap called the synaptic cleft. Nerve signals cannot propagate across the synaptic cleft. However, a chemical signal in the form of a neurotransmitter, such as acetylcholine, can diffuse across the synaptic cleft and stimulate the receptors on the post-synaptic neuron. The post-synaptic neuron receives the signal and generates an action potential.

A typical chemical synapse transmits as follows:

- The action potential arrives at a synaptic end bulb of a pre-synaptic neuron.
- The depolarising action potential activates Ca^{2+} channels causing an influx of Ca^{2+} into the neuron.
- The Ca^{2+} triggers exocytosis of the synaptic vesicles.
- The vesicles fuse with the plasma membrane to cause a release of the neurotransmitter into the synaptic cleft.
- The neurotransmitter diffuses across the synaptic cleft and binds to neurotransmitter receptors on the post-synaptic membrane.
- This interaction between the neurotransmitter and the receptor causes activation of the ion channels and a resultant inward flow of ions.
- The influx of ions into the neuron causes depolarisation of the post-synaptic membrane.
- If polarisation reaches threshold, an action potential occurs.

The neuromuscular junction

Whereas neurons communicate with each other at synapses, the neuromuscular junction (NMJ) is the site where a motor neuron communicates with a skeletal muscle fibre. At the NMJ the axon terminals divide into a cluster of synaptic end bulbs. Each synaptic end bulb contains hundreds of membrane enclosed sacs called synaptic membrane-bound vesicles, containing the excitatory neurotransmitter acetylcholine (ACh). ACh is used for communication between the neuron and muscle cell. It is thought that Ca^{2+}, being in close proximity to the regions that release the neurotransmitter inside the terminal, is the trigger for neurotransmitter release. Ca^{2+} causes fusion of the vesicular membrane with the terminal membrane resulting in a release of ACh from the vesicles. Ca^{2+} influx into the cell can be graded and therefore there is also a graded release of quantal units of ACh. The region of the muscle fibre membrane adjacent to the synaptic end bulbs is termed the motor end plate. The motor end plate contains between 30–40 acetylcholine receptors (integral transmembrane proteins that bind specifically to ACh). The enzyme acetylcholinesterase (AChE) is located in the synaptic cleft and is used to break down ACh following completion of synaptic transmission.

A nerve impulse elicits a muscle action potential in the following way:

- An action potential travels down the axon and reaches the axon terminal.
- This causes Ca^{2+} channels in the synaptic end bulb to open and Ca^{2+} to flow into the nerve cell.
- Influx of Ca^{2+} stimulates exocytosis of ACh into the synaptic cleft.
- ACh diffuses across the synaptic cleft at the NMJ and binds to acetylcholine receptors at the motor end plate.
- On binding of ACh to the receptor sites, Na^+ channels in the plasma membrane of the motor end plate open and Na^+ enters the post-synaptic sarcolemma (muscle membrane).
- The resulting change in Na^+ concentration causes depolarisation of the sarcolemma.
- This causes depolarisation of the adjacent plasma membrane, which reaches threshold causing an action potential to be initiated.
- The action potential propagates over the surface of the entire muscle fibre and continues into the fibre along specialised invaginations of the sarcolemma called transverse or T-tubules. These T-tubules form a tunnel from the surface towards the centre of each muscle fibre allowing the action potential to reach all parts of the muscle fibre virtually simultaneously.
- The transverse tubules come into contact with a system of tubules containing Ca^{2+} ions which encircle each myofibril and is called the sarcoplasmic reticulum (SR).
- The action potential reaches the SR via the T-tubules causing the release of Ca^{2+} from the SR resulting in a muscle contraction.

Muscle contraction

There are three ways in which a myofibril (muscle fibre) contracts or is activated. These are termed: isometric, eccentric and concentric contractions. Isometric contraction occurs when both ends of the muscle fibre are fixed, with no movement occurring in the joints and hence the muscle length remains unaltered. In dynamic exercise a shortening of the muscle fibre is called concentric contraction, whereas fibre lengthening is termed eccentric contraction. Both types are classed as isotonic contractions. Maximal force generation by a muscle occurs during a fast eccentric contraction with force declining when the fibre is activated in a concentric contraction at high speed. Although eccentric contractions produce the highest force output this type of contraction is also associated with skeletal muscle damage, presumably due to mechanical stresses occurring during lengthening. A large number of studies have used the appearance of biochemical markers such as lactate dehydrogenase, myoglobin and phosphocreatine kinase in the blood to confirm the occurrence of muscle damage.

Muscle contraction occurs in the following way:

- Ca^{2+} released from the SR binds to troponin on the actin filament.
- The binding of Ca^{2+} to troponin moves the tropomyosin from its blocking position and the active binding site on actin is exposed.
- Myosin 'heads' are then able to bind to actin and rotate.
- As the myosin heads rotate, they pull the actin along so that myosin and actin myofilaments slide past each other.
- Actin myofilaments from opposite ends of the sarcomere move toward each other and the muscle contracts.
- This process is known as the sliding filament theory of muscle contraction.
- Muscle relaxation occurs when Ca^{2+} is sequestered (bound) by the SR. Troponin and tropomyosin once again block the binding sites and the sarcomeres return to regular resting length. The re-uptake of Ca^{2+} by the SR depends on the action of a calcium pump and therefore requires the presence of ATP.

Skeletal muscle strength and endurance

Muscle strength

Muscle strength is typically defined as the maximal force that a muscle can generate. Gains in muscular strength are largely the result of increases in muscle size (hypertrophy), and adaptations to the neuromuscular system, combined to a lesser degree with muscle hyperplasia (increase in number of fibres per unit of volume). Prior to visual changes in muscle, there are a number of neurogenic changes that occur, which contribute to an overall increase in muscular strength. Indeed, it has been suggested that gains in strength may be achieved without structural changes to muscle, but not without neuromuscular adaptations. Thus, strength is not entirely a property of the muscle, rather it is a property of the motor system.

The neuromuscular adaptations that occur from strength training include:

- A more efficient neural recruitment pattern
- Increased central nervous system activation
- Improved synchronisation of motor units
- Inhibition of Golgi tendon organs

In addition to the neuromuscular adaptations, strength training stimulates an increase in the size of predominately, fast-twitch glycolytic fibres (hypertrophy). Such hypertrophy of muscle tissue is readily caused by exercise that emphasises isometric or slow isotonic contractions. The modifications to fibre size are mainly a consequence of increased synthesis of the filament proteins myosin and actin, which permit a greater opportunity for cross-bridge interaction and thus substantial increases in muscular force. It has been reported that the diameter of skeletal muscle increases by approximately 30% as a result of frequent resistance training (hypertrophy), while work has shown a 46% increase in the number of nuclei within the muscle fibres (McArdle et al., 2001). Increased cross-sectional area occurs as a result of new myofilaments being added to the external layers of the myofibril, creating a cumulative effect of fibre enlargement. These alterations with intense muscular overload are associated with a marked upregulation in DNA synthesis and a proliferation of connective tissue cells. This proliferation strengthens and thickens the connective tissue of the muscle, thereby improving the functional integrity of both tendons and ligaments. These modifications to the structure of the muscle provide some protection from joint and muscle damage. Importantly, this offers clear justification for the use of resistance training in preventive and therapeutic rehabilitation programmes. Changes to energy-generating compounds within the muscle cell have also been observed as a result of resistance training. These biochemical modifications include an increase in the enzymes creatine phosphokinase, phosphofructokinase, phosphorylase and Krebs cycle enzyme activity as well as increases in various intramuscular fuels such as adenosine triphosphate, phosphocreatine and glycogen (McArdle et al., 2001).

Aside from an increase in the cross-sectional area of muscle fibres, research also suggests that intensive strength training can cause the actual number of muscle cells to divide (Antonio and Gonyea, 1993). This phenomenon is termed hyperplasia, and occurs through the development of some new muscle fibres from satellite cells (precursor muscle cells), or through a process of longitudinal splitting. Satellite cells lie between the basement layer and plasma membrane and are predominately dormant. However, they can be activated to develop new muscle fibres under conditions of stress such as that brought about by resistance training, muscle damage and in some disease states, for example, neuromuscular disease (McArdle et al., 2001). The mechanism of activation of satellite cells, once muscle damage has occurred, involves a movement of the satellite cells into the damaged portion of the muscle tissue. Following several mitotic episodes the new cells form a multi-nucleated tube of cells called myotubes. The myotubes develop into a myofibre and become innervated by nerve cells. In the case of longitudinal splitting, a relatively large hypertrophied muscle fibre splits into two or more smaller individual daughter fibres. See Chapter 6 for assessment of muscular strength.

Muscle endurance

Local muscle endurance can be defined as the ability of a muscle to perform repeated contractions against a sub-maximal resistance. Muscle endurance can be increased through gains in:

- Muscular strength
- Metabolic efficiency (increases in myoglobin, mitochondrial function and oxidative enzymes)
- Circulatory function (changes in heart size, stroke volume, heart rate, cardiac output, blood flow and blood volume) (see Chapter 6 for measurement of muscular endurance)

Skeletal muscle adaptations to aerobic exercise training

The study of adaptations to exercise training demonstrates a diverse range of integrative approaches, from the peripheral to the molecular level. This section is concerned only with localised skeletal muscle adaptations caused as a result of aerobic exercise training.

Myoglobin content

Myoglobin is an oxygen binding protein, similar to the structure of haemoglobin, which acts as a storage site for oxygen within muscle. The main function of myoglobin is to facilitate the transportation of oxygen from the cell membrane to the mitochondria. Animal studies have shown an increase in skeletal muscle myoglobin content following endurance training (Chaikovski et al., 1987), whilst a recent study in human skeletal muscle by Masuda et al. (2001) has concluded that eight weeks of endurance training does not alter myoglobin content.

Mitochondrial volume, size and enzymes

An increase in the number and size of mitochondrial proteins is perhaps the most important effect of exercise training. These changes will greatly increase capacity of myofibrillar muscle to generate ATP aerobically. Along with a substantial increase in mitochondrial volume comes a parallel increase in oxidative enzyme activity. The predominant mitochondrial enzymes to increase include those of the citric acid cycle (NADH dehydrogenase, succinate dehydrogenage, pyruvate-malate oxidase) and mitochondrial electron transport chain (cytochrome oxidase, cytochromes a and c).

Substrate utilisation

It is widely accepted that trained muscles, exercising at the same relative intensity as untrained muscles rely on fatty acids as the main energy source, whereas in untrained muscle their efficiency in utilising fat as a fuel is compromised. In the main, fatty acids are oxidised due to:

- An upregulation of fat oxidative enzymes
- Increased intramuscular triglyceride stores
- Increased lipolysis

This preferential oxidation of fats results in a carbohydrate sparing effect and increased muscular endurance. In addition, research has shown that aerobic exercise can be extremely effective in preventing and/or treating some of the most common metabolic diseases of the modern era. For example, endurance trained muscle can rapidly clear plasma lipids, thus decreasing susceptibility to cardio-vascular disease (Durstine et al., 2002).

Skeletal muscle, oxidative stress and antioxidants

Oxidative stress and exercise

Free radicals are molecules with one or more unpaired electrons that are often highly reactive and are capable of independent existence. They can cause damage to DNA, proteins, lipids and sugars when formed in muscle cells. Common types of free radicals found in vivo include:

- superoxide anion ($O_2^{\cdot-}$)
- nitric oxide ($NO^{\cdot}$)
- hydroxyl ($OH^{\cdot}$)
- hydroperoxyl radical ($HOO^{\cdot}$)

In addition, other compounds can cause oxidative damage in vivo but are not strictly free radicals because they do not possess an unpaired electron. Examples include hydrogen peroxide (H_2O_2) and hypochlorous acid (HOCl) the common ingredient in household bleach.

Importantly these oxidants are formed at rest as by-products of normal energy metabolism and it has been estimated that for every 25 oxygen molecules reduced by normal cellular respiration, one free radical is formed (McCord, 1979). However, given the fact that the rate of oxygen uptake by the body during exercise may increase up to approximately 35-fold and that oxygen flux through active skeletal muscle tissue may reach 200-fold above resting values (Aw et al., 1986), it is conceivable that any rise in metabolism may well increase free radical production leading to damage to surrounding muscle tissue. This hypothesis was investigated and confirmed by two recent studies using electron spin resonance (ESR) spectroscopy (the most direct and sensitive method to measure free radical species) to measure free radical concentration in the venous circulation of male university students following exhaustive aerobic exercise (Ashton et al., 1998; Davison et al., 2002a).

Both studies also observed an increase in lipid hydroperoxide concentration, suggesting that exhaustive exercise causes cell membrane damage. This paradoxical 'oxygen' relationship between an apparently healthy act (such as exercise) and the occurrence of harmful biological reactions, prompted Jenkins (1993) to state that: 'elemental and gaseous oxygen presents a conundrum in that it is simultaneously essential for and potentially destructive to human life'.

Among the most widely reported sources of exercise-induced free radical production in skeletal muscle are:

Mitochondrial electron leakage

The mitochondia are the major site of oxidation and reduction of molecular oxygen (O_2) to water (H_2O). The mitochondrial electron transport chain is possibly the main source of cellular free radical formation.

In a normally functioning mammalian respiratory chain, electrons are passed from substrates in the citric acid cycle either directly from succinate or by the electron carrier nicotinamide adenine di-nucleotide (NAD^+). The electrons pass through a sequence of protein or non-protein transporters to the catalytic site of cytochrome oxidase, where 4 electrons together with 4 hydrogen ions tetravalently reduce molecular oxygen to H_2O. A proportion of the O_2 reduced by normal respiration is converted to O_2^- at intermediate steps of the mitochondrial respiratory chain. This production may occur at the level of the NADH dehydrogenase (Turrens and Boveris, 1980) and/or at the level of ubiquinone-cytochrome bc_1 segment of complex III (Raha et al., 2000). There seems to be a disruption in the transfer of electrons from ubisemiquinone to the non-protein quinone, where electrons become dislodged and are 'freed' into the mitochondrial matrix where they bind with O_2 to form O_2^- (univalent reduction).

Estimates of resting percent leakage with the mitochondria can vary from 1–15%. However, if O_2 flux in active mammalian skeletal muscle increases 200-fold, an increase in electron flux through rapidly respiring mitochondria could possibly lead to an enhancement of electron leakage and the formation of free radicals such O_2^- and OH^-. Therefore a greater biochemical demand from exercise may cause an increase in free radical production and surrounding skeletal tissue damage.

Xanthine oxidase activation

Xanthine is an intermediary product of adenine nucleotide (purine) metabolism and exists primarily in two enzymatic forms in vivo: xanthine dehydrogenase (XDH) and xanthine oxidase (XO). In normal tissue, it is estimated that between 70–90% of the total enzyme activity exists in the dehydrogenase form, located primarily in the vessel walls of many tissues including cardiac and skeletal muscle (Hellsten, 1996). Under normal resting metabolic conditions, XDH catalyses the oxidation of hypoxanthine to xanthine, and xanthine to uric acid, using NAD^+ as the sole electron acceptor. However, when the body is subjected to heavy stress and ischaemia, it is thought that the configuration of the XDH enzyme changes to the irreversible oxidase form (XO). Upon reperfusion XO uses molecular oxygen as the final electron acceptor, univalently forming O_2^- radicals. The conversion mechanism of XDH to XO is largely unknown. However, a number of theories have been put forward, including the oxidation of critical sulphydryl (–SH) groups or proteolysis (Halliwell and Gutteridge, 1999). It is suggested that the proteolytic cleavage of XDH during ischaemia is due to a lack of ATP regeneration, causing a malfunction to the ATP-dependent calcium pumps. The subsequent rise in intracellular calcium may activate calcium proteases (calpin) causing enzymatic cleavage (Sjödin et al., 1990). A theoretical mechanism has been proposed linking intense exercise, at or above maximum oxygen uptake ($\dot{V}O_2$max) with XO activated free radical production in skeletal muscle tissue (Witt et al., 1992). It is suggested that during exhaustive exercise the decrease in blood flow to various organs and tissues (especially the kidneys and gut) could result in hypoxia. Upon cessation of exercise the return of re-oxygenated blood (reperfusion) to these regions may lead to an excess of O_2^{-} production.

Excessive calcium accumulation

Increased intracellular calcium (Ca^{2+}) concentration has been implicated in free radical production. The mechanisms known to induce cellular damage to skeletal muscle tissue have been the subject of much debate, and it is thought that a disruption in Ca^{2+} homeostasis is the primary reason for exercise-induced muscle damage (Jackson, 1994).

Hypoxic cells are known to deplete ATP, which may cause the ATP-dependent Ca^{2+} pumps to malfunction. This occurrence may raise intracellular free Ca^{2+} content which may activate Ca^{2+} proteases, causing enzymatic cleavage to xanthine oxidase, and as a consequence produce O_2^{-} radicals. This increased production of O_2^{-} leads to tissue damage and exercise-induced oxidative stress. Research by Jackson et al. (1984) and Claremont et al. (1984) showed that the amount of cellular damage (as measured by extracellular lactate dehydrogenase) observed in isolated soleus muscle tissue in response to hypoxic exposure, was directly proportional to extracellular calcium concentration. Similar observations have been highlighted in cardiac tissue, where the degree of cellular damage induced by periods of ischemia-reperfusion also appears to be dependent on extracellular Ca^{2+} levels (Supinski et al., 1999). It is thus evident that cellular deformation and disruption of Ca^{2+} homeostasis are closely associated with oxidative stress and are important components of the damage caused by free radicals. As with other mechanisms there still remains the challenge in determining cause and effect with reference to the relationship between intracellular Ca^{2+} accumulation and exercise-induced oxidative stress.

The previous sections have examined the various sources of these harmful free radicals to which we are continuously exposed, particularly during exercise. Fortunately, the muscle cell is not defenceless against the generation of free radicals. All mammalian aerobic organisms utilise a series of antioxidant defences in an attempt to protect against oxidative stress. The main function of antioxidants in the muscle cell is to prevent free radical formation or intercept free radical attack by scavenging the reactive species and converting them to less harmful molecules. Antioxidant defences within skeletal muscle cells may be divided into enzymatic and non-enzymatic antioxidants.

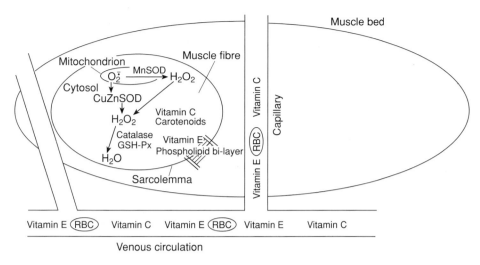

Figure 4.2 Antioxidant activity within skeletal muscle.

Enzymatic antioxidant defences

Enzymatic antioxidants include:

- Catalase (CAT)
- Glutathione peroxidase (GPX)
- Superoxide dismutase (SOD) (including manganese SOD found within the mitochondria and copper-zinc SOD found in the cytosol)

SOD, CAT and GPX are thought to provide the first line of defence against free radical formation in the muscle cell (see Figure 4.2). Therefore it is inevitable that exercise per se may increase these enzymes. Various exercise-training studies have shown an increase in muscle content of MnSOD, CuZnSOD and GPX. For example, Miyazaki et al. (2001) recently exercised nine untrained male subjects for 12 weeks, and found an increase in erythrocyte total SOD and glutathione peroxidase activity. This work suggests that in order to combat cell damage induced by free radicals, a structured exercise-training programme is particularly beneficial for a protective adaptation to occur.

Non-enzymatic antioxidant defences

The most important non-enzymatic antioxidants, include, but are not limited to, antioxidant vitamins, such as:

- Ascorbic acid (vitamin C)
- Tocopherols (vitamin E)
- Carotenoids (beta carotene, lycopene)

These antioxidants are located at specific sites within a muscle cell (see Figure 4.2), and all serve to decrease free radical formation and subsequent cellular damage. A number of studies have examined the role of antioxidant supplementation in the prevention of exercise-induced free radical production. The general consensus being that supplementation decreases oxidative stress induced by physical exercise. For example, the effect of an antioxidant mixture on oxidative stress during exercise was examined by Viguie et al. (1989). Twenty-three trained male volunteers exercised at 65% $\dot{V}O_2$max following eight weeks of supplementation with 10 mg β-carotene, 800 IU vitamin E and 1000 mg of vitamin C. The findings show a reduction in skeletal muscle damage as measured by creatine kinase following exercise. Instead of examining the effect of long-term supplementation, others have examined the effects of short-term supplementation. Ashton and colleagues (1999) were the first to use ESR spectroscopy to directly measure free radical concentration and hence determine the effect of vitamin C supplementation on exercise-induced free radical production. Subjects ingested either 1000 mg of vitamin C or a placebo two hours prior to performing a $\dot{V}O_2$max test. The vitamin C decreased free radicals and cell membrane damage following exercise in comparison to that observed in the placebo group. In a follow-up study using patients with type 1 diabetes mellitus, Davison et al. (2002b) observed a decreased free radical concentration following supplementation with 1000 mg of vitamin C. These latter studies demonstrate the effective use of vitamin C in combating cell damage.

It is widely accepted that exercise is beneficial to health and can lead to considerable health benefits. However, even a brief overview of the oxidative stress literature, would suggest that strenuous exercise, especially by untrained individuals, causes damage to cell membranes. Furthermore, recent evidence has shown that exercise can modify DNA molecules (Poulsen et al., 1996). If exercise causes DNA damage then the possibility for cellular mutation exists with potentially serious consequences. Jenkins (2000) has recently asked a pertinent question: can exercise induce an oxidant stress that might exert potentially adverse effects on human health? Undoubtedly, much more research applying a broader spectrum of analytical tools is needed to make conclusive statements relating exercise and oxidative stress to pathology. However, there is a wealth of information suggesting that regular moderate exercise training can increase the antioxidant enzymes, leading to important muscular adaptations which protect the cells against the damage caused by increased production of free radicals and hence oxidative stress. In addition, it is well documented that ingesting at least five portions of fresh fruit and vegetables per day should provide the necessary antioxidant vitamins the body requires for good health.

Summary

Striated muscle, especially skeletal muscle, is a remarkable organ system. It is virtually the only organ system that can undergo substantial increases in size and can change from complete rest to maximum effort within a few seconds. It can generate enormous force, yet also allow the most delicate of movement. Witness the phenomenal force generated by Olympic power lifters to lift spectacularly heavy weights compared to the most delicate of movements by the hand of a surgeon. It consumes vast quantities of molecular oxygen during cellular respiration and can be severely damaged by molecular species such as free radicals and mechanical stress during exercise. Yet it can continue to function and even repair itself. Muscle wasting is a feature of bed rest in hospital patients and of pathologies such as Duchenne muscular dystrophy and contributes to poor clinical outcomes following surgery. Thus the ability to deliver a comprehensive, well thought out plan of muscular exercise for therapeutic purposes and general health is an essential skill required by virtually all physiotherapists.

BONES AND JOINTS

Bone and joint structure

The main functions of bone within its role in the musculoskeletal system are support and assistance with movement. Bones serve as a framework providing attachment points for skeletal muscle. Where two bones come into contact with each other they form a joint. Skeletal muscle is positioned across joints between long bones. Contraction of this skeletal muscle therefore allows movement of the long bones.

Anatomy of a bone

A typical long bone consists of several parts. The diaphysis is the long cylindrical main portion of the bone. The epiphyses are the proximal and distal ends of the bone. These are covered on the external surface by articular cartilage, which allows friction free movement at joints. The metaphyses are the regions where the diaphysis and the epiphyses join. In the growing bone this region is made of cartilage, which allows the bone to grow in length. In the mature adult bone this is replaced by bone forming the epiphyseal line. The outer surface of the bone is made of dense irregular tissue known as the periosteum and enclosed within this periosteum, along the length of the diaphysis, is the medullary cavity containing bone marrow. The lining of this medullary cavity is called the endosteum and this membrane contains bone forming cells.

Bone histology

The bony matrix is made up of about 25% water, 25% protein fibres and 50% crystallised mineral salts, in addition to bone forming and bone re-sorbing cells called osteoblasts and osteoclasts respectively. The main mineral salts found in bone are hydroxyapetite (calcium phosphate) and some calcium carbonate. These are scattered through the matrix of collagen fibres and as they crystallise, the matrix hardens, a process known as calcification. Osteoblasts are the bone forming cells and secrete the collagen fibres required for the matrix of the bone; they also initiate the calcification process. Bone is not completely solid but has many channels for nerves and blood vessels that supply the bone cells with nutrients. Depending on the volume of these spaces, bone is classified as either compact (80% of bone) or spongy (20% of bone). Compact bone contains few spaces and forms the external layer of all bones. It functions in protection and support. Spongy bone is made up of an irregular lattice of thin columns of bone called trabeculae. The spaces between are filled with bone marrow, which produces red bone cells. Spongy bone makes up most of the structure of short, flat and irregular shaped bones and the epiphyses of long bones. It is lighter than compact bone and therefore makes movement easier.

Bone is constantly undergoing a process of renewal called remodelling, whereby the bone tissue redistributes its matrix along lines of mechanical stress. A balance exists between the action of osteoblasts and osteoclasts, which remove minerals and collagen from the bone. The main mechanical stresses on bones result from the contraction of skeletal muscle. Bones of athletes, which are repetitively and highly stressed, become notably thicker than those of non-athletes. Thus weight-bearing exercise is important in protecting and promoting bone health, and can be used in therapeutic and rehabilitation programmes, such as in the treatment of osteoporosis.

Joint structure

The structure of a joint determines its combination of strength and flexibility. Some joints permit no movement such as those between the bones of the skull. Those associated with the bones in the limbs and thereby associated with movement of the body are mainly synovial joints. These joints have a space called a synovial cavity between the articulating bones, allowing the joints to move freely. The bones at a synovial joint are covered by hyaline cartilage, providing a smooth slippery surface for the articulating bone. The joint itself is enclosed in a capsule consisting of an outer fibrous layer, providing mobility and strength, and an inner synovial membrane. The synovial membrane secretes synovial fluid, consisting of interstitial fluid and hyaluronic acid. The primary function of this fluid is to reduce friction by lubricating the joint and to supply nutrients to the cells of the joint. The joint is held together by fibrous bundles called ligaments.

Bone and joint adaptations to exercise

In general, studies have found an increase in the density of weight-bearing long bone with exercise training. However, the mechanism behind this observation is not well understood. This adaptation appears to be regardless of gender and age. Males and females that participate in strength and power activities have a greater bone mass than endurance athletes (Robinson et al., 1995). This beneficial effect of exercise is thought to occur at the particular site of the working muscles and bones to which they are attached. For example, the lower limb bones of endurance athletes have a greater bone mineral content when compared to a less active group (McArdle et al., 2001), and tennis players show on average 20–25% greater bone mineral content in the humeral shaft and proximal humerus of the playing arm when compared with the non-dominant arm (Kontulainen et al., 1999). Research has also demonstrated that bone mineral density correlates to measures of muscular strength (Nichols et al., 1995) and that the lumbar spine and proximal femur bone densities of elite junior weightlifters are greater than adult mature bone values (Conroy et al., 1993).

The beneficial effects of exercise as a prophylactic measure against bone loss is well documented in post-menopausal women. The menopause makes women extremely susceptible to osteoporosis. Osteoporosis is a disease of near epidemic proportions (particularly in women above age 60) and is characterised by decreased bone mineral content. The aetiology of osteoporosis in post-menopausal women is due to three primary factors:

- Oestrogen deficiency
- Inadequate physical exercise
- Inadequate calcium and vitamin D status

Although exercise is not as effective as hormone replacement therapy in preventing bone loss in post-menopausal women, exercise can maintain and even increase bone mass. An early study by White and colleagues (1984) suggests that mechanical loading due to aerobic dancing, that is, weightbearing exercise, may be effective in preventing post-menopausal osteoporosis. Importantly, the bone mineral content of normally menstruating runners is higher than that of normally menstruating non-running females, suggesting that female athletes have a greater bone mineral content than untrained, when matched by menstrual status (Wilmore and Costill, 1999) (see also Chapter 9).

McArdle et al. (2001) outline five principles for promoting bone health through exercise:

- *Specificity*: exercise provides a local osteogenic effect.
- *Overload*: progressively increasing exercise intensity promotes continued bone deposition.
- *Initial values*: individuals with the smallest total bone mass show the greatest potential for bone deposition.
- *Diminishing returns*: as one approaches the biologic ceiling for bone density, further density gains require greater effort.
- *Reversibility*: discontinuing exercise overload reverses the positive osteogenic effects gained through appropriate exercise stress.

Perhaps one of the most important side effects of performing stretching exercises is an increase in joint flexibility. In 1995 the American College of Sports Medicine (ACSM) suggested that a balanced fitness programme should incorporate both static and dynamic range of motion exercises of the body's main muscle groups in order to increase joint flexibility. This has proven to be the case in a recent study, where ankle joint stiffness decreased by 35% after static stretching (Bressel and Nair, 2002).

Summary

It is clear, then, that bone is a dynamic fully functioning organ of the human body. It is not merely a solid form that does not change. Bone has a strong network of nerve and blood vessels and constantly remodels itself to maintain its integrity. It can repair itself when broken and support phenomenal loads during exercise. For example, a load of several tons is placed upon the bones of the heel during running and jumping. If this is extrapolated to a long-distance run, such as a marathon or ultra-marathon, then an appreciation of the extraordinary properties of bone is apparent. Similarly, when bone deteriorates, such as during osteoporosis, its impact on functional health can be devastating. Thus the preservation of optimal bone health should be a priority of health professionals, including physiotherapists.

References

American College of Sports Medicine (1995). American College of Sports Medicine position stand on osteoporosis and exercise. *Medicine and Science in Sports and Exercise* **27**, I.

Antonio, J. and Gonyea, W.J. (1993). Skeletal muscle fiber hyperplasia. *Medicine and Science in Sports and Exercise* **25**, 1333.

Ashton, T., Rowlands, C.C., Jones, E., Young, I.S., Jackson, S.K., Davies, B. and Peters, J.R. (1998). Electron spin resonance spectroscopic detection of oxygen-centred radicals in human serum following exhaustive exercise. *European Journal of Applied Physiology* **77**, 498–502.

Ashton, T., Young, I.S., Peters, J.R., Jones, E., Jackson, S.K., Davies, B. and Rowlands, C.C. (1999). Electron spin resonance spectroscopy, exercise and oxidative stress: an ascorbic acid intervention study. *Journal of Applied Physiology* **87**, 2032–6.

Aw, T.Y., Andersson, B.S., Kennedy, F.G. and Jones, D. (1986). Intracellular O_2 supply to support mitochondrial function. In *Biochemical Aspects of Physical Exercise* (Benzi, G., Packer, L. and Siliprandi, N. eds). Elsevier, Amsterdam.

Bressel, E. and Nair, P.J. (2002). The effect of prolonged static and cyclic stretching on ankle joint stiffness, torque relaxation and gait in people with stroke. *Physical Therapy* **82** (9), 880–87.

Buller, A.J., Eccles, J.C. and Eccles, R.M. (1960). Interaction between motoneurons and muscles in respect of their characteristic speeds of their responses. *Journal of Physiology* (London) **150**, 417–39.

Chaikovski, V.S., Basharina, O.B., Shaliapina, I.V. and Rogozkin, V.A. (1987). Effect of physical exercise on myoglobin and tropomyosin levels in skeletal muscle of rats. *Voprosy Meditsinskoi Khimii* **33** (4), 79–83.

Claremont, D., Jackson, M.J. and Jones, D.A. (1984). Accumulation of calcium in experimentally damaged mouse muscles *in vitro*. *Proceedings of Physiological Society* March, 57P.

Conroy, B.P., Kramer, W.J., Marsh, C.M., Fleck, S.J., Stone, M.H., Fry, A.C., Miller, P.D. and Dalsky, G.P. (1993). Bone mineral density in elite junior Olympic weightlifters. *Medicine and Science in Sports and Exercise* 25, 1103–9.

Davison, G.W., George, L., Jackson, S.K., Davies, B., Young, I.S., Peters, J.R., Bailey, D.M. and Ashton, T. (2002a). Exercise, free radicals, and lipid peroxidation in type I diabetes mellitus. *Free Radical Biology and Medicine* 33 (11), 1543–51.

Davison, G.W., Young, I.S., George, L., Jackson, S.K., Davies, B., Bailey, D.M., Peters, J.R. and Ashton, T. (2002b). Oxidative stress in type I diabetes mellitus: the effect of ascorbic acid supplementation. *Free Radical Biology and Medicine* 33, Suppl. 1, S110.

Durstine, J.L., Grandjean, P.W., Cox, C.A. and Thompson, P.D. (2002). Lipids, lipoprotein and exercise. *Journal of Cardiopulmonary Rehabilitation* 22 (6), 385–98.

Halliwell, B. and Gutteridge, J.M.C. (1999). *Free Radicals in Biology and Medicine.* Oxford University Press, USA.

Hamilton, M.T. and Booth, F.W. (2000). Skeletal muscle adaptation to exercise: a century of progress. *Journal of Applied Physiology* 88, 327–31.

Hellsten, Y. (1996). Adenine nucleotide metabolism – a role in free radical generation and protection. In: *Human Muscular Function During Dynamic Exercise. Medicine and Sports Science.* (Marconnet, P., Saltin, B., Komi, P. and Poortmans, J. eds), 41, pp. 102–20. Karger, Basel.

Jackson, M.J. (1994). Exercise and oxygen radical production by muscle. In: *Exercise and Oxygen Toxicity* (Sen, C.K., Packer, L. and Hanninan, O. eds). Elsevier, Amsterdam.

Jackson, M.J., Jones, D.A., Edwards, R.H.T. (1984). Experimental muscle damage: the nature of the calcium activated degenerative processes. *European Journal of Clinical Investigation* 14, 369–74.

Jenkins, R.R. (1993). Exercise, oxidative stress, and antioxidants: a review. *International Journal of Sports Nutrition* 3, 356–75.

Jenkins, R.R. (2000). Exercise and oxidative stress methodology: a critique. *American Journal of Clinical Nutrition* 72, 670S–74S.

Kontulainen, S., Kannus, P., Haapalasalo, H., Heinonen, A., Sievanen, H., Oja, P. and Vuori, I. (1999). Changes in bone mineral content with decreased training in competitive young adult tennis players and controls. A prospective follow up study. *Medicine and Science in Sports and Exercise* 31, 646–52.

McArdle, W.D., Katch, F.I. and Katch, V.L. (2001). *Exercise Physiology: Energy, Nutrition and Human Performance.* Lippincott Williams and Wilkins, USA.

McCord, J.M. (1979). Superoxide, superoxide dismutase and oxygen toxicity. *Reviews in Biochemical Toxicology* 1, 109–24.

Masuda, K., Okazaki, K., Kuno, S., Asano, K., Shimojo, H. and Katsuta, S. (2001). Endurance training under 2500 m hypoxia does not increase myoglobin content in human skeletal muscle. *European Journal of Applied Physiology* 85 (5), 486–90.

Miyazaki, H., Oh-ishi, S., Ooakawara, T., Kizaki, T., Toshinai, K., Ha, S., Haga, S., Ji, L.L. and Ohno, H. (2001). Strenuous endurance training in humans reduces oxidative stress following exhausting exercise. *European Journal of Applied Physiology* 84, 1–6.

Nichols, D.L., Sandorn, C.F., Bonnick, S.L., Gench, B. and DiMarco, N. (1995). Relationship between regional body composition to bone mineral density in college females. *Medicine and Science in Sports and Exercise* 27, 178–82.

Poulsen, H.E., Loft, S. and Vistisen, K. (1996). Extreme exercise and oxidative DNA modification. *Journal of Sports Science* 14, 343–6.

Raha, S., McEachern, G.E., Myint, A.T. and Robinson, B.H. (2000). Superoxides from mitochondrial complex III: the role of manganese superoxide dismutase. *Free Radical Biology and Medicine* 29 (2), 170–80.

Robinson, T.L., Snow-Hartery, C., Taaffe, D.R., Gillis, D., Shaw, J. and Marcus, R. (1995). Gymnasts exhibit higher bone mass than runners despite similar prevalence of amenorrhea and oligomenorrhea. *Journal of Bone and Mineral Research* **10**, 26–35.

Sjödin, B., Westing, Y.H. and Apple, F.S. (1990). Biochemical mechanisms for oxygen free radical formation during exercise. *Sports Medicine* **10** (4), 236–54.

Supinski, G., Nethery, D., Stofan, D. and DiMarco, A. (1999). Extracellular calcium modulates generation of reactive oxygen species by the contracting diaphragm. *Journal of Applied Physiology* **87** (6), 2177–85.

Turrens, J.F. and Boveris, A. (1980). Generation of superoxide anion by the NADH dehydrogenase of bovine heart mitochondria. *Biochemistry Journal* **191**, 421–7.

Viguie, C.A., Packer, L. and Brooks, G.A. (1989). Antioxidant supplementation affects indices of muscle trauma and oxidant stress in human blood during exercise. *Medicine and Science in Sports and Exercise* **21**, S16.

White, M.K., Martin, R.B., Yeater, R.A., Butcher, R.L. and Radin, E.L. (1984). The effects of exercise on the bones of post-menopausal women. *International Orthopaedics* **7** (4), 209–14.

Wilmore, J.H. and Costill, D.L. (1999). *Physiology of Sport and Exercise*. Human Kinetics, Champaign Ill.

Witt, E.H., Reznick, A.Z., Viguie, C.A., Starke-Reed, P. and Packer, L. (1992). Exercise, oxidative damage and effects of antioxidant manipulation. *Journal of Nutrition* **122**, 766–73.

Chapter 5

EXERCISE IN DIABETES AND OBESITY

Donal O'Gorman and John Nolan

Key words: obesity, diabetes, type 1 (insulin dependent), type 2 (non-insulin dependent diabetes), body composition, insulin resistance.

Introduction

The incidence of chronic disease has increased dramatically in the latter half of the twentieth century. During this time we have also had tremendous technological development that has drastically changed our lifestyles. Dietary habits have changed with the advent of processed foods, prepackaged foods and fast foods. In addition, our physical activity levels have been curtailed directly by automated systems such as motorised transport and indirectly by leisure time activities including television and computers. The combination of altered dietary habits and physical inactivity indicates that our lifestyle may contribute to the increased incidence of chronic disease.

Obesity, according to the World Health Organization, has increased to epidemic proportions in recent times. In the United States 64.5% of the population are considered overweight, with 30.5% obese (Flegal et al., 2002) and some 300 000 deaths each year are attributed to unhealthy dietary habits and inactive lifestyles (Allison et al., 1999). This trend is not exclusive to the United States and most developed countries across the globe are experiencing increased rates of obesity (Flegal, 1999).

Type 2 diabetes is another chronic disease associated with poor dietary habits and inactivity. An increase in weight of 5–10 kg doubles the risk of developing type 2 diabetes. The prevalence of type 2 diabetes is rapidly increasing, particularly in regions undergoing urbanisation and industrial development. In 1985 the World Health Organization estimated that 30 million people around the world had diabetes. By 2000 it was estimated that 130 million had the disease, and this is expected to rise to 300 million by 2020 (Amos et al., 1997). Type 2 diabetes is thought to account for approximately 90% of these figures.

Obesity

Classification of obesity

The classification of a person as overweight or obese must be carefully and sensitively done. Individuals who are overweight or obese are more likely to have poor self-image and self-esteem. The purpose of classification is not to label people, but to identify those who are at greatest risk of disease. These individuals should be targeted in order to prevent the development of associated diseases such as type 2 diabetes and cardiovascular disease.

Obesity is defined in terms of body composition, the amount of body fat relative to lean body mass, and clinically by the body mass index (BMI), which is the relationship between body mass and body height. In addition, body fat distribution can be determined from the ratio between waist and hip circumference.

Body mass index (BMI)

The BMI is calculated by dividing the person's weight in kilograms by their height in metres squared (kg/m^2). The BMI is used as a clinical tool to determine if an individual has a healthy weight for their height, or if they are under or overweight. Table 5.1 outlines the range of BMI categorising individuals from underweight to morbidly obese.

Waist-to-hip ratio

The waist-to-hip ratio (WHR) is calculated by dividing the waist circumference by the hip circumference. Waist circumference has also been shown to be a good independent predictor of obesity, type 2 diabetes and hypertension. Table 5.2 outlines the values corresponding to increased risk for males and females.

Table 5.1 Body mass index (BMI) classification of health and disease.

Classification	BMI (kg/m^2)
Underweight	< 18.5
Normal	< 18.5–24.9
Overweight	25.0–29.9
Obese	30.0–39.9
Morbidly obese	≥ 40

Table 5.2 Risk thresholds for body circumferences.

	Male	Female
Waist-to-hip ratio	> 1.00	> 0.90
Waist circumference (cm)	> 102	> 88

Body composition

Being overweight or obese refers to an excess accumulation of body fat. There are a number of methods for estimating the percentage of fat and non-fat tissue in the body. The gold standard methods include underwater weighing and dual energy X-ray absorptiometry (DEXA). However, skinfold measurement and bioelectrical impedance analysis have been used for screening large groups. A young, healthy male should have a body fat between 15–20% while a young female should be 25–30%.

How to use the classification measures

In general the body mass index is used to classify individuals. However, it is important not to use this measure as the sole criterion and the combination with either the waist-to-hip measure or body composition is the best approach. It is possible that an individual could have a normal body mass index but have a high waist-to-hip ratio. These individuals may have excess central fat mass but lean limbs. However, a high WHR also increases the risk for hypertension, type 2 diabetes and cardiovascular disease. It may also be possible that an individual may have a BMI greater than 25 kg/m^2 but their body fat percentage may be low.

Aetiology of obesity

A minimum amount of body fat is essential for physiological homeostasis, not only as a source of energy but also to synthesise cell membranes and facilitate intracellular reactions. Fat, or fat derivatives, such as those derived from cholesterol are also essential for regulating reproductive function and steroid synthesis. Fat is an energy dense substrate and consequently there is a limit to the amount that is functionally useful. An excess of energy intake over expenditure is associated with an increase in plasma triglycerides and free fatty acids (FFA), an increase in the synthesis of low density lipoprotein (LDL) cholesterol and the accumulation of subcutaneous and visceral adipose tissue.

Physiological factors associated with obesity

The regulation of body weight, appetite and energy balance is extremely complex and not fully understood. It is thought that the brain, as a central regulator, plays a vital role in stabilising body weight and controlling appetite. There now appears to be a strong link between the central nervous system and the digestion and metabolism of food. The discovery of the hormone leptin, in 1994, heralded a new era in obesity research. It was important for two reasons. First, leptin administration resulted in appetite suppression and weight reduction in obese animals. Second, it was secreted from adipose tissue and, for the first time, described adipose as a neuroendocrine tissue and not just a fat storage depot. However, the success of leptin in animals was not found to be as effective in humans, except in cases of human leptin deficiency.

Further research identified the arcuate nucleus in the hypothalamus as a key regulator of appetite. It was found to have two opposing sets of neurons, one to stimulate appetite through neuropeptide Y (NPY) and agouti-related peptide (AgRP) and the other to suppress appetite through α-melanocyte-stimulating hormone (α-MSH) released by POMC/CART neuron activation. Understanding the regulation of these opposing neuronal pathways is important for the regulation of body weight and the prevention of weight gain.

It has been demonstrated that leptin inhibits NPY and therefore suppresses appetite, contributing to weight loss. Ghrelin, a hormone secreted for the stomach, is a potent appetite stimulator and activator of NPY/AgRP neurons. It is thought that the overproduction of ghrelin may contribute to the development of obesity. PYY, a hormone secreted from the intestine, is thought to suppress appetite as it has been demonstrated to downregulate NYP/AgRP and upregulate POMC/CART activation. A more traditional hormone in metabolic regulation, insulin, is also thought to play a role in appetite regulation and has been shown to inhibit NPY signalling. These and probably other, yet unidentified, neuroendocrine pathways are very important in the regulation of body weight and the development of obesity.

Obesity, type 2 diabetes and cardiovascular disease

Obesity is associated with a number of chronic diseases, including cardiovascular disease (CVD), type 2 diabetes, and hypertension. Cardiovascular disease has been the single greatest cause of mortality in the twentieth century. According to the *Surgeon General's Call to Action to Prevent and Decrease Overweight and Obesity* a 5–8 kg weight gain is associated with a 2-fold increased risk of developing type 2 diabetes while a 20 kg weight gain increases the risk 4-fold (US Department of Health and Human Services, 2001). Similarly, a 4.5–9.0 kg increase in weight increases the risk of cardiovascular disease 1.25 fold in women and 1.6 fold in men.

Type 2 diabetes

Diabetes is the result of an increase in the concentration of circulating blood glucose. Our fasting blood glucose is very well regulated and unless we do not eat for a long time it will remain close to 4–5 mmol/l. Blood glucose concentrations are balanced between glucose production and glucose use, both processes are continually taking place. Blood glucose levels will increase after ingesting food, when the carbohydrate components of the food are metabolised to glucose. As a result of the increase in glucose concentration insulin is released from the β-cell of the pancreas. Insulin release is necessary for glucose transport through the cell membranes of most tissues. Insulin, through a series of intracellular signalling cascades, facilitates glucose transport into cells by recruiting glucose transporter molecules to the cell surface. As blood glucose concentrations return toward 5 mmol/l, the amount of insulin released from the pancreas also decreases. Under normal circumstances this process works effectively to regulate circulating blood glucose concentrations.

Table 5.3 Diagnosis of impaired glucose tolerance and type 2 diabetes.

	Fasting glucose (mmol/l)	**2-hr OGTT glucose (mmol/l)**
IGT	6.1–7.0	7.8–11.1
Type 2 diabetes	> 7.0	> 11.1

Impaired glucose tolerance (IGT) and type 2 diabetes

However, when blood glucose concentrations are not well regulated the fasting plasma glucose concentration increases. A high blood glucose value will come under two broad categories, impaired glucose tolerance (IGT) and type 2 diabetes. Table 5.3 outlines the diagnostic classification for IGT and type 2 diabetes. While a fasting blood glucose greater than 7 mmol/l is diagnostic for type 2 diabetes, a value greater than 6.1 mmol/l is impaired fasting glucose. An oral glucose tolerance test (OGTT) is also used for the diagnosis and monitoring of type 2 diabetes. After an overnight fast a fasting blood sample is taken and a 300 ml drink containing 75 g of glucose is consumed. Blood samples are taken every 30 minutes for two hours. The two-hour value is also used to diagnose type 2 diabetes and impaired glucose tolerance. The identification of IGT is important as it confers a significant risk for the development of type 2 diabetes.

Symptoms of type 2 diabetes

Type 2 diabetes may be present for many years before a diagnosis is made. The development of this disease is a gradual process. It is quite common for a diagnosis to be made by chance, with the patient having a routine blood test or being in hospital for another reason. The common symptoms to be aware of include:

- Polydipsia: chronic thirst and the craving for fluids. A person with diabetes who has high blood glucose concentrations will constantly crave water.
- Polyuria: frequent urine excretion. In addition to being thirsty the patient will make frequent visits to the bathroom, even throughout the night.
- Weight loss may be an additional symptom, especially weight lost over a short period of time.
- Blurred vision. In some cases, where blood glucose concentrations are very high, vision may become blurred.

Aetiology of type 2 diabetes

Blood glucose is used as an energy source by most tissues in the body. The majority of glucose is used as energy in the brain or in skeletal muscle. There is also a store of glucose, glycogen, in the liver and skeletal muscle. As glucose can pass directly across the blood brain barrier, skeletal muscle is the largest site for insulin mediated glucose disposal. Patients with type 2 diabetes have lower insulin stimulated glucose disposal when compared to a normal control population. The decreased glucose disposal and high blood glucose concentration can be explained by: (i) insulin resistance at the level of skeletal muscle and liver, (ii) β-cell dysfunction.

Insulin resistance refers to the decreased effectiveness of insulin. As insulin is a multi-functional hormone, many metabolic processes are affected. Insulin is responsible for the suppression of gluconeogenesis (the biochemical process in which glucose is synthesised from non-carbohydrate sources such as amino acids (*Oxford Medical Dictionary*, 1996)), or glucose production by the liver. Increased hepatic glucose production is thought to contribute significantly to the elevated blood glucose in type 2 diabetes. In addition, insulin suppresses lipolysis, or the release of FFA from adipose tissue. Therefore, insulin resistance is also associated with increased circulating FFA. Insulin is also a key regulator of transcription and protein synthesis. Many of the proteins under the regulation of insulin influence metabolism and, therefore, decreased protein expression resulting from insulin resistance causes further metabolic disturbance. However, insulin is probably best known for the transport of glucose into skeletal muscle to be oxidised for energy production or stored as glycogen. Decreased insulin mediated glucose transport, oxidation and muscle glycogen storage are common characteristics of type 2 diabetes.

Muscle cells contain transporters that facilitate diffusion into the cytoplasm. Glut-4 is an insulin responsive glucose transporter that is translocated from cytoplasmic stores to the plasma membrane following a signalling cascade initiated when insulin is bound to its receptor on the cell surface. In type 2 diabetes the rate of glucose transport is decreased, though the affinity for glucose and the amount of Glut-4 protein in skeletal muscle remain unchanged. However, the translocation of Glut-4 is decreased, suggesting a defect in the insulin signalling pathway. The regulation of Glut-4 translocation is not fully understood but is essential to the prevention and treatment of type 2 diabetes.

Insulin resistance develops progressively and is associated with an increase in body weight, especially central or visceral adiposity. As nutrient intake and physical activity contribute to body weight regulation they play a key role in the development of insulin resistance. However, first degree relatives of people with type 2 diabetes also have a significantly impaired rate of glucose disposal, and insulin resistance, indicating a genetic predisposition to the development of diabetes.

The initial physiological response to insulin resistance is for the pancreas to increase insulin secretion. The increased availability of insulin counteracts the downregulation in function, allowing blood glucose concentrations to remain within the normal range. Though this may continue for a number of years, the progressive deterioration of insulin sensitivity results in a greater state of hyperinsulinemia, until the physiological effect can no longer control blood glucose. As blood glucose continues to rise, the ability of the pancreas to secrete enough insulin also becomes impaired and insulin responsiveness decreases. The combination of insulin resistance and decreased pancreatic function contribute to the development of type 2 diabetes.

Complications associated with type 2 diabetes

Cardiovascular disease has been the single greatest cause of mortality in the twentieth century. Patients with type 2 diabetes are at increased risk of cardiovascular disease and the majority of people with type 2 diabetes die of cardiovascular complications. In addition, approximately 70% of type 2 diabetes patients have hypertension. The relationship between type 2 diabetes and cardiovascular disease is not fully understood but insulin resistance is thought to play a key role in both.

Type 2 diabetes is also associated with other complications:

- *Retinopathy.* The risk of developing eye disease either by cataracts or haemorrhaging of blood vessels in the back of the eye is increased in type 2 diabetes.
- *Neuropathy.* Nerve damage can cause decreased blood flow and pain in the hands and feet which may even result in amputation.
- *Nephropathy.* Damage to the nephrons of the kidney result in proteinurea that could lead to progressive renal failure.
- *Foot ulcers.* Neuropathy and ischaemia are the chief factors that cause foot ulcers in type 2 diabetes, with the latter being the more serious of the two. Diabetes is the greatest non-traumatic cause of amputation.

It is important to note that all of these complications, including the increased risk of cardiovascular disease, may be prevented. Glycaemic control, or the maintenance of normal blood glucose concentrations, is essential to long-term health. When glycaemic control is good, the risk of developing complications is no greater than for the general population.

Young type 2 diabetes

Though the age of presentation for type 2 diabetes has typically been greater than 40 years, it is decreasing and the incidence of adolescent and young adult (< 25 years) onset type 2 diabetes is increasing (American Diabetes Association, 2000a). A study from Cincinnati showed that the incidence of type 2 diabetes in children increased from 4% in 1982 to 16% in 1994. These patients tend to be obese, with an abnormal blood pressure and blood lipid profile. They typically have a two-to-three generation family history of diabetes and appear to be extremely insulin resistant. As the prevalence of obesity and diabetes is increasing and the onset age is decreasing, medical services are going to be put under tremendous pressure in the coming years. As the duration of diabetes is also greater, there is an increased risk for developing complications. Strategies to address the prevention of obesity and type 2 diabetes are essential for the long-term health of our society.

Exercise for obesity and type 2 diabetes

Obesity and type 2 diabetes are diseases with similar causes and many similar characteristics. Most patients with type 2 diabetes are overweight or obese, with a high waist-to-hip ratio, while most obese patients are also insulin resistant, though not as severely as those with type 2 diabetes. Both groups usually have altered lipid metabolism with high triglycerides, LDL cholesterol, total cholesterol and low HDL cholesterol and an increased risk of cardiovascular disease. Therefore, there are many related benefits exercise may confer on both diseases.

Body weight and energy balance

Stable body weight is maintained by balancing energy intake, by food consumption, with energy expenditure. While metabolic systems can adjust for short-term changes in equilibrium, a long-term imbalance of energy intake over expenditure results in weight gain and obesity. Successful weight loss is achieved by reducing caloric intake and increasing energy expenditure.

Energy expenditure

Energy expenditure can be subdivided into three categories.

(1) Resting metabolic rate (RMR) refers to the energy necessary to sustain all of the physiological processes in the body at rest.
(2) Thermic effect of food (TEF) is the energy we require to metabolise the food we ingest on a daily basis. The digestion, absorption and metabolism of food all require energy.
(3) Physical activity refers to the energy we utilise for all body movements throughout the day.

Therefore, when looking to increase energy expenditure for the purpose of weight loss, the basal metabolic rate and daily physical activity are most important. Exercise is also thought to potentiate the TEF, though the results are inconclusive and the relative contribution, if any, is small, as it contributes approximately 10% to total energy expenditure.

RMR is the most significant contributor to total energy expenditure accounting for approximately 60–70%. It should be possible to increase RMR in two ways: (i) by increasing muscle mass, or (ii) by increasing the activity and number of mitochondrial enzymes in muscle cells. Resistance training results in muscle hypertrophy and protein synthesis, which contribute to an increase in fat free mass and RMR. Aerobic exercise upregulates the activity of key enzymes such as citrate synthase and succinate dehydrogenase in muscle mitochondria as well as the number of mitochondria. However, most, but not all, studies conclude that aerobic exercise does not confer a significant benefit to RMR. It appears that increasing muscle mass is the best mechanism for increasing RMR though the overall benefit is usually about 5% of baseline values. Therefore, daily physical activity, which accounts for approximately 20–30% of total energy expenditure, is the best way of modifying total energy expenditure.

All daily movement related to work, leisure or formal exercise contributes to daily physical activity. Therefore, the manner by which we decide to undertake daily tasks will determine our physical activity. It is now recommended that we accumulate at least 30 minutes of physical activity on all, or most, days of the week for health related benefits. The more physical activity we participate in during the day, the greater the energy expenditure. Increasing physical activity may occur by including formal exercise, like a 30-minute brisk walk, or may be accumulated by lifestyle changes, like walking to the shop. Therefore, energy expenditure is mostly effectively increased by daily physical activity that will increase caloric expenditure and RMR.

Exercise and weight loss

Epidemiological studies indicate that low levels of physical activity are associated with greater body weight when compared to more active individuals (Jakicic et al., 2001). These studies also indicate that the percentage of stored body fat is greater in less active individuals and they are at a greater risk of weight gain. Therefore, it would appear that physical activity is a robust regulator of body weight and composition. It is surprising, therefore, that the use of exercise as a weight loss strategy has not yielded impressive results when used alone. In fact, many of the research studies indicate that caloric restriction is more effective in weight loss than exercise alone, on average approximately 3% greater weight reduction. This may be explained in two ways.

First, there is a large degree of variability in research design of exercise trials. The frequency of exercise from 3–7 days per week, the intensity from 40–75% $\dot{V}O_2$max, the duration from 30–60 minutes and the length of study from a few weeks to more than 12 months. Therefore, it is very difficult to obtain consistent and comparable results. Also, while some studies supervise the exercise programme, others rely on subject adherence and compliance.

Second, it makes sense that many of the exercise trials do not show significant differences. Most studies base their design on the recommended physical activity guidelines for health, 30 minutes of exercise on 5–7 days per week. A brisk walking speed will expend approximately 7 kcal/min. Over 30 minutes that accumulates to approximately 210 kcal. There are 9000 kcal in 1 kg of body fat; therefore it would take approximately 8.5 weeks to lose 1 kg of body fat if exercising five times per week. The recommended caloric restriction for weight loss is approximately 500–1000 kcal/day; therefore caloric restriction is going to be more effective when compared in this manner.

Exercise training does alter the balance between carbohydrate and fat utilisation and therefore has benefits for body composition. During exercise of a moderate intensity carbohydrate will be the primary source of energy. However, when exercise finishes, fat oxidation increases in the muscle mitochondria. Exercise training will lead to enhanced whole body fat oxidation and favourably decrease body fat stores.

When exercise and dietary restriction are combined, the resulting weight loss and benefits to body composition are greater than either strategy alone. While caloric restriction may form the major source of the energy deficit, exercise will increase energy expenditure and favourably decrease fat mass. Caloric restriction alone is known to decrease RMR but exercise can help maintain or enhance RMR when aerobic and resistance exercise is combined, as muscle mass is maintained or increased.

Insulin resistance

Insulin resistance is prevalent in obesity and type 2 diabetes but while obesity compensates by increasing insulin secretion and maintaining normal or impaired glucose tolerance, in type 2 diabetes insulin secretion is impaired. As insulin has multi-functional intracellular actions, an improvement in tissue sensitivity for insulin has many positive health-related benefits.

Tissue sensitivity to insulin appears to be very responsive to physical activity. There is a direct relationship between insulin sensitivity and aerobic fitness, measured by oxygen consumption, indicating that the trained individual will have a greater insulin sensitivity and capacity to transport and utilise glucose in skeletal muscle (Kirwan et al., 2000). Conversely, insulin sensitivity is inversely related to intra-abdominal fat. The greater the amount of abdominal fat the lower the insulin sensitivity.

Exercise, even a single bout, has been shown to improve insulin sensitivity in lean, obese and type 2 diabetes patients. As a result glucose utilisation is greater and glucose production by the liver is decreased. This improvement is associated with an increase in the content of Glut-4 mRNA and protein in skeletal muscle cells, facilitating the transport of glucose across the plasma membrane. Therefore, insulin sensitivity can be improved in obese and type 2 diabetes patients, independently of weight loss. However, this effect is transient and lasts approximately 24–72 hours. Therefore, regular exercise is important for the long-term enhancement of insulin sensitivity.

While exercise improves insulin sensitivity, it also increases glucose transport during exercise, independently of insulin. Insulin secretion is reduced during exercise and though Glut-4 is translocated to the plasma membrane, the insulin-mediated mechanisms are not active. Studies have also been conducted where insulin and glucose were infused during exercise. Results from these studies indicate that glucose disposal is increased in a synergistic manner. Therefore, exercise has an insulin independent mechanism for glucose transport (Wallberg-Henriksson et al., 1998). In lean, control subjects blood glucose concentrations remain constant unless the exercise is of sufficient duration to significantly decrease muscle glycogen stores. When blood glucose is elevated, as in type 2 diabetes, exercise has a glucose lowering effect and can help to maintain blood glucose in the recommended range of 5–7 mmol/l.

Persistent exercise over time also increases insulin sensitivity, though the increase is not proportional. Therefore, many of the benefits of exercise on insulin sensitivity are associated with the last bout of exercise. This has implications for exercise prescription in terms of the amount and frequency of exercise to sustain and maintain improvements in insulin sensitivity. Glucose tolerance is also known to benefit from exercise training. The glucose and insulin response to an oral glucose load is significantly lower following exercise training, indicating the positive effect exercise has on metabolic regulation and substrate utilisation.

One of the primary treatment goals for type 2 diabetes is to control plasma glucose. Exercise has been shown to increase insulin sensitivity and lower blood glucose, but do these changes influence long-term glucose control? The results of training studies are dependent on the duration, frequency and intensity of the exercise protocol and have not always yielded consistent results. However, a meta-analysis using the data from 14 well controlled studies revealed that glucose control had improved.

Both acute and chronic exercise have significant benefits on insulin resistance in obese and type 2 diabetes patients. Exercise appears to have an impact on insulin sensitive tissues, improving glucose utilisation and decreasing endogenous glucose production. It also influences the oxidation of carbohydrate and fat, creating a more efficient metabolic profile. These changes can occur independently of weight loss, signifying the importance of exercise prescription in the treatment of these conditions, but reinforcing the importance of combined dietary and exercise treatment, as weight loss also improves insulin sensitivity. Long-term exercise can have other benefits which improve the health and risk profile of both obese and type 2 diabetes patients.

Exercise in obesity, type 2 diabetes and cardiovascular disease

The fact that the risk of cardiovascular disease is significantly greater in obese and type 2 diabetes patients has been well established. In addition to the metabolic changes relating to weight loss and insulin resistance, exercise also confers many benefits to the cardiovascular system. Regular exercise increases oxygen delivery, uptake and utilisation in the muscle cells. Oxygen is necessary for energy generation in the mitochondria and while the size and number of mitochondria increase in response to aerobic exercise, greater oxygen availability will also facilitate energy expenditure. The oxidation of a mole of FFA requires approximately 2.5 times the amount of oxygen more than for a mole of glucose. Therefore, increased oxygen availability will also facilitate greater lipid oxidation and long-term changes in body composition.

Chronic exercise is also associated with increases in the number of capillaries supplying blood, and therefore oxygen and nutrients, to the working muscles. The increased capillary-to-fibre ratio increases the distribution of blood to a larger volume of muscle. The enhanced glucose availability should increase glucose disposal.

Cardiac muscle responds to exercise in a similar fashion to skeletal muscle. Regular exercise training increases the size of the heart, the force of muscular contraction and therefore, the volume of blood ejected by each beat. The increase in stroke volume helps to explain why the heart rate response, at rest or during the same absolute exercise intensity, is lower in a trained individual. Exercise also improves arterial dilation and blood pressure, further reducing the stress placed on heart and reducing the risk of myocardial disease.

The majority of obese and type 2 diabetes patients have an abnormal blood lipid profile with elevated triglycerides and FFA, with or without increased total cholesterol and LDL cholesterol, with decreased HDL cholesterol. Exercise training has a positive impact on triglycerides and FFA in obese and type 2 diabetes though the results on cholesterol are less well established. Exercise does increase

HDL cholesterol and decrease total cholesterol, though not many well controlled studies have been conducted in patients with type 2 diabetes. The results of these studies also depend on the frequency, intensity, and duration of exercise. However, the risk of developing cardiovascular disease is reduced 35–55% by maintaining an active compared to sedentary lifestyle (see also Chapter 7).

In general, exercise has a positive influence on the prevention and treatment of cardiovascular disease. As obesity and type 2 diabetes are risk factors for cardiovascular disease the combined benefits of improved insulin sensitivity, metabolic functioning, cardiorespiratory endurance and vascular health support the role of exercise as an effective strategy for the prevention and treatment of obesity and type 2 diabetes.

Prevention strategies

The physiological changes in obesity and type 2 diabetes associated with physical activity have been outlined. These recommendations, along with dietary modification, are effective in the treatment and also the prevention of obesity and type 2 diabetes. The prevention of these diseases has to become a key strategic goal in health care policy. The exponential increase in the incidence of obesity and type 2 diabetes will have major implications for global health care. The main focus for prevention must centre on three core areas: (i) physical activity, (ii) dietary habits, (iii) behaviour. Education programmes are key to changing attitudes toward obesity and type 2 diabetes as well as informing people of the severe health consequences.

In a recent policy document the United States Surgeon General (US Department of Health and Human Services, 2001) identified families and communities, schools, health care, media and communications, and worksites as key settings for activities and interventions designed to prevent obesity. Their vision for the future involves:

- Communicating to and educating the American people about the health issues related to overweight and obesity.
- Assistance to balance healthy eating with regular physical activity.
- Investing in research to improve the understanding of causes, prevention and treatment of obesity.

The epidemiological evidence supporting the role of physical activity as an effective preventative tool is also strong, with a 50% risk reduction when reducing body weight and increasing physical activity. Recently, a number of studies examining the role of diet and physical activity modifications in the prevention of type 2 diabetes have been published. Of these, the Finnish Diabetes Prevention Study (Tuomilehto et al., 2001) and the Diabetes Prevention Program (Diabetes Prevention Program Research Group, 2002) in the United States are most widely referenced.

The Finnish Diabetes Prevention Study

A total of 522 subjects with impaired glucose tolerance were randomised to a control group or a lifestyle modification group. The control group were given the general recommendations associated with diet and physical activity but were not provided with any formal intervention. The intervention goals were:

- Reduce body weight ≥ 5% body weight
- Reduce total fat intake < 30% energy consumed
- Reduce saturated fat intake < 10% energy consumed
- A fibre intake of 15 g per 1000 kcal consumed
- Moderate physical activity ≥ 30 minutes per day

Subjects were followed for four years and the results showed that the risk of developing diabetes was 58% lower in the intervention group than the control group, demonstrating the positive impact of lifestyle modification. Interestingly, if the five key goals were achieved, whether subjects were in the intervention group or in the control group, where they were only given oral and written information, the incidence of type 2 diabetes was zero.

The Diabetes Prevention Program

In 27 centres across the United States, 3234 individuals with impaired glucose tolerance were recruited into the study. Subjects were randomly assigned into three groups:

(1) Standard lifestyle recommendations with placebo twice daily. The standard lifestyle recommendations emphasised the importance of a healthy lifestyle and were in written format with an annual individual session. The control group took a placebo tablet twice daily.
(2) Standard lifestyle recommendations with metformin twice daily. Metformin suppresses glucose production by the liver and by so doing, helps to reduce and control plasma glucose concentrations. The dose of 850 mg of metformin twice daily with recommendations for lifestyle modification is a standard treatment for type 2 diabetes.
(3) Intensive lifestyle intervention. The intensive lifestyle intervention group were to achieve and maintain weight reduction of at least 7% of initial body weight through a healthy low calorie diet and at least 150 minutes of moderate intensity exercise per week. They received regular dietary advice and were provided with an exercise prescription to help achieve these goals.

The programme was stopped one year early because of the positive results. Over three years the estimated cumulative incidence of diabetes was 29% in the control group, 22% in the metformin group and only 14% in the intensive lifestyle group. This represents a 58% lower incidence rate and was a major advancement for strategies designed to prevent the onset of type 2 diabetes.

Exercise prescription for obese and type 2 diabetes patients

Needs analysis and goal setting

Up to 50% of individuals who undertake an exercise programme will default within the first six months. Therefore, it is important to establish the needs of the individual and to set realistic and attainable goals based on their health profile. Some individuals undertake an exercise programme with the expectation that they will lose a large amount of weight in a short period of time. When the progress is not as they expected, motivation may be lost and adherence to the exercise programme decreases. The expectation of the patient is often different to that of the health care professional.

For obese patients a weight reduction of 5–10% significantly decreases the risk of co-morbidities such as type 2 diabetes and cardiovascular disease. Therefore, for the exercise professional and dietician, this becomes the primary goal. Making the patient aware of this goal and the supporting evidence can help with motivation and adherence. Once this initial goal has been achieved, further weight loss strategies may be implemented.

Research has also shown that weight reduction improves insulin sensitivity in patients with type 2 diabetes and therefore as a strategy is very important. However, the primary role of an exercise prescription for patients with type 2 diabetes is to help control blood glucose by improving insulin sensitivity and concurrently decrease the risk of complications. It is possible to improve insulin sensitivity in the absence of weight loss, though most strategies will also aim for weight reduction. The primary aim for the exercise professional is to help control and reduce blood glucose and, secondary, to work with the dietician for weight reduction. There is a greater chance of compliance to a programme if the patient accepts that improvements are occurring in the short term, even if weight reduction has not yet been significant.

It is also important to be aware that patients with type 2 diabetes may also have some of the complications previously outlined. In this case, and especially for cardiovascular disease, the goal of the exercise programme will again be different. As exercise is a physiological stress the primary goal for a patient with type 2 diabetes and cardiovascular disease will focus on improving the cardiovascular system, then glycaemic control and weight loss.

Therefore, careful characterisation of the patient, to determine their needs and to set realistic goals, is important for developing an effective programme. Also evident is the fact that these individuals are at greater risk than the general population and that screening prior to exercise prescription and monitoring during exercise is very important.

Screening prior to exercise prescription

Exercise is a physiological stress that results in an increased heart rate and blood pressure. Physician clearance should be obtained for obese and type 2 diabetes patients prior to prescribing exercise. A detailed medical history and physical examination should be performed to search for any co-morbidities or complications. In the case of type 2 diabetes it is important to check for glucose control, as well as neurological and vascular complications. The American Diabetes Association (2000b) recommends that an exercise stress test should be performed on those that have known or suspected cardiovascular disease, are older than 35 years, have had diabetes for longer than 10 years and have any other risk factor for cardiovascular disease, microvascular disease, peripheral vascular disease or autonomic neuropathy.

Exercise prescription in type 2 diabetes

Guidelines for health-related physical activity focus on maintaining health status and preventing the development of hypokinetic diseases. The American College of Sports Medicine (ACSM, 2000) recommends accumulating 30 minutes of moderate physical activity on all, or most, days of the week. The guidelines for exercise prescription are discussed in Chapter 7. Exercise prescription for patients with obesity and diabetes is based on the FITT principles, but in addition there are a few important points that need consideration.

- In its position stand 'appropriate intervention strategies for weight loss and prevention of weight regain in adults' the American College of Sports Medicine recommends an energy expenditure of greater than 2000 kcal/week from leisure time physical activity for weight loss and maintenance (Jakicic et al., 2001). In order to improve glycaemic control in patients with type 2 diabetes, ACSM recommends a minimum of 1000 kcal/week energy expenditure. It is important to structure exercise sessions throughout the week taking the frequency, intensity and duration of exercise into account (see Chapters 7 and 10).

- For patients with type 2 diabetes, similar guidelines can be adhered to, so long as the patient has no complications. However, research has shown that the improvement in insulin sensitivity associated with one bout of exercise lasts between 24–72 hours. Therefore, exercise must be performed on a regular basis to maintain the improvements. It is recommended that patients should exercise a minimum of every second day, or seven sessions in two weeks, to improve insulin sensitivity.

- Research has shown that those who exercise at 75% $\dot{V}O_2$max have a greater increase in insulin-mediated glucose disposal than those who exercise at 50% $\dot{V}O_2$max. However, exercise at 75%+ should only be prescribed in supervised facilities with appropriate emergency equipment. If the patient also has cardiovascular disease the intensity of exercise starts lower, close to 50% $\dot{V}O_2$max. As training progresses the intensity may be gradually increased.

- A recent study looking at the dose response relationship between exercise and weight loss demonstrated that while the general recommendations did produce a modest 3.5 kg reduction in body weight after 18 months, physical activity greater than 150 minutes was more effective. In fact, an average exercise time of 280 minutes per week had the greatest effect, resulting in a weight loss of approximately 13 kg, which was maintained for between 6 and 18 months. These individuals had energy expenditure in excess of 2000 kcal/week of leisure time physical activity. This duration of exercise is approximately double the general guidelines and has implications for the exercise prescription of adults undertaking a weight loss strategy.

● Overweight and obese patients may not have a full range of movement at their joints, compromising their functional capacity. The use of certain pieces of exercise equipment is not practical. In the patient with type 2 diabetes the mode of exercise is important, bearing in mind their complication profile. Peripheral neuropathy is common in type 2 diabetes and is strongly linked to the development of foot ulcers. Often, the patient may not be aware because of the dulled sensation in the foot. However, weight bearing exercise, especially if the ulcer is in the base of the foot, can further aggravate the ulcer. In these circumstances it would be recommended that the patient undertake non-weightbearing exercise. The foot pressure when cycling a stationary bicycle is significantly less than when walking.

A case study of exercise prescription and type 2 diabetes

The subject is a 44-year-old male with a three-year history of type 2 diabetes. He was morbidly obese with a BMI of 42 kg/m^2 and a weight of 115.8 kg. He had recently returned to clinic after defaulting, and his glycaemic control, measured by HbA$_{1c}$, was 10.9% (normal range 4.9–6.9%), and his fasting blood glucose was 15 mmol/l. Up until the point of defaulting he was not on pharmacological treatment for diabetes but was on antihypertensives and had an elevated blood lipid profile. Even on his medication his blood pressure was 136/101 mmHg.

Though he was a candidate for glucose lowering treatment he was hesitant, but very keen to undertake an exercise programme. He had a physical examination, an exercise stress test and an oral glucose tolerance test. He did not have ketones and his blood glucose was below the 16.67 mmol/l contraindicated for exercise, so he was deemed appropriate. Prior to exercise he had a graded exercise test on a bicycle ergometer and had a $\dot{V}O_2$peak of 2.16 litres/min. Subsequently a heart rate range of 123–133 beats per minute was calculated to correspond to 70% $\dot{V}O_2$peak.

The subject was asked to exercise four times per week for 60 minutes at this intensity, with a ten-minute warm up and a five-minute cool down built in. Prior to each session, he performed some stretching exercises and had a seated resting blood pressure taken. The preferred mode of exercise was on a bicycle ergometer. During exercise his heart rate was constantly monitored by radiotelemetry and his blood pressure was checked every ten minutes. For the first four weeks of the exercise programme all sessions were supervised. After this time he joined a local gym and performed two supervised sessions and the other sessions in the gym.

In the following four months his weight dropped from 115.8 kg to 106.4 kg, corresponding to a decrease of 8.1% body weight, and his BMI to 38.6 kg/m². His fasting glucose was in the 5–7 mmol/l range, his fasting triglycerides were within the normal range. Maximal oxygen consumption had increased by 21% to 2.61 litres/min. Importantly, his blood pressure had decreased to 132/84 mmHg and he was off his medication.

Though this person is still obese, he has reduced the risk of disease progression immensely and no longer receives treatment. Exercise can have positive benefits on body weight, glycaemic control and cardiovascular health.

References

Allison, D.B., Fontaine, K.R., Manson, J.E., Stevens, J. and Van Itallie, T.B. (1999). Annual deaths attributable to obesity in the United States. *Journal of the American Medical Association* **282** (16), 1530–38.

American College of Sports Medicine (2000). *Guidelines for Exercise Testing and Prescription*, 6th edn. Lippincott, Williams and Wilkins, Philadelphia.

American Diabetes Association (2000a). Type 2 diabetes in children and adolescents. *Diabetes Care* **22** (12), 381–9.

American Diabetes Association (2000b). Diabetes mellitus and exercise. *Diabetes Care* **23** (Suppl. 1), S50–S54.

Amos, A., McCarthy, D.J. and Zimmet, P. (1997). The rising global burden of diabetes and its complications: estimates and projections to the year 2010. *Diabetic Medicine* **14**, S7–S85.

Diabetes Prevention Program Research Group (2002). Reduction in the incidence of type 2 diabetes with lifestyle intervention or metformin. *New England Journal of Medicine* **346** (6), 393–403.

Flegal, K.M. (1999). The obesity epidemic in children and adults: current evidence and research issues. *Medicine and Science in Sports and Exercise* **31** (11 Suppl.), S509–14.

Flegal, K.M., Carroll, M.D., Ogden, C.L. and Johnson, C.L. (2002). Prevalence and trends in obesity among US adults, 1999–2000. *Journal of American Medical Association* **288**, 1723–7.

Jakicic, J.M., Clark, K., Coleman, E., Donnelly, J.E., Foreyt, J., Melanson, E., Volek, J. and Volpe, S.L. (2001). American College of Sports Medicine position stand on the appropriate intervention strategies for weight loss and prevention of weight regain for adults. *Medicine and Science in Sports and Exercise* **33** (12), 2145–56.

Kirwan, J.P., del Aguila, L.F., Williamson, D.L., O'Gorman, D.J., Lewis, R.M. and Krishnan, R.K. (2000). Regular exercise enhances insulin activation of IRS-1 associated PI 3-kinase in human skeletal muscle. *Journal of Applied Physiology* **88**, 797–803.

Oxford Medical Dictionary (1996). Oxford University Press, Oxford.

Tuomilehto, J., Lindstrom, J., Eriksson, J.G., Valle, T.T., Hamalainen, H., Ilanne-Parikka, P., Keinanen-Kiukaanniemi, S., Laakso, M., Louheranta, A., Rastas, M., Salminen, V. and Uusitupa, M. (2001). Finnish Diabetes Prevention Study Group. Prevention of type 2 diabetes mellitus by changes in lifestyle among subjects with impaired glucose tolerance. *New England Journal of Medicine* **344** (18), 1343–50.

US Department of Health and Human Services (2001). *The Surgeon General's Call to Action to Prevent and Decrease Overweight and Obesity*. Public Health Service, Office of the Surgeon General, Rockville, Maryland.

Wallberg-Henriksson, H., Roncon, J. and Zierath, J.R. (1998). Exercise in the management of non-insulin-dependent diabetes mellitus. *Sports Medicine* 25 (1), Jan., 25–35.

Bibliography

Albright, A., Franz, M., Hornsby, G., Kriska, A., Marrero, D., Ullrich, I. and Verity, L.S. (2000). American College of Sports Medicine position stand on exercise and type 2 diabetes. *Medicine and Science in Sports and Exercise* 32 (7), 1345–60.

American Diabetes Association (2003). Economic costs of diabetes in the US in 2002. *Diabetes Care* 26 (3), 917–32.

SECTION 2

Chapter 6

MEASUREMENT OF PHYSICAL FITNESS AND HABITUAL PHYSICAL ACTIVITY

Juliette Hussey

Key words: maximal exercise testing, sub-maximal exercise testing, clinical/field exercise testing, assessment of physical activity.

Introduction

This chapter will concentrate on the measurements of physical fitness and habitual physical activity. The first section of the chapter will discuss the measurement of physical fitness and the second section will consider the assessment of physical activity.

Physical fitness may be defined in terms of cardiovascular endurance, muscular strength and endurance and flexibility of joints. Objectives of measuring physical fitness include diagnostic evaluation, deriving data for individualised exercise prescription, the education of participants about their fitness status, stratifying risk and motivating subjects as regards exercise habits. The objective of exercise testing is to increase total body and myocardial oxygen demand in safe increments within a short time period.

Exercise testing

Exercise testing in the laboratory

The 'gold standard' criterion of cardiovascular fitness is maximal oxygen uptake ($\dot{V}O_2max$), which is defined as the maximal volume of oxygen the body musculature can take up and use. $\dot{V}O_2max$ depends on the strength of the heart, the amount of oxygen the blood can carry and the amount of oxygen the muscles can extract from the blood. There are a number of factors which affect $\dot{V}O_2max$, including genetic make-up, age, gender and the amount and intensity of activity and exercise that are regularly performed. The most accurate assessment of $\dot{V}O_2max$ is by the measurement of expired air composition and respiratory volume during maximal exertion (Haskell et al., 1992). This approach involves open circuit spirometry, where the subject breathes through a low resistance valve with the nose occluded, while pulmonary ventilation and expired fractions of O_2 and CO_2 are measured.

In the laboratory setting measurable workloads can be imposed while monitoring ventilation per minute (minute ventilation), oxygen consumption, carbon dioxide production, heart rate, blood pressure, oxygen saturation and cardiac rate and rhythm (ECG). Measurement procedures are considerably simpler now, with modern automated systems compared to collecting expired gas in Douglas bags and using chemical analysers to determine O_2 and CO_2 content. The cost of directly measuring $\dot{V}O_2$max is considerable in terms of equipment and space, and therefore its use is often confined to research purposes or to the diagnosis of patients with suspected cardiovascular or pulmonary conditions. Furthermore, trained personnel are required to conduct the test and to ensure the safety of the participant at all times.

The measurement of $\dot{V}O_2$max in the laboratory yields a large volume of clinically useful data. $\dot{V}O_2$max is usually expressed in one of two ways: in absolute terms as litres per minute (l/min) or relative to a person's body mass in millilitres per kilogram per minute (ml/kg/min) (see Chapter 3).

Dynamic exercise using the major muscle groups is performed usually using either cycle ergometry or treadmill walking/running (Figures 6.1, 6.2) but can also be

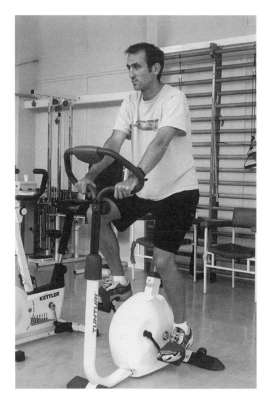

Figure 6.1 Cycle ergometer.

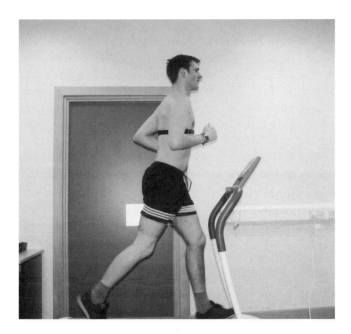

Figure 6.2 Running on a treadmill.

done with arm ergometry. A cycle ergometer is less expensive than a treadmill and occupies less space. During cycling, as the upper limb is relatively stable, it is easier to measure blood pressure and record ECG. On electronically braked cycle ergometers workload is accurate and expressed in watt or kg/min. An advantage of the treadmill is that most subjects are more accustomed to walking than cycling. Maximal oxygen uptake and maximal heart rate have been found to be higher using the treadmill compared to cycle ergometry (Wasserman et al., 1994). Dynamic arm exercise testing may be useful in patients who have neurological or orthopaedic conditions of the lower limbs which interfere with walking or cycling. As the upper limbs have a smaller muscle mass than the lower limbs the peak workload achieved is therefore lower and for any matched work rate, heart rate and systolic blood pressure tend to be higher (due to a comparatively higher peripheral resistance in the working muscles).

The protocol chosen needs to be appropriate for the subject being tested. Many protocols exist and individual laboratories often have their own preference. Protocols used in clinical testing should include a low-intensity warm-up phase followed by progressive, continuous exercise, where the subject reaches his/her maximal levels in 8–12 minutes (Wasserman et al., 1994).

There are both one stage and multi-stage sub-maximal exercise tests available to estimate $\dot{V}O_2$max from heart rate and work rate measurements. As heart rate can be influenced by a number of factors such as heat, smoking, previous activity and caffeine intake these must be controlled so that heart rate is as reliable as possible. Some common protocols are described below, but for explicit detail of extrapolating $\dot{V}O_2$max the reader is referred to the ACSM guidelines for exercise testing and prescription (2000).

Cycle ergometer tests

The Astrand-Rhyming cycle ergometer test is a single stage test which takes six minutes on a standard cycle ergometer, where work rate can be accurately measured in watts (Astrand and Rhyming, 1954). Heart rate is taken at the end of each minute. The pedal rate is set at 50 rpm and the goal is to achieve HR values between 125 and 170 bpm. Heart rate during the fifth and sixth minute are averaged and used to estimate $\dot{V}O_2$max from the Modified Astrand-Ryhming nomogram. (ACSM, 2000).

The YMCA protocol uses two to four three-minute stages of continuous exercise. The test is designed to raise the steady state HR of the subject to between 110 bpm and 85% of the age-predicted maximal heart rate, for at least two consecutive stages. Each work rate is performed for three minutes and heart rates are recorded during the final 15–30 seconds of the second and third minutes. If these heart rates are not within 6 bpm of each other then the last work rate is maintained for another minute. Heart rate measured during the last minute of each stage is plotted against work rate (ACSM, 2000).

Treadmill tests

Treadmill testing provides a common form of physiological stress (such as walking) and subjects are more likely to achieve a higher $\dot{V}O_2$ and peak heart rate than during cycle ergometer testing. The treadmill should have front and side rails for safety, which may be used if a subject has poor balance. A safety belt should also be available and if activated can stop the treadmill. An emergency stop button should also be incorporated.

The Bruce treadmill test is a frequently used protocol. The Bruce protocol begins with three-minute stages of walking at 1.7 mph at 0%, 5% or 10% gradient (the 0% and 5% grades are omitted in fitter individuals). The grade is then increased by 2% every three minutes and the speed is increased by 0.8 mph every three minutes until the treadmill reaches 18% and 5 mph, whereafter the speed is increased by 0.5 mph every three minutes. It is commonly used for the detection of myocardial ischaemia. Protocols that are suitable for clinical exercise testing should include a low intensity warm-up phase followed by progressive, continuous exercise where the demand is increased to the patient's maximal level within 8–12 minutes.

Full laboratory exercise testing is costly in terms of personnel (clinical supervision/technical assistance), space and equipment and this may inhibit its use in many places. In addition, when performing these tests physician attendance is often required, as participants exercise to fatigue. The protocols used for full laboratory tests can also be used without full gas analysis and the $\dot{V}O_2$max can be estimated, for example, Bruce, Balke and Naughton protocols (Wasserman et al., 1994). Because maximal exercise testing is not always feasible for many situations in health/fitness testing, sub-maximal tests are commonly used. The aim of the sub-maximal test is to determine the heart rate at specific work rates and use the result to predict $\dot{V}O_2$max. As heart rate varies linearly with $\dot{V}O_2$max it is argued that maximal testing is not necessary to predict $\dot{V}O_2$max. Sub-maximal exercise tests make several assumptions (ACSM, 2000):

- 'A steady state heart rate is obtained for each exercise work rate
- A linear relationship exists between heart rate and work rate
- The maximal heart rate for a given age is uniform
- Mechanical efficiency ($\dot{V}O_2$ at a specific work rate) is the same for all.'

Exercise tests in the field/clinical setting

Laboratory methods of measuring cardiovascular fitness are not suitable, in the main, for field work, where simple tests requiring little equipment are needed. Field tests consist of walking or running a distance in a given time, for example, 12-minute run test or a given distance, for example, 1.5-mile test. In field tests many subjects can be tested at the same time and little equipment is needed. The Cooper 12-minute test, the 1.5-mile test, the Rockport One-Mile Fitness Walking Test and the multi-stage shuttle fitness test are commonly used for assessing cardiorespiratory fitness. Exercise tests such as the incremental shuttle walking test, the modified shuttle walking test and step tests used in the assessment of patients with respiratory disease are discussed in Chapter 9.

The Cooper 12-minute run field test: On a flat course or lapped track the subject walks/runs as far as possible in 12 minutes and the distance covered is recorded. A corresponding $\dot{V}O_2$max is obtained by the formula $\dot{V}O_2$max − 22.351 × distance (km) − 11.288 (ml/kg/min) (Cooper, 1968). This test has been used extensively for assessing disability in patients with respiratory disease. A marked area on a hospital corridor can be used. The participant is instructed to try and keep going but not to be concerned if he/she needs to slow down or stop and rest. At the end of the test the patient should feel that he/she could not have covered any more ground. However, despite the 12-minute walk being a simple and practical measure of exercise tolerance in patients with respiratory disease (McGavin et al., 1976) it depends on a variety of factors, including motivation, judgement of pace as well as cardiovascular fitness and neuromuscular function.

The Rockport Walking Test (1-mile walk) and 1.5-mile Run Test: The subject walks or runs the set distance and the times achieved are recorded and put into specific equations to estimate $\dot{V}O_2$max. In the Rockport Walking Test the subject walks one mile as fast as possible and heart rate is measured in the final minute during the last one quarter mile. The 1.5-mile test involves the subject running the distance in the shortest time possible.

Calculation for $\dot{V}O_2$max using The Rockport Walking Test

$\dot{V}O_2$max = 132.853 − (0.0769 × weight) − (0.3877 × age) + (6.315 × gender) − (3.2649 × time) − (0.1565 × heart rate)
Weight in pounds (lb)
Gender: male = 1, female = 0
Time expressed in minutes
Heart rate in bpm
Age in years

The Multishuttle Test (MST): The multi-stage shuttle test was originally developed by Leger and Lambert (1982) and consists of incremental stages of running back and forward between two markers set 20 metres apart with the pace set by bleeps from a cassette tape. The initial velocity is 8.5 km/hr and increases by 0.5 km/hr every minute. The test is terminated when the subject cannot reach the end lines concurrent with the audio signals on two consecutive occasions. The $\dot{V}O_2$max is predicted from a chart of the stage achieved and number of further shuttles completed. As the test is standardised and externally paced the subject's level of motivation is less likely to affect the test result.

Level 8 = 40 ml/kg/min
Level 10 = 47 ml/kg/min
Level 12 = 54 ml/kg/min
Level 14 = 61 ml/kg/min
Level 16 = 68 ml/kg/min
Level 18 = 75 ml/kg/min

The MST has been found to be a valid estimate of $\dot{V}O_2$max (Ramsbottom et al., 1988; Leger and Gadourg, 1989). The test can be carried out individually or in small groups, on most gymnasium surfaces.

Monitoring exercise responses

Heart rate

Heart rate can be monitored during exercise by the use of a pulse monitor, electro-cardiograms or a wireless chest strap heart rate monitoring system such as the *Polar* or *Cardiosport* systems. Pulse monitors use a fingertip or earlobe and work on the principle that when the pulse of blood travels through a light or infrared beam it is registered on the monitor. Accuracy depends on keeping the part still which is easier during stationary cycling than treadmill walking. The electro-cardiogram (ECG) is the most accurate tool for measuring heart rate. However, special training is required to apply and interpret an ECG. The wireless chest strap personal heart rate monitors are probably the easiest to use and permit monitoring of heart rate during almost all forms of activity. The chest strap has two electrodes which work on the same principle as the ECG, by directly picking up the electrical impulses controlling the heart. The chest strap contains a radiotransmitter that sends a signal to a receiver on a wrist watch which calculates and displays heart rate in beats per minute. Many of these watches can store many hours of heart rate which can be downloaded to a PC. Personal heart rate monitors are used by many individuals, from elite athletes to patients during cardiac rehabilitation (Figure 6.3).

Rating of perceived exertion

A rating of perceived exertion is explained as the detecting and interpreting sensations from the body during physical exertion. RPE tracks perception of intensity

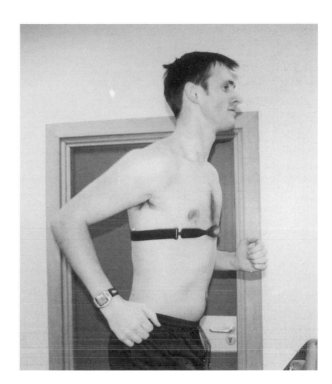

Figure 6.3 Personal heart rate monitor strapped on the chest.

of exercise. The use of Borg's RPE scale is a well accepted measure in sports and exercise science and in the rehabilitation of patients with cardiac and respiratory disease. The RPE was devised by Borg in the 1950s. It has been extensively researched by testing its relationship with physiological and psychological responses in both athletes and patient populations (Borg, 1982). The 15 point scale is probably the most often used (from 6 (no exertion at all) to 20 (maximal exertion)) (Box 6.1). RPE is strongly associated with breathing rate, oxygen consumption, lactic acid level, and Dishman (1994) has reported that RPE is more closely linked with oxygen consumption than with heart rate. The RPE can be used for estimating intensity of exercise. The subject performs a specific task or predetermined work rate and they give a rating of their feeling of exertion in response to performing the task. Another use of the RPE is that the subject exercises to a predetermined/prescribed RPE, thus the RPE becomes the focus of establishing one's effort.

The patient needs to understand that perceived exertion is a method to determine the intensity of effort felt during exercise. The sensation experienced needs to correspond to the scale and the individual must understand the descriptors used.

Blood pressure

During exercise systolic blood pressure should rise in proportion to the amount of effort. The pressure rise depends on the intensity of the activity and the resting systolic blood pressure. Systolic blood pressure can rise to 200 mmHg but a failure

Box 6.1 The Borg scale.

6	No exertion at all
7	Extremely light
8	
9	Very light
10	
11	Light
12	
13	Somewhat hard
14	
15	Hard (heavy)
16	
17	
18	
19	Extremely hard
20	Maximal exertion

Reproduced with permission of G. Borg. For correct usage of the scale the exact design and instructions given in Borg's folders must be followed. See *Borg's RPE Scale*, Borg, G., 1994 and *The Borg CR10 Scale*, Borg, G., 2003. For applied usage in medicine, sports, ergonomy, etc., you have to pay to get a special licence. In scientific work and teaching you are encouraged to use the scale without paying a fee. The folders together with scales can be obtained from Borg Perception, Radisvagen 124, 165 73 Hasselby, Sweden. borg.08271426@telia.com.

of systolic pressure to rise with exercise may be an indication of heart failure. Diastolic blood pressure should remain unchanged and an increase of more than 15 mmHg during progressive exercise testing may be an indicator of severe ischaemic heart disease or hypertension. Exercising blood pressure is easier to measure during cycle ergometry than treadmill walking/running as the arm can be kept virtually still.

Screening and safety

Prior to all tests, full history and pretest screening is important to identify risk factors or symptoms for many chronic cardiovascular, pulmonary and metabolic disorders to optimise safety during exercise testing and exercise prescription.

Preparticipation health screening allows:

- The identification and exclusion of subjects with medical contraindications to exercise.
- The identification of subjects at increased risk for disease who need to undergo medical evaluation and exercise testing before starting an exercise programme.
- The identification of subjects with clinical disease who need medically supervised exercise programmes.

The Physical Activity Readiness Questionnaire (PAR-Q)(see Appendix 6.1) (Canadian Society for Exercise Physiology, 1994) is often used as a minimal standard for entry into moderate-intensity exercise programmes and was devised by the Canadian Society for Exercise Physiology in order to identify adults in whom medical advice concerning type of activities is required. The PAR-Q asks questions on heart conditions, chest pain, balance/dizziness, bone/joint problems, prescription drugs or any other reasons why physical activity may be not be advised.

In the absence of cardiac pathology, symptom limited exercise testing is generally a safe procedure with a very small risk. A physician experienced in handling cardiovascular emergencies should be available if required. The risks of sub-maximal exercise testing are even lower than for maximal and are therefore safely supervised by non-medical staff (for example, sports/fitness clubs) in subjects without clinical symptoms who have completed the PAR-Q successfully. Staff involved in exercise testing need to be proficient in cardiopulmonary resuscitation (CPR) and emergency drills. A defibrillator and appropriate emergency drugs should be checked daily. Risk stratification has been devised by the American Association of Cardiovascular and Pulmonary Rehabilitation (Box 6.2). Contraindications to exercise testing are listed in Box 6.3. Details of stress testing in patients with cardiac disease are discussed in Chapter 8.

Box 6.2 Stratification for risk of event (not specific only to exercise). With permission from the American Association of Cardiovascular and Pulmonary Rehabilitation (AACVPR, 1999).

Low No significant left ventricular dysfunction (EF > 50%).
No exercising or exercise induced complex dysrhythmias.
Uncomplicated MI; coronary artery bypass grafting; angioplasty, atherectomy or stent; absence of CHF or signs/symptoms indicating post event ischaemia.
Normal haemodynamics with exercise or recovery.
Asymptomatic including absence of angina with exertion or recovery.
Functional capacity ≥ 7.0 METS*.
Absence of clinical depression.

Lowest risk classification is assumed when each of the risk factors in the category is present

Moderate Moderately impaired left ventricular function (EF − 40–49%).
Signs/symptoms including angina at moderate levels of exercise (5–6.9 METs)* or in recovery.

Moderate risk is assumed for patients who do not meet the classification of either high risk or low risk

High Decreased left ventricular function (EF < 40%).
Survivor of cardiac arrest or sudden death.
Complex ventricular dysrhythmia at rest or with exercise.
MI or cardiac surgery complicated by cardiogenic shock, CHF, and/or signs/symptoms of post procedure ischaemia.
Abnormal haemodynamics with exercise (especially flat or decreasing systolic blood pressure or chronotropic incompetence with increasing workload.
Signs/symptoms including angina pectoris at low levels of exercise (< 5.0METS)* or in recovery.
Functional capacity < 5.0 METS*.
Clinically significant depression.

Highest risk classification is assumed with the presence of any one of the risk factors included in this category

* If measured functional capacity is not available, this variable is not considered in the risk stratification process.

Box 6.3 Contraindications to exercise testing. Reproduced with permission of the ACC/AHA from the ACC/AHA Guidelines (2002).

Absolute contraindications

- Acute myocardial infarction (within 2 days)
- High-risk unstable angina
- Uncontrolled cardiac arrhythmias causing symptoms or haemodynamic compromise
- Symptomatic severe aortic stenosis
- Uncontrolled symptomatic heart failure
- Acute pulmonary embolus or pulmonary infarction
- Acute myocarditis or pericarditis
- Acute aortic dissection

Relative contraindications

- Left main coronary artery stenosis
- Moderate stenotic valvular heart disease
- Electrolyte abnormalities
- Severe arterial hypertension (systolic BP of > 200 mmHg and/or a diastolic BP of > 110 mmHg) at rest
- Tachyarrhythmias or bradyarrhythmias
- Hypertrophic cardiomyopathy and other forms of outflow tract obstruction
- Mental or physical impairment leading to inability to exercise adequately
- High-degree atrioventricular block

The subject should be advised to wear loose clothing which is comfortable to exercise in and facilitates the application of ECG electrodes and a blood pressure cuff. He/she should abstain from coffee, alcohol or smoking for at least three hours before testing and should not engage in other vigorous activity on the day of testing. Patients should continue taking any prescribed medication unless directed otherwise by their physician. Informed consent must be obtained as it has important legal and ethical implications and ensures that the patient is aware of the purpose and risks associated with testing. This is to prevent claims by the participant of breach of contract or negligence by the health professional by providing the subject with full knowledge of the procedure, the relevant risks and benefits and any alternative procedures that may be available for the same objective. The subject of safety will also be discussed in Chapter 7.

Muscle strength

Muscular strength refers to the maximal force that can be generated by a specific muscle or muscle group. Static or isometric muscle strength can be measured easily by using a handgrip dynamometer. However, the measurement of isometric muscle strength is then specific to strength at the joint angle where tested and only measures muscle strength at that point in the range in movement. For dynamic

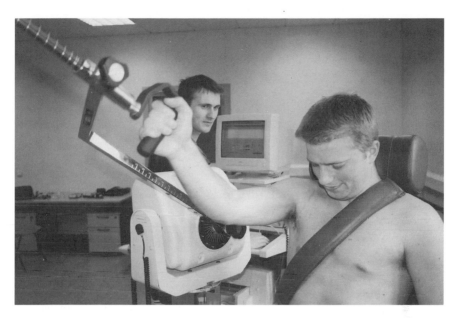

Figure 6.4 Isokinetic dynamometer to measure muscle strength.

muscle strength testing an external load is used. The traditional gold standard method is the 1-RM (1 Repetition Maximum): the heaviest weight that can be lifted once. However, this measurement is limited by the weakest point in the range. Isokinetic testing involves the assessment of maximal muscle tension throughout the range. Peak torque is obtained (Figure 6.4). However, isokinetic muscle testing is expensive and time consuming and many clinical departments would not have the facilities for this.

Muscle endurance is the ability of a muscle group to execute repeated contractions over a period of time, sufficient to cause muscle fatigue or to maintain a specific percentage of the maximum voluntary contraction for a prolonged period of time.

Flexibility

Flexibility is the ability to move a joint through its complete range of motion (ROM). Flexibility depends on the distensibility of the joint capsule, adequate warm up and muscle viscosity. The compliance of various other tissues, such as ligaments and tendons, affects the range of movement. Joint motion is measured as part of evaluations of fitness or work capacity. In rehabilitation, measuring joint ranges is used to assess status and for goal settings and patient motivation. Children generally have larger ROMs than adults. After the age of 40 years there is a gradual decline in ROM in many joints.

Flexibility is joint specific and is measured by goniometry, inclinometry, tape measures and flexible rules. Goniometers consist of two arms, are inexpensive and portable, and commonly used for measuring ROM, especially in the larger joints. The reliability of goniometers is high if standard techniques are used (Rothstein et al., 1983). Inclinometers may be mechanical or electronic and use gravity to track the arc of motion during movement of the head, trunk or extremity. Strong reliability has been demonstrated when using inclinometry in the lumbar and cervical spine (Protas, 1998). Tape measures can be used to measure spinal and finger movements. The skin distraction technique can be used in the measurement of trunk flexion by comparing differences in position of two marks placed on the skin prior to and after the movement. A flexible rule can be used to measure spinal movements with the tangent of the arc described by applying the rule to the contours of the back during movement.

Anthropometry

Measurement of height, weight, hip and waist circumferences and skinfolds are used to estimate body composition. Body mass index (BMI) is used to assess weight relative to height by dividing body weight in kilograms by height in meters squared (kg/m^2). See Table 5.1 for descriptions of classes of BMI. Obesity standards, based on BMI, have been developed and increased BMI is associated with increased risk of chronic disease. However, BMI is not always a good predictor of body fat and can incorrectly classify subjects as obese if they have above average muscularity and/or skeletal mass, rather than excess fat. While BMI is a useful measurement, results do need to be interpreted with a degree of caution. The range of normal on the BMI scale is between 20 and 25. A result below 20 is considered underweight whereas over 25 is considered overweight, with a score of over 30 being considered obese.

Skinfolds give accurate estimates of percentage fat and FFM (fat free mass) since they are direct measurements of subcutaneous fat. The procedure for measuring fatfold thickness involves grasping the fold between the thumb and first two fingers. It is pulled away from the bone, ensuring that no muscular tissue is included. The jaws of the measuring callipers are then released into the fold and after two seconds the measurement is read from the dial. The average of three measurements is taken for each site. Fatfold measurements can be utilised by calculating the total millimetre score of all sites measured to give a raw value of skinfold thickness (Durin and Rahman, 1967) or by putting this raw value into mathematical equations (Jackson and Pollock, 1985). Skinfolds and circumferences are also useful in assessing fat pattern and fat distribution. The ratio of subscapular to triceps skinfolds has been used to reflect a central versus peripheral fat pattern and the ratio of waist-to-hip circumferences (WHR) is a common index of upper versus lower body fat distribution. WHR has been identified as a predictor of chronic disease risk in epidemiological studies. In adults the absolute value of waist circumference along with BMI is predictive of risk of disease (Table 11.1). To measure waist circumference the top of the iliac crest is located and a measuring tape is placed in a horizontal plane around the abdomen at this level. The tape should be snug but should not compress the skin. The measurement should be taken at end expiration.

Measurement of habitual physical activity

Regular participation in physical activity is associated with health benefits which include a reduced risk of cardiovascular disease, non-insulin dependent diabetes mellitus, obesity, hypertension, osteoporosis, some cancers, anxiety and depression. In the last 30 years much research has focused on the relationship between low levels of physical activity and the development of chronic diseases and health conditions. Due to this large interest many methods of measuring physical activity have been investigated. Accurate assessment of physical activity is necessary in order to objectively evaluate the health benefits related to physical activity and to understand the dose-response relationship between physical activity and health.

Physical activity is defined as body movement produced by skeletal muscles and resulting in energy expenditure (Caspersen et al., 1985). Its measurement is particularly difficult as it is a multidimensional variable, which includes type, frequency, duration and intensity. A further problem is that habitual levels of activity vary during the day, with different days of the week and different times of the year. Physical activity is a variable and unstable behaviour.

For the purpose of this review, measurements of habitual physical activity will be divided into four areas (observation, self recall/diaries/questionnaires, heart rate monitoring and the use of motion sensors) and the relative merits and difficulties of each will be discussed. One of the greatest obstacles to validating field methods of assessing habitual physical activity is a lack of an adequate criterion to which techniques may be compared. Doubly labelled water (DLW) is considered the gold standard for the measurement of physical activity, but its limitations include expense and the requirement of sophisticated equipment. The method uses stable isotopes of hydrogen and oxygen, ingested as water, and is based on the assumption that oxygen atoms in expired carbon dioxide are in isotopic equilibrium with the oxygen atoms in total body water. DLW provides information on total daily energy expenditure and cannot be used to examine acute patterns of physical activity such as time spent in specific activities or intensity of specific exercise sessions.

Observation

Observation studies of levels of physical activity have mainly been used in children and in workers in specific jobs. Observers are trained to note behavioural information on types of activities, the time spent in each activity and its frequency of performance. The cost of data collection in these studies is high, due to the need for trained observers, and therefore numbers in these studies are often small. Accuracy is improved with the use of prepared forms for recording of activities and categories need to be clearly established, for example, sitting quietly, sitting with small movements (Montoye et al., 1996). Recording of data over long periods is tedious and can lead to inaccuracies, but if observations are confined to time periods that are too short they may not be reflective of habitual physical activity. Videoing increases the reliability of measurements as well as providing a permanent record. Adults may alter their usual patterns of activity if they are aware of being watched but it is possible that this may occur less so in children. In very young children many other methods of assessing physical activity are not suitable, for example, self report or use of equipment (for example, heart rate monitors or accelerometers, which may be difficult to attach for prolonged periods of time, or in very small children may be too cumbersome to wear during activity). Observation methods also allow data to be collected on intervals between activity, such as inactivity.

O'Hara et al. (1989) have described and validated a system which can discriminate between different levels of energy expenditure using an activity points system to predict heart rate from four different levels of intensity. The highest intensity level is called MVPA (moderate to vigorous physical activity), which is defined as an activity of sufficient intensity to lift heart rate above 139 bpm, for example, brisk walking. Points are given for each minute in each category which is then converted to a predicted heart rate for that level. Information on the physical surroundings which may influence physical activity levels can be easily obtained in observation studies.

Other activity rating scales include the CARS (Children's Activity Rating Scale) as described by Puhl et al. (1990) and the SOFIT (System for Observing Fitness Instruction Time) (McKenzie et al., 1991a). With CARS, activity levels which are measured every minute are classified into five levels according to a rating system. In level 1 activities are sedentary, in level 2 activities are sedentary but there is movement of the limbs or torso, in levels 3–5 there is movement of the body and the speed/intensity of the activity determines the level. The SOFIT is a system for observing the strenuousness of activities in a physical education (PE) class. It consists of a five-point activity scale from level 1: lying on the floor with minimal movement to level 5: jogging around the gym. In BEACHES the activity component requires an observer to use a series of codes to describe a child's physical activity level and physical and social environment (McKenzie et al., 1991b). While observation studies are successful where subjects are confined to a defined space, they are time consuming as they require many observers and intense training. Expense may be prohibitive in epidemiological or large-scale studies.

Self report/diaries/questionnaires

Measures of physical activity used in large-scale studies need to be simple and inexpensive. Where time and manpower are limited questionnaires are used and they are the only real method of collecting data on physical activity in epidemiological studies. There are several survey procedures which Laporte et al. (1985) have classified as:

- Short-term diary (previous 24 hours)
- Past week recall surveys (1–7 days)

- Quantitative over past 1–5 years
- General survey regardless of time reference

Questionnaires measuring physical activity need to include questions specific to the purpose of the survey. Questions can be self administered or interviewer administered (in person or by telephone) using a prepared form to record answers. Self administered questionnaires need to be suited to respondents' ages and education levels. A number of physical activity questionnaires have been developed for national surveys, which are simple to administer and often suitable for telephone surveys requiring less than ten minutes to administer. Objective rather than subjective responses should be sought, to help provide consistent interpretation and scoring. In most adult studies on physical activity, questions on occupational and leisure time activity need to be included.

The procedure of measuring levels of physical activity by questionnaires does not influence subjects' activities and by using energy expenditure tables may give an estimated total energy expenditure. Limitations to the use of questionnaires for assessing overall physical activity levels are that subjects do not necessarily recall all their activities and may overestimate the time spent in activity or its intensity. Validity for all questionnaires is difficult to establish due to the lack of a gold standard criterion against which to compare the measurement in question. Moderate intensity activity is more difficult to assess than vigorous bouts of exercise as it is generally less structured and therefore more difficult to recall.

Children's activity is often unplanned and spontaneous (Armstrong et al., 1990) with a far more diverse range of activities than adults. The more diffused, unorganised and spontaneous the activity the more difficult it is to recall. Many physical activity questionnaires have been developed for populations in geographic areas and others have been devised for the assessment of activity in relation to the incidence of specific disease processes, such as coronary heart disease. Questionnaires for use in adults assess work related and leisure time activities and the timeframes vary from days to the past year.

A number of questionnaires have been devised assessing the relationship between physical activity and the development of specific conditions where inactivity is a clear risk factor. The British Civil Servant Questionnaire was used in studies on heart disease in British male executive civil servants (Yasin et al., 1967). Only leisure time activities were recorded in the interview, which required about one hour. Respondents were asked to recall all activity lasting five minutes or more during the previous two days. Points were awarded per five minutes of reported activity, ranging from one point for sedentary activities such as reading, to five points for sports such as tennis. The daily activity score is the sum of the points. Occupational physical activity was not included as it was designed for subjects in sedentary occupations.

The Paffenbarger/Harvard Alumni Questionnaire is a simple self administered questionnaire that was designed to study the relationship between physical activity and disease among a population of Harvard University alumni. Questions included: stairs climbed, city blocks walked, sports activities and light activities (Paffenbarger et al., 1993).

An example of a questionnaire that assesses activity over a longer timeframe is the Minnesota Questionnaire. It is self administered and estimates physical activity during the past year (leisure time and occupational). The total time taken to complete the questionnaire is one hour and as it was designed to study activity patterns of males in an entire community it is suitable for subjects with a wide educational range. Good reliability has been reported over a short timeframe with test retest over one month for the Minnesota correlation coefficient being 0.88 (Folsom et al., 1986). As the timeframe respondents are questioned on spans from the previous year adequate representation of seasonal variation is obtained.

The use of questionnaires in children

The use of questionnaires in children is more limited than in adults as many factors can contribute to measurement error when using self report methods in children. Below the age of 10–12 years, children can only give limited information about their activity patterns. Even in children aged 11–13 years, recall of activities can be inaccurate with Wallace et al. (1985) reporting only 46% of activities during the previous seven days being recalled and 55–65% during the previous 24 hours, when compared to those documented by three observers. Parents, teachers or other adults may give details of the child's physical activity but this information may be secondary, especially for outside activities. Questionnaires designed for adults are usually not suitable for children because of the differences in their activity patterns. Adults tend to perform activity in readily identifiable sessions whereas children tend to be active much of the day. As children engage in physical activity that is sporadic in time and in intensity they find the task of recalling activities difficult. Much activity in young children is spontaneous, non-organised and occurs due to the situations and opportunities found and may not be 'memorable' in terms of frequency, duration and intensity (information commonly asked for in questionnaires). Generally, children have difficulties estimating the duration of activities, as intensity and preference are important for the duration of time spent in specific activities. However, despite the recognition that questionnaires may not be entirely suitable for children, they are the only method at present for collecting a broad range of data from large numbers. In children the most reliable values are obtained from questions about participation in sports, which is probably due to the regular character of this type of activity. Timeframes need to be provided for the child in terms of 'on the way to school, break time, way home from school, before dinner' etc. Inquiries should be made about participation in physical education (PE), number of PE sessions per week, organised sports, transportation to and from school, recreational activities after school or during weekends. A recall list of activities is useful.

Questionnaires for assessing physical activity levels in children include the Netherlands Health Education Project Questionnaire, Northern Ireland Questionnaire, Amsterdam Growth Study Questionnaire and Modifiable Activity Questionnaire for Adolescents. Informed consent from parents/guardians is essential prior to obtaining information from minors.

The use of questionnaires in the elderly

In the elderly, questionnaires such as the Baecke have been modified, with additional questions added which ask about household activities. Most elderly people are retired, so leisure time activity is most important. Many elderly people do not participate in moderate or strenuous physical activity and at this age may have physical or medical conditions that restrict physical activity considerably.

Questionnaires/surveys on physical activity are usable over a wide age range but with moderate reliability over a longer timeframe. In the young and middle-aged it is necessary to investigate occupational and leisure time activity. Vigorous activity is more reliably recalled than light activity, and timeframes of the day need to be clearly outlined for children whose activity is not as organised and identifiable as adults.

Motion sensors

Motion sensors have evolved from mechanical devices like pedometers to electronic accelerometers, which reflect not only the occurrence of body movement but also the intensity of movement.

Accelerometers

Present day accelerometers are small, easy to use and incorporate interval based time sampling and computer downloading facilities. They allow measurement of quantity and intensity of movement. They are non-obtrusive and cost effective. The assessment of physical activity by accelerometers is based on the measurement of body movement, that is, the dynamic component of physical activity. The validation of accelerometers is performed against energy expenditure by direct or indirect calorimetry (measuring gas exchange associated with the oxidation of energy substrates or measuring TEE breathing through a mouthpiece). Accelerometer output is influenced by the place of attachment to the body, as different body sites are differentially active depending on the behaviour engaged in and movements of one site are not necessarily correlated with movements of other sites.

The first generation of accelerometers were uniaxial, for example, Caltrac and the CSA. Triaxial accelerometers include the RD3 and more recently the RT3 (Figure 6.5). The Caltrac is a one axial accelerometer measuring vertical movement, and energy expenditure is estimated by entering the subject's age, height, weight and gender. Activity counts are displayed. The first generation of accelerometers were capable of detecting motion in only one plane, which may have caused a limitation of their ability to accurately estimate energy expenditure for activities that had motion in more than one plane, as most activities do. The Computer Science Application (CSA) accelerometer uses integrated circuitry and memory to provide a continuous recording of minute by minute movement counts. A uni-dimensional (vertical axis) activity monitor may be just as valid as a three-dimensional monitor because most movements in the saggital and horizontal planes are accompanied by movement in the vertical plane. However, activity in children is highly sporadic and may involve

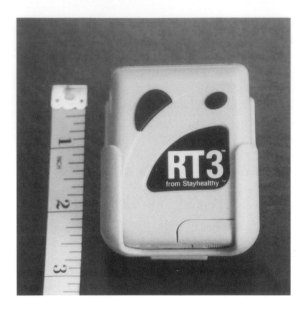

Figure 6.5 Accelerometer.

more non-vertical movements (climbing, crawling) than typical activities performed by adults (Welk and Corbin, 1995).

Triaxial accelerometers such as the Tritrac-R3D can assess activity in three dimensions. Activity counts and energy expenditure are displayed. The Tritrac R3D is designed to be worn clipped to a belt at the waist. It can be worn for up to two weeks and then data downloaded to a PC to give minute by minute values for activity in three planes. It thus has the potential for a relatively long assessment of activity patterns which relate to habitual physical activity. The Tritrac measures acceleration in three individual planes and integrates acceleration to yield one value called the vector magnitude. Vector magnitude is calculated as the square root of the sum squared of activity counts in each vector. The energy expenditure is estimated by entering the subject's age, weight, height and gender, and data can be downloaded to a PC and used for the calculation of body acceleration by subtracting the calculated resting energy expenditure from the registered energy expenditure. The Tritrac has been shown to be highly reliable from day to day and is sensitive to changes in speed of movement but not to any incline. It accurately distinguishes the various intensities of walking and jogging on level ground and could lead to categorisation of light, moderate and vigorous levels of physical activity and can estimate energy expenditure.

In highly sedentary subjects with COPD, who have severe limitations to physical activity, the Tritrac has been found to be a reliable, valid and stable measure of walking and daily physical activity (Steele et al., 2000). If the energy cost of an activity is related to muscular loading from isometric contractions, upper body movement, graded surfaces or carrying, lifting or pushing a weight (lawnmowing, pushing a buggy) there will not be an increase in counts registered on the accelerometer. Accelerometers placed at the hip appear unable to detect increased energy cost of upper body movement, load carriage or changes in surface or terrain (Fehling et al., 1999). These activities are probably more typical in adults, where they contribute to overall daily activity levels, than in children. The effects of vehicular transportation need to be assessed as these could be a confounding source of error when used in assessing daily activity in free living situations. For a more complete assessment of overall activity and, in particular, where lifting, carrying and walking uphill are concerned, it may be advisable to complement the use of the accelerometer with a questionnaire.

Accelerometry is an objective and reliable method for assessment of activity. It is a suitable method to measure physical activity in large populations over relatively long and representative periods, with minimal discomfort to individuals, and the small size and unobtrusiveness would probably not influence activity patterns. Accelerometers cannot be used to measure the static components in exercise such as weightlifting or carrying heavy loads. It is assumed that in normal daily life the effect of static exercise on the total level of physical activity is negligible. Sedentary activities are probably better reflected by triaxial accelerometry than uniaxial accelerometry.

Pedometers

Pedometers are designed to count steps and the first was devised over 500 years ago by Leonardo da Vinci (Haskell et al., 2001). The pedometer records acceleration and deceleration of the waist in the vertical direction. It does not record intensity of movement during walking/running and, when cycling, no movement counts are registered. For large studies where only total activity is of interest, the pedometer may be useful (Eston et al., 1998; Louie et al., 1999).

Heart rate monitoring

Heart rate is an objective but an indirect method of measuring physical activity. It can operate by telemetry and can be interfaced with a PC. The interpretation of heart rate monitoring is based on the linear relationship between oxygen uptake and heart rate. The relative stress placed on the cardiopulmonary system due to physical activity is assessed. Heart rate monitoring is a common objective method used to assess physical activity, due to its relatively low cost and ability to record values over time. The advancement of microelectronics has made it possible to detect and store impulses over long time periods using unobtrusive equipment and the use of these monitors by athletes has led to the development of reliable heart rate recorders with minimal size and weight but maximal storage capacity.

Heart rate monitoring has been used in many studies assessing physical activity in children (Armstrong et al., 1990; Van den Berg-Emons et al., 1996; Coleman et al., 1997) and adults (Wareham et al., 1997). The volume of physical activity (frequency, duration and intensity) can be estimated from continuous heart rate monitoring, and monitors such as the Polar Vantage can store information on heart rate each minute for up to seven days. When the data is downloaded, via an interface onto a PC, heart rates above a percentage maximum (for example, 70%) can be readily identified and the time spent at specific heart rates can be obtained.

There is some day-to-day variation in heart rate for any particular energy expenditure and heart rate can also be elevated by emotional stress independent of any change in oxygen uptake. The return of heart rate to baseline may lag behind the rate of oxygen uptake to baseline. Training lowers the heart rate at which work at a specific energy cost is performed. Physical fitness levels are a limiting factor, as the fitter the child the higher the stroke volume and hence a lower heart rate for any given workload. Other sources of error include ambient temperature and humidity. Upper body work elicits higher heart rates for work of the same oxygen cost performed by the lower limbs. Heart rate telemetry is frequently used to validate other methods of measuring daily activity in children as it has minimal interference with the child's activity and reflects moderate to vigorous activity.

Summary

Observation methods, while prohibitive in population studies, can be highly accurate and provide a validation criterion for other methods. Recall may provide a valid measure of vigorous physical activity, but is less useful in measuring light to moderate or sedentary activity. Children's activities are probably less easily remembered as they accumulate activity via a large number of short sessions which are often not predetermined. Equipment, when used, such as heart rate monitoring or accelerometry, should not influence activity patterns. While heart rate monitoring is of value in measuring moderate to vigorous activity it does not provide an accurate prediction of energy expenditure during periods of low activity. Triaxial accelerometry does predict energy expenditure during periods of inactivity as well as light and moderate activity. The range and variety of movements experienced by children are probably well reflected by triaxial accelerometry.

There is a lack of strong correlations between different instruments used in validity studies as the instruments may assess different dimensions of physical activity. Self report methods correlate weakly with heart rate monitoring or motion sensors. Motion sensors have received increased attention over the last few years and appear to have good potential. It appears that cost is inversely related to precision and the final decision of choice is often a trade-off between precision, subject characteristics, cost, time, subject numbers and feasibility.

Appendix 6.1

The Physical Activity Readiness Questionnaire (PAR-Q; Canadian Society for Exercise Physiology, 2002). Reprinted with permission of the Canadian Society for Exercise Physiology.

Physical Activity Readiness
Questionnaire - PAR-Q
(revised 2002)

PAR-Q & YOU

(A Questionnaire for People Aged 15 to 69)

Regular physical activity is fun and healthy, and increasingly more people are starting to become more active every day. Being more active is very safe for most people. However, some people should check with their doctor before they start becoming much more physically active.

If you are planning to become much more physically active than you are now, start by answering the seven questions in the box below. If you are between the ages of 15 and 69, the PAR-Q will tell you if you should check with your doctor before you start. If you are over 69 years of age, and you are not used to being very active, check with your doctor.

Common sense is your best guide when you answer these questions. Please read the questions carefully and answer each one honestly: check YES or NO.

YES	NO		
☐	☐	1.	Has your doctor ever said that you have a heart condition <u>and</u> that you should only do physical activity recommended by a doctor?
☐	☐	2.	Do you feel pain in your chest when you do physical activity?
☐	☐	3.	In the past month, have you had chest pain when you were not doing physical activity?
☐	☐	4.	Do you lose your balance because of dizziness or do you ever lose consciousness?
☐	☐	5.	Do you have a bone or joint problem (for example, back, knee or hip) that could be made worse by a change in your physical activity?
☐	☐	6.	Is your doctor currently prescribing drugs (for example, water pills) for your blood pressure or heart condition?
☐	☐	7.	Do you know of <u>any other reason</u> why you should not do physical activity?

If you answered

YES to one or more questions

Talk with your doctor by phone or in person BEFORE you start becoming much more physically active or BEFORE you have a fitness appraisal. Tell your doctor about the PAR-Q and which questions you answered YES.

- You may be able to do any activity you want — as long as you start slowly and build up gradually. Or, you may need to restrict your activities to those which are safe for you. Talk with your doctor about the kinds of activities you wish to participate in and follow his/her advice.
- Find out which community programs are safe and helpful for you.

NO to all questions

If you answered NO honestly to <u>all</u> PAR-Q questions, you can be reasonably sure that you can:
- start becoming much more physically active – begin slowly and build up gradually. This is the safest and easiest way to go.
- take part in a fitness appraisal – this is an excellent way to determine your basic fitness so that you can plan the best way for you to live actively. It is also highly recommended that you have your blood pressure evaluated. If your reading is over 144/94, talk with your doctor before you start becoming much more physically active.

DELAY BECOMING MUCH MORE ACTIVE:
- if you are not feeling well because of a temporary illness such as a cold or a fever – wait until you feel better; or
- if you are or may be pregnant – talk to your doctor before you start becoming more active.

PLEASE NOTE: If your health changes so that you then answer YES to any of the above questions, tell your fitness or health professional. Ask whether you should change your physical activity plan.

Informed Use of the PAR-Q: The Canadian Society for Exercise Physiology, Health Canada, and their agents assume no liability for persons who undertake physical activity, and if in doubt after completing this questionnaire, consult your doctor prior to physical activity.

No changes permitted. You are encouraged to photocopy the PAR-Q but only if you use the entire form.

NOTE: If the PAR-Q is being given to a person before he or she participates in a physical activity program or a fitness appraisal, this section may be used for legal or administrative purposes.

"I have read, understood and completed this questionnaire. Any questions I had were answered to my full satisfaction."

NAME _____

SIGNATURE _____   DATE_____

SIGNATURE OF PARENT _____   WITNESS _____
or GUARDIAN (for participants under the age of majority)

Note: This physical activity clearance is valid for a maximum of 12 months from the date it is completed and becomes invalid if your condition changes so that you would answer YES to any of the seven questions.

 © Canadian Society for Exercise Physiology   Supported by: Health Santé
Canada Canada

continued on other side...

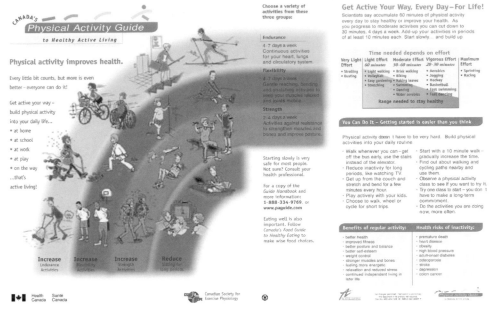

Source: Canada's Physical Activity Guide to Healthy Active Living, Health Canada, 1998 http://www.hc-sc.gc.ca/hppb/paguide/pdf/guideEng.pdf
© Reproduced with permission from the Minister of Public Works and Government Services Canada, 2002.

FITNESS AND HEALTH PROFESSIONALS MAY BE INTERESTED IN THE INFORMATION BELOW:

The following companion forms are available for doctors' use by contacting the Canadian Society for Exercise Physiology (address below):

The **Physical Activity Readiness Medical Examination (PARmed-X)** – to be used by doctors with people who answer YES to one or more questions on the PAR-Q.

The **Physical Activity Readiness Medical Examination for Pregnancy (PARmed-X for Pregnancy)** – to be used by doctors with pregnant patients who wish to become more active.

References:
Arraix, G.A., Wigle, D.T., Mao, Y. (1992). Risk Assessment of Physical Activity and Physical Fitness in the Canada Health Survey
   Follow-Up Study. **J. Clin. Epidemiol.** 45:4 419-428.
Mottola, M., Wolfe, L.A. (1994). Active Living and Pregnancy. In: A. Quinney, L. Gauvin, T. Wall (eds.), **Toward Active Living: Proceedings of the International
   Conference on Physical Activity, Fitness and Health.** Champaign, IL: Human Kinetics.
PAR-Q Validation Report, British Columbia Ministry of Health, 1978.
Thomas, S., Reading, J., Shephard, R.J. (1992). Revision of the Physical Activity Readiness Questionnaire (PAR-Q). **Can. J. Spt. Sci.** 17:4 338-345.

For more information, please contact the:

Canadian Society for Exercise Physiology
202-185 Somerset Street West
Ottawa, ON K2P 0J2
Tel. 1-877-651-3755 • FAX (613) 234-3565
Online: www.csep.ca

The original PAR-Q was developed by the British Columbia Ministry of Health. It has been revised by an Expert Advisory Committee of the Canadian Society for Exercise Physiology chaired by Dr. N. Gledhill (2002).

Disponible en français sous le titre «Questionnaire sur l'aptitude à l'activité physique - Q-AAP (revisé 2002)».

© Canadian Society for Exercise Physiology   Supported by: Health Canada Santé Canada

References

ACC/AHA (2002). *Guideline Update for Exercise Testing*. American College of Cardiology American Heart Association. www.americanheart.org

American Association of Cardiovascular and Pulmonary Rehabilitation (1999). *Guidelines for Cardiac Rehabilitation and Secondary Prevention Programs*, 3rd edn. Human Kinetics, Champaign, Ill.

American College of Sports Medicine (2000). *Guidelines for Exercise Testing and Prescription*, 6th edn. Lippincott Williams and Wilkins, Baltimore.

Armstrong, N., Balding, J., Gentle, P. and Kirby, B. (1990). Patterns of physical activity among 11 to 16-year-old British children. *British Medical Journal* 301, 203–5.

Astrand, P.O. and Rhyming, I.A. (1954). Nomogram for calculation of aerobic capacity (physical fitness) from pulse rate during sub-maximal work. *Journal of Applied Physiology* 7, 218–21.

Baecke, J.A.H., Burema, J. and Frijters, J.E.R. (1982). A short questionnaire for the measurement of habitual physical activity in epidemiological studies. *American Journal of Clinical Nutrition* 36, 936–42.

Borg, G. (1982). The psychophysical bases of perceived exertion. *Medicine and Science in Sports and Exercise* 14: 377–81.

Canadian Society for Exercise Physiology (1994). *PAR-Q and You*. pp. 1–2. Canadian Society for Exercise Physiology Inc, Ontario.

Caspersen, C.J., Powell K.E. and Christenson, G.M. (1985). Physical activity, exercise, and physical fitness: definitions and distinctions for health-related research. *Public Health Reports* 100, 126–31.

Coleman, K.J., Saelens, B.E., Wiedrich-Smith, M.D., Finn, J.D. and Epstein, L.H. (1997). Relationships between TriTrac-R3D vectors, heart rate, and self report in obese children. *Medicine and Science in Sports and Exercise* 29, 1535–42.

Cooper, K.M. (1968). A means of assessing maximal oxygen intake. *Journal of American Medical Association* 203, 201–4.

Dishman, R.K. (1994). Prescribing exercise intensity for healthy adults using perceived exertion. *Medicine and Science in Sports and Exercise* 26, 1087–94.

Durin, J.V.G.A. and Rahaman, M.M. (1967). The assessment of the amount of fat in the human body from measurements of skinfold thickness. *British Journal of Nutrition* 21, 681–9.

Eston, R.G., Rowlands, A.V. and Ingledew, D.K. (1998). Validity of heart rate, pedometry and accelerometry for predicting the energy cost of children's activities. *Journal of Applied Physiology* 84, 362–71.

Fehling, P.C., Smith, D.L., Warner, S.E. and Dalsky, G.P. (1999). Comparison of accelerometers with oxygen consumption in older adults during exercise. *Medicine and Science in Sports and Exercise* 31, 171–75.

Folsom, A.R., Jacobs, D.R., Casperen, C.J., Gomez-Martin, O. and Knudsen, J. (1986). Test-retest reliability of the Minnesota Leisure Time Physical Activity Questionnaire. *Journal of Chronic Diseases* 39, 505–11.

Haskell, W.L., Leon, A.S., Casperen, C.J., Froelicher, V.F., Hagberg, J.M., Harlan, W., Holloszy, J.O., Regensteiner, J.G., Thompson, P.D. and Washburn, R.A. (1992). Cardiovascular benefits and assessment of physical activity and physical fitness in adults. *Medicine and Science in Sports and Exercise* 24 (6 Suppl.), June, S201–20.

Jackson, A.S. and Pollock, M.L. (1985). Practical assessment of body composition. *Physician Sport Medicine* 13, 76–90.

Laporte, R.E., Montoye, H.J. and Caspersen, C.J. (1985). Assessment of physical activity in epidemiologic research: problems and prospects. *Public Health Reports* 100, 131–46.

Leger, L. and Lambert, J. (1982). A maximal 20 meters shuttle run test to predict $\dot{V}O_2$max. *European Journal of Applied Physiology* 49, 1–12.

Leger, L. and Gadoury, C. (1989). Validity of the 20-minute shuttle run test with one-minute stages to predict $\dot{V}O_2$max in adults. *Canadian Journal of Sports Science* 14 (1), March, 21–6.

Louie, L., Eston, R.G., Rowlands, A.V., Tong, K.K., Ingledew, D.K. and Fu, F.H. (1999). Validity of heart rate, pedometry and accelerometry for estimating the energy cost of activity in Hong Kong Chinese boys. *Pediatric Exercise Science* 11, 229–39.

McGavin, C.R., Gupta, S.P. and McHardy, G.J.R. (1976). Twelve-minute walking test for assessing disability in chronic bronchitis. *British Medical Journal* 1, 822–3.

McKenzie, T.L., Sallis, J.F. and Nader, P.R. (1991a). SOFIT: System for observing fitness instruction time. *Journal of Teaching in Physical Education* 11, 195–205.

McKenzie, T.L., Sallis, J.F., Nader, P.R., Patterson, T.L., Elder, J.P., Berry, C.C., Rupp, J.W., Atkins, C.G., Bucno, M.J. and Nelson, J.A. (1991b). BEACHES: an observational system for assessing children's physical activity behaviours and associated events. *Journal of Applied Behaviour Analysis* 24, 141–51.

Montoye, H.J., Kemper, H.C.G., Saris, W.H.M. and Washburn, R.A. (1996). *Measuring Physical Activity and Energy Expenditure*. Human Kinetics, Champaign, Ill.

O'Hara, N.M., Baranowski, T., Simons-Morton, B.G., Wilson, B.S. and Parcel, G. (1989). Validity of the observation of children's physical activity. *Research Quarterly for Exercise and Sport* 60, 42–7.

Paffenbarger, R.S., Blair, S.N., Lee, I.M. and Hyde, R.T. (1993). Measurement of physical activity to assess health effects in free-living populations. *Medicine and Science in Sports and Exercise* 25, 60–70.

Protas, E.J. (1998). Flexibility and range of motion. In: *Guidelines for Exercise Testing and Prescription* (ACSM, 2001), 3rd edn. Williams and Wilkins, Baltimore.

Puhl, J., Greaves, K., Hoyt M. and Baranowski, T. (1990). Children's activity rating scale (CARS): description and calibration. *Research Quarterly for Exercise and Sport* 61, 26–36.

Ramsbottom, R., Brewer, J. and Williams, C. (1988). A progressive shuttle run test to estimate maximal oxygen uptake. *British Journal of Sports Medicine* 22 (4), Dec., 141–4.

Rothstein, J.M., Miller, P.J. and Roettger, R.F. (1983). Goniometric reliability in a clinical setting. *Physical Therapy* 63, 1611.

Steele, B.G., Holt, L., Belza, B., Ferris, S., Lakshminaryan, S. and Buchner, D.M. (2000). Quantitating physical activity in COPD using a triaxial accelerometer. *Chest* 117, 1359–67.

Van den Berg-Emons, R.J.G., Saris, W.H.M., Westerterp, K.R. and Van Baak, M.A. (1996). Heart rate monitoring 431 to assess energy expenditure in children with reduced physical activity. *Medicine and Science in Sports and Exercise* 28, 496–501.

Wallace, J.P., Mckenzie, T.L. and Nader, P.R. (1985). Observed versus recalled exercise behaviour: a validation of a seven-day exercise recall for boys 11 to 13 years old. *Research Quarterly for Exercise and Sport* 56, 161–5.

Wareham, N.J., Hennings, S.J., Prentice, A.M. and Day, N.E. (1997). Feasibility of heart-rate monitoring to estimate total level and pattern of energy expenditure in a population-based epidemiological study: the Ely young cohort feasibility study 1994–5. *British Journal of Nutrition* 78, 889–900.

Wasserman, K., Hansen, J.E., Sue, D.Y., Whipp, B.J. and Casaburi, R. (1994). *Principles of Exercise Testing and Interpretation*, 2nd edn. Lea and Febiger, Philadelphia.

Welk, G.J. and Corbin, C.B. (1995). The validity of the Tritrac-R3D activity monitor for the assessment of physical activity in children *Research Quarterly for Exercise and Sport* **66** (3), 202–9.

Yasin, S., Alderson, M.R., Marr, J.W., Paltison, D.C. and Morris, J.N. (1967). Assessment of habitual physical activity apart from occupation. *British Journal of Preventive and Social Medicine* **21**, 163–9.

Chapter 7

GUIDELINES FOR EXERCISE PRESCRIPTION

Juliette Hussey

Key words: safety, screening, exercise prescription intensity, duration and frequency.

Introduction

This chapter discusses considerations when prescribing exercise. The prescription of exercise in the young, the elderly and those with conditions that are not discussed in other chapters in the book will also be addressed.

Safety and pre-participation screening

The risk of death during exercise is extremely slight. Vigorous exercise increases the risk of myocardial infarction and sudden death in those with heart disease (diagnosed or undiagnosed) (Thompson et al., 2003). In younger adults or children, vigorous activity may be associated with sudden death in those with a variety of congenital or acquired conditions, for example, aortic stenosis or cardiomyopathies. Atheroslerotic CAD is the main reason for exercise related deaths in adults, with an estimated incidence of 1 per 15 000–18 000. While this risk is very low it does support the recommendation that those unaccustomed to vigorous physical activity should increase physical activity levels gradually (Thompson et al., 2003). Other cardiovascular complications of vigorous physical activity are also rare, but could include cerebrovascular accidents, aortic dissection and symptomatic cardiac arrythmias (Haskell et al., 1992). Vigorous exercise involves risks which include musculoskeletal injury as well as cardiovascular complications. The risk of adverse events is reduced through screening and risk stratification procedures (Chapter 6), exercise prescription techniques and safety standards.

Appropriate pre-participation medical screening identifies those at risk either from previously undiagnosed congenital cardiac defects or those with ischaemic heart disease.

People with chronic health conditions such as heart disease or diabetes, or those at high risk for these conditions should first consult with a physician and have a full medical assessment prior to commencing an exercise programme. Men over 40 and women over 50 years of age who plan to begin a programme involving high intensity exercise should consult a physician to ascertain whether they have undiagnosed health problems. The general principles for pre-exercise testing screening would apply to those about to become involved in an exercise programme. A basic lifestyle questionnaire will give data on current levels of activity, medication, smoking habits and risk factors for CHD. The PAR-Q (Chapter 6) may also be used. Well written emergency plans for medical complications need to be formulated. Contact numbers for emergency response need to be clearly detailed and staff need to be trained in first aid and cardiopulmonary resuscitation (CPR).

Exercise prescription

Exercise prescription can be designed to: (i) improve or maintain aerobic fitness, muscle strength, body composition, flexibility, balance, coordination and proprioception, or (ii) promote health by reducing the risk factors for chronic disease. The outcome required will influence the exercise prescribed. The approach will differ and may be thought of as a hierarchy, with the lower requirements of activity necessary for health required by all. At a higher level the requirements necessary for increasing aerobic capacity will be undertaken by those with a specific interest in this outcome. It could be argued that a greater proportion of the population should have this aim, due to the evidence that higher levels of aerobic fitness are associated with lower mortality, etc. However, the greatest benefits in terms of health gain are seen when those previously sedentary engage in physical activity recommended for general health.

Both physical activity and physical fitness are associated with a reduction in coronary heart disease and all causes of mortality. Traditionally exercise prescription was based on the objective of increasing or maintaining cardiovascular fitness and was determined as exercise using the large muscle groups for 3–4 times per week for at least 20 minutes at 65–80% $\dot{V}O_2max$. With increasing evidence demonstrating that regular participation in moderate intensity physical activity is associated with health benefits even in the absence of changes in aerobic fitness the Centers for Disease Control and Prevention (CDC) and the American College of Sports Medicine (ACSM) recommended in 1995 that: 'every adult should accumulate at least 30 minutes of moderate intensity physical activity on most, preferably all, days of the week'. This general message can be applied to all for health benefits but many individuals may still need help in achieving this level of exercise in their daily lives. For improvements in aerobic fitness individualised prescription is needed.

In 1998 the ACSM produced a position stand 'The recommended quantity and quality of exercise for developing and maintaining cardiorespiratory and muscular fitness, and flexibility in healthy adults', which states:

'The combination of frequency, intensity and duration of chronic exercise has been found to be effective for producing a training effect. The interaction of these factors provide the overload stimulus. In general, the lower the stimulus the lower the training effect, and the greater the stimulus the greater the effect. As a result of specificity of training and the need for maintaining muscular strength and endurance, and flexibility of the major muscle groups, a well rounded training programme including aerobic and resistance training, and flexibility exercises is recommended. Although age in itself is not a limiting factor to exercise training, a more gradual approach in applying the prescription at older ages seems prudent. It has also been shown that aerobic endurance training of fewer than two days per week, at less than 40–50% $\dot{V}O_2R$ and for less than ten minutes is generally not a sufficient stimulus for developing and maintaining fitness in healthy adults. Even so, many health benefits from physical activity can be achieved at lower intensities of exercise if frequency and duration of training are increased appropriately. In this regard, physical activity can be accumulated through the day in shorter bouts of ten minute durations.'

The British Heart Foundation (2001) recommend that:

'. . . regular, frequent aerobic physical activity of moderate intensity is desirable. This can be achieved by regular walking, cycling or swimming for an average of 30 minutes per day on at least five days of the week. Such activity makes people feel warm and mildly out of breath. Those who are initially sedentary should start at a lower exercise level and increase this gradually in terms of duration, frequency and intensity . . .'

Many people need to be shown how they can be more active in their daily lives. These ideas need to be discussed with the individual and may include the following:

- Parking a distance away from the shop/supermarket, allowing a five minute walk from and back to the car
- Using stairs rather than lifts/escalators
- Using manual rather than power tools for gardening
- Washing the car rather than taking it to a garage
- Washing windows and doing other housekeeping activities
- Using public transport, as this will invariably result in a walk either end of the total journey
- Walking with children to and from school and after school activities
- Walking rather than taking the car for short journeys
- Going for a walk at lunchtime

In starting an achievable programme it is hoped that many, once they enjoy the health benefits of moderate activity, may then go on to become involved in a more formal exercise programme for fitness benefits.

Principles of exercise prescription for increasing and/or maintaining fitness

The principle of overload and specificity are followed in exercise prescription.

Overload: For a tissue to improve its function it must be exposed to a load to which it is not normally accustomed. Exposing the tissue to this load repeatedly, results in an adaptation that leads to increased functional capacity. The interaction of intensity, frequency and duration of exercise results in the cumulative overload required.

Specificity: The effects gained are specific to the type of exercise performed and muscles involved, for example, low resistance, high repetition exercises cause an increase in the number of mitochondria in the active muscles leading to increased muscle endurance with little change in strength, whereas heavy resistance exercises lead to increases in muscle strength.

The optimal exercise prescription is determined from $\dot{V}O_2$ measured directly or estimated. For improvements in $\dot{V}O_2$max exercise should usually involve the large muscle groups in periods of activity that are aerobic in nature, for example, walking, running, swimming, dancing, cycling, or endurance games. There is a wide range of activities which helps individual choice of preference. The prescribed amount of any type of exercise is based on intensity, duration and frequency. The ultimate goal with exercise prescription is to enable people to exercise safely, obtaining health and/or fitness benefits which they will maintain throughout their lives.

Intensity

The intensity of an exercise is the degree of difficulty experienced during the exercise.

Intensity and duration of an exercise session determine energy expenditure and are inversely related, that is, a similar kilocalorie expenditure can be obtained by a low intensity, long duration as with a high intensity, short duration. The total volume of training (kcal) is an important factor in obtaining cardiovascular fitness. The kcal concept appears to hold independently of whether the activity is continuous or performed in bouts (with ten minutes being a minimum) accumulated throughout the day. Higher intensity exercise is associated with lower adherence rates than lower intensity exercise and is associated with higher cardiovascular risk and musculoskeletal injury.

Generally, exercise should be prescribed at an intensity of between 40 and 50% to 85% of oxygen uptake reserve ($\dot{V}O_2R$) or heart rate reserve, or between 55 and 65% to 90% of maximum heart rate (ACSM, 2000). The $\dot{V}O_2R$ is the difference between $\dot{V}O_2$max and resting $\dot{V}O_2$, and heart rate reserve (HRR) is the difference between maximum heart rate and resting heart rate. The broad range of given intensities is to accomadate for all levels of baseline fitness and those with low baseline levels can increase fitness with exercise intensities of only 40–49% HRR or 55% to 64% of HRmax. Those with initial high levels of fitness would require intensities much higher in order to further increase cardiorespiratory fitness.

Heart rate is used as a guide for exercise intensity due to the relatively linear relationship between heart rate and percentage $\dot{V}O_2$max. If maximal heart rate is not measured during a progressive exercise test it may be estimated by subtracting the person's age from 220. As a method the use of percentage maximum heart rate is simple to calculate and generally the range of 70–85% of HRmax is prescribed for fitness benefits. Heart rate can be measured by heart rate monitors (see Chapter 6) or by palpation. However, during an exercise session measurement by palpation is difficult and may lead to stopping exercise in order to count heart rate. Heart rate can be affected by temperature, altitude, infection and certain medications. In patients on beta blockers the use of heart rate to guide exercise intensity would be inappropriate and other methods to prescribe intensity need consideration.

Exercise intensity can also be prescribed in terms of RPE (rating of perceived exertion). The subject can learn to rate his/her exercise intensity on a scale during a supervised exercise session and this rating of perceived exertion can be used when exercising at home. Scales such as the Borg (Chapter 6) can be used. The RPE response to graded exercise correlates highly with $\dot{V}O_2$ and HR (Dishman et al., 1987). Okura et al. (2001) found the RPE method to be a valid and useful tool in various settings of exercise prescription. Using the RPE or HR as a means of measuring intensity does facilitate easy progression of the programme because as the individual becomes 'fitter' their physiological adaptations will require them to work harder to elicit the required RPE or heart rate.

Workloads can be expressed as an estimation of oxygen uptake using METS. A MET is the unit equal to resting metabolic rate and is approximately 3.5 ml oxygen per kilo body weight. The energy requirements of specific activities have been defined and are presented in tables (Ainsworth et al., 1993). This approach to exercise prescription is easily understood and in most cases appropriate activities can be selected. It should be appreciated that individual subjects can expend different amounts of energy in specifically defined MET activities due to the vigour and skill employed.

Walking 3.5 mph, level surface = 4.0 MET
Cycling < 10 mph, general leisure to work/pleasure = 4.0 MET
Running 5 mph = 8.0 MET
Swimming, leisurely = 6.0 MET
Swimming, crawl fast = 10.0 MET

Duration

Duration and intensity together result in the energy expended in an exercise session. Thus, if a low intensity exercise is performed it will need to be done for a longer time than a high intensity exercise in order to achieve the same energy expenditure. The general health message is to accumulate 30 minutes of exercise preferably each day and this can be achieved in three accumulated bouts of ten minutes. The minimum number of days per week recommended for health benefits is four.

In subjects who have a history of very little activity or very low exercise tolerance it is best to start with as little as a few 5–10 minute bouts of exercise with rest periods between bouts and the duration of the exercise increased gradually as the subject becomes accustomed and does not demonstrate injury or excess fatigue. Short bouts of exercise may enhance exercise adherence (Jakicic et al., 1995) and in obese women it has been found that there is no difference in terms of changes in cardiorespiratory fitness when compared to long bouts.

Frequency

Health recommendations as regards frequency of activity state 'on most, but preferably every day of the week'. If the subject wants to increase his/her aerobic fitness then exercising for three to five days per week is advised. If an individual engages in a high intensity training programme then in the early stages at least two days may be needed between training sessions to allow the body to recover. In a subject who has previously been sedentary it may be advisable to begin exercising 2–3 days per week and building up from there.

FITT principles

The overall training stimulus can be described in terms of frequency (F), intensity (I), duration or time (T) and type of exercise (T). Recommended frequency (F) of exercise is usually 3–5 days per week, intensity (I) is set at 50–85% of $\dot{V}O_2$ max or 60–90% of maximal heart rate and time (T) of each exercise bout is 20–60 minutes. The type (T) of activity should be aerobic in nature, involving large muscle groups, such as walking, brisk walking, jogging, cycling or swimming. It is important to select an activity appropriate to the preferences and abilities of the individual for whom it is prescribed. The emphasis in exercise for weight loss should be on longer times, whereas the athlete will need to increase intensity for higher levels of cardiovascular fitness. The total volume of work calculated from frequency, intensity and time can be expressed in kilocalories per week.

Warm up, cool down and stretching

Both warm up and cool down should be included in any exercise session and may just commence with a few stretching exercises and gentle aerobic activity such as walking/gentle jogging if about to commence a running session. The warm up gently prepares the body for the activity about to be undertaken. Warm-up exercises cause an increase in myocardial blood flow and muscle temperature, thus preparing the body for exercise. Increasing muscle temperature improves the elasticity of the intramuscular connective tissue, which helps protect against injury. A cool down should be performed at the end of the exercise session. The last few minutes of a session should involve a reduction in intensity of the activity allowing heart rate to gradually lower. Cool down includes light exercise followed by stretching to maintain range of movement.

Muscle strengthening exercises

The principles of specificity and overload are the principles used in resistance training. Overload occurs when a greater than normal demand is placed on the muscles. Overload can be achieved by increasing the resistance or weight, increasing the repetitions, the number of sets and shortening the rest period between sets. An intensity of approximately 40–60% of 1RM is required for muscle strengthening. The one repitition maximum (1RM) test measures the greatest amount of weight that can be lifted one time for a specific weight. Usually testing begins with a weight that can be lifted with relative ease. After a 2–3 minute rest the weight to be lifted is increased. The 1RM value is the amount of weight in the last trial that can be completed successfully. For increases in muscle strength, more resistance and fewer repetitions are emphasised, in contrast to endurance, where low to moderate resistance and more repetitions is the goal. General guidelines for muscle strengthening include a warm up, performing 8–12 repetitions of each exercise throughout range of motion, increases in resistance should be made gradually with at least 48 hours between resistance training sessions.

Guidelines for exercise prescription in the elderly and children

Elderly

Regular exercise is associated with decreased mortality and morbidity in older people (Nied and Franklin, 2002), with health benefits such as a significant reduction in the risk of coronary heart disease, diabetes mellitus and insulin resistance, and hypertension (Mazzeo and Tanaka, 2001). Exercise prescription for this group should involve aerobic exercise, strength training and flexibility. The quantity of exercise prescribed depends on whether it is being prescribed for general health benefits or for improvements in fitness.

The general principles of exercise prescription hold in the elderly, but specific conditions more common in the elderly, such as osteoarthritis, may need to be taken into consideration when designing an exercise programme.

The advice of at least 30 minutes of moderate intensity exercise a day on most, and preferably all, days of the week holds. Walking is an excellent type of exercise and is convenient and inexpensive. Swimming may be particularly beneficial to those with problems with weight-bearing activity. However, gardening and housework, if performed with sufficient vigour, are activities that may contribute to the overall 30 minutes. The intensity of activity should be of a moderate intensity using a guide of the RPE scale, as many elderly may be on medication that can affect heart rate. Exercise does not need to be continuous to be of benefit and in the elderly it may be preferable to recommend three periods of ten minutes of exercise throughout the day rather than 30 minutes in one session. To minimise the risk of injury it is prudent to advise on increasing the duration of activity rather than the intensity in this age group.

Muscle strength may be increased by resistance training. Ades et al. (1996) found that participation in a resistance training programme for three months increased walking endurance and leg strength in elderly persons. As these measures are essential components of physical functioning it is vital that efforts are made to maintain them and prevent disability.

Children and adolescents

Young children are naturally quite active, given the opportunity. Their patterns of activity involve short bursts of high intensity interspersed with low intensity, rather than sustained activities. The optimum amount of physical activity for young children has not been defined but the Centre for Disease Control (CDC) and National Institute of Health (NIH) advocate that children over six years of age should accumulate at least 30 minutes of moderate intensity activity on most and preferably all days of the week. However, in young children activity through play is important and children need to be encouraged in a wide variety of activities, to promote bone formation and optimise bone mineral content (especially weight-bearing activities), skill acquisition, weight management and aerobic fitness (Figures 7.1, 7.2). In 1994 the consensus statement 'Physical activity guidelines for adolescents' (Sallis and Patrick, 1994) recommended that all adolescents

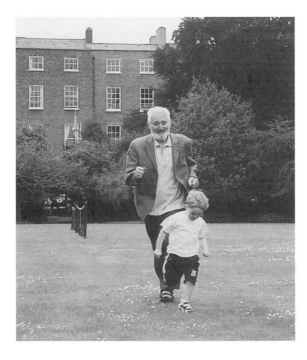

Figure 7.1 Elderly subject enjoying exercise with child.

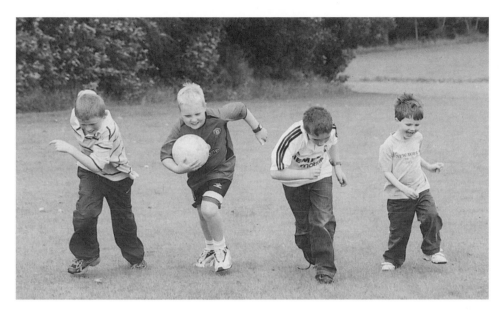

Figure 7.2 Activity through play.

should be physically active daily or nearly every day as part of their lifestyle and that they should engage in three or more sessions per week of activities that last 20 minutes or more and that require moderate to vigorous levels of exertion.

In view of increasing obesity seen in children in the last part of the twentieth century, in tandem with increasing levels of sedentary activities and less time in physical activity, it is important to establish regular activity patterns in children. The amount of time spent sedentary each day is of concern because of the relationship between the amount of time spent sedentary and body fat (Andersen et al., 1998). Time spent sedentary by children may be at the expense of unorganised spontaneous activity rather than regular activities such as swimming, ballet or rugby. These tend to be planned and timetabled in advance, whereas TV is watched at times when the child is free from school or organised activities.

An increasing prevalence of childhood obesity is evident. Current data suggests that 20% of children in the US are overweight (Goran, 2001), with the prevalence of obesity set to rise from 12.5% to 25.3% in third and fifth grade students (Morrison et al., 1999). Trends indicate that Canadian children aged between 7–13 are becoming progressively more overweight and obese (Tremblay and Willms, 2000), and data from the UK suggests that obesity exists in 9% of boys and 13% of girls. This rise in obesity brings with it an increase in obesity related diseases, as more than 60% of overweight children have at least one additional risk factor for cardiovascular disease (Freedman et al., 1999). There is evidence that tracking of activity exists from childhood to adulthood (Telema et al., 1996). Safety for children exercising should always be a primary consideration. If exercise is excessive then damage to the epiphyseal growth plates or overuse injuries can occur.

Exercise prescription for diseases/conditions not referred to elsewhere in this book

Renal disease

Patients with end stage renal disease may have cardiovascular changes, anaemia and skeletal muscle weakness which lead to poor exercise tolerance. This results in these patients becoming deconditioned and adopting a sedentary lifestyle. Modifications in coronary risk factors (improvements in aerobic capacity, blood glucose, hypertension and serum lipid levels) and beneficial effects on muscle structure and function occur with exercise training in these patients (Kouidi, 2001). Ideally exercise training should be done on non-dialysis days (Konstantinidou et al., 2002) and prescription should include measures to minimise risks to the cardiovascular and musculoskeletal systems (Copley and Lindberg, 1999). Prolonged warm up, cool down and exercise commenced at low intensity should minimise the risks.

Chronic fatigue syndrome

Chronic fatigue syndrome is also known as myalgic encephalomyelitis (ME) and involves profound fatigue in addition to symptoms of pain in the joints and muscles. There is currently no concensus on exercise prescription for these patients as exertion beyond the patient's tolerance usually results in a worsening of symptoms. However, Clapp et al. (1999) found that 30 minutes of intermittent walking (ten three-minute bouts) did not cause an exacerbation of symptoms. In the acute stages of the condition exercise may not be indicated, but as soon as the condition allows exercise with the goal of re-establishing normal function should be encouraged. Fulcher and White (1998) recommend assessing aerobic capacity in these patients by a graded incremental and continuous exercise test performed on a treadmill or cycle ergometer in two-minute stages, with the patient exercising to a symptom limited maximum or exhaustion. Contrary to the belief of many patients with this condition, testing to the point of exhaustion does not cause a lasting deterioration (Mullis et al., 1999). Exercise prescription then follows the basic principles, with most subjects able to begin at 40% of aerobic capacity or 50% of individual maximum heart rate reserve. The aim, to begin with, is to establish a regular pattern of activity, for example, walking, which may start with as little a five minutes a day. The patient needs to be reminded to pace themselves and not to do too much on days when not feeling well.

HIV

Due to advances in treatment HIV may now present as a chronic infection, with periods of the person being well, alternated with periods of illness. The needs of this patient group have therefore changed. A Cochrane review on the topic of aerobic exercise interventions for people with HIV/AIDS found that performing constant or interval aerobic exercise for at least 20 minutes three times per week for four weeks may lead to an increased CD4 count, improved cardiopulmonary fitness and improved psychological status (Nixon et al., 2001).

Cancer

Exercise has a positive effect on quality of life in patients diagnosed with cancer (Courneya et al., 2000). The general exercise prescription is moderate intensity exercise, three to five days per week of 20 to 30 minutes per session. Specific attention needs to be paid to fatigue periods during treatment, the presence of acute or chronic physical impairments due to surgery or treatment and the presence of bone cancer.

Psychological well-being

Positive effects of exercise have been documented in terms of depression, anxiety, mood state and self-esteem, both in healthy populations and those with clinical symptoms of mental health problems (Scully et al., 1998). Donaghy and Mutrie (1999) present clear evidence that exercise should be prescribed for those with alcohol problems. Studies found that exercise is a beneficial adjunct to the rehabilitation of problem drinkers, in terms of improving fitness and physical self perceptions. Three to four weeks of moderate intensity exercise of 30–40 minutes, undertaken three times per week has been found to result in the above described benefits. To develop this area and discuss the vast amount of evidence in the area of exercise and psychological well-being is beyond the scope of this book.

Learning disability

A sedentary lifestyle is seen in many adults with learning disabilities (Messent et al., 1998). Obesity is seen more often in those with sensory, physical and mental health conditions when compared to those without disabilities (Weil et al., 2002). These individuals often do not have the opportunity to engage in physical activity as they lack choice and require accompaniment in going to local leisure facilities. Physiotherapists working in this area need to address the problems of inactivity and its adverse health consequences in this population. Exercise classes and organised leisure time activities would help to address this problem.

References

Ades, P.A., Ballor, D.L., Ashikaga, T., Utton, J.L. and Nair, K.S. (1996). Weight training improves walking endurance in healthy elderly persons. *Annals of Internal Medicine* **124**, 568–72.

Ainsworth, B.E., Haskell, W.L., Leon, A.S., Jacobs, D.R., Montoye, H.J., Sallis, J.F. and Paffenbarger, R.S. (1993). Compendium of physical activities: classification of energy costs of human physical activities. *Medicine and Science in Sports and Exercise* **25**, 71–80.

American College of Sports Medicine (1998). The recommended quantity and quality of exercise for developing and maintaining cardiorespiratory and muscular fitness, and flexibility in healthy adults. *Medicine and Science in Sports and Exercise* 30, 975–91.

American College of Sports Medicine (2000). *Guidelines for Exercise Testing and Prescription*, 6th edn. Lippincott Williams and Wilkins, Philadelphia.

Andersen, R.E., Crespo, C.J., Bartlett, S.J., Cheskin, L.J. and Pratt, M. (1998). Relationship of physical activity and television watching with body weight and level of fatness among children. *Journal of American Medical Association* 279, 938–42.

British Heart Foundation (2001). www.bhf.org.uk

Clapp, L.L., Richardson, M.T., Smith, J.F., Wang, M., Clapp, A.J. and Pieroni, R.E. (1999). Acute effects of thirty minutes of light-intensity, intermittent exercise on patients with chronic fatigue syndrome. *Physical Therapy* 79, 749–56.

Copley, J.B. and Lindberg, J.S. (1999). The risks of exercise. *Advances in Renal Replacement Therapy* 6, 165–71.

Courneya, K.S., Mackey, J.R. and Jones, L.W. (2000). Coping with cancer: can exercise help? *Physican and Sports Medicine* 28 (5), 49–51.

Dishman, R.K., Patton, R.W., Smith, J., Weinberg, R. and Jackson, A. (1987). Using perceived exertion to prescribe and monitor exercise training heart rate. *International Journal of Sports Medicine* 8, 208–13.

Donaghy, M.E. and Mutrie, N. (1999). Is exercise beneficial in the treatment and rehabilitation of the problem drinker? A critical review. *Physical Therapy Reviews* 4, 153–66.

Freedman, D., Dietz, W., Srinivasan, S. and Berenson, G. (1999). The relation of overweight to cardiovascular risk factors among children and adolescents: the Bogalusa Heart Study. *Pediatrics* 103, 1175–82.

Fulcher, K.Y. and White, P.D. (1998). Chronic fatigue syndrome: a description of graded exercise treatment. *Physiotherapy* 84 (5), May, 223–6.

Goran, M.I. (2001). Metabolic precursory and effects of obesity in children: a decade of progress, 1990–1999. *American Journal of Clinical Nutrition* 73 (2), Feb., 158–71.

Haskell, W.L., Leon, A.S., Caspersen, C.J., Froelicher, V.F., Hagberg, J.M., Harlan, W., Holloszy, J.O., Regensteiner, J.G., Thompson, P.D. and Washburn, R.A. (1992). Cardiovascular benefits and assessment of physical activity and physical fitness in adults. *Medicine and Science in Sports and Exercise* 24 (6 Suppl.), June, S201–20.

Jakicic, J.M., Wing, R.R., Butler, B.A. and Robertson, R.J. (1995). Prescribing exercise in multiple short bouts versus one continuous bout: effects on adherence, cardiorespiratory fitness, and weight loss in overweight women. *International Journal of Obesity and Related Metabolic Disorders* 19, 893–901.

Konstantinidou, E., Koukonval, G., Kouidi, E., Deligiannis, A. and Tourkantonis, A. (2002). Exercise training in patients with end-stage renal disease on hemodialysis: comparison of three rehabilitation programmes. *Journal of Rehabilitation Medicine* 34 (1), Jan., 40–5.

Kouidi, E.J. (2001). Central and peripheral adaptations to physical training in patients with end-stage renal disease. *Sports Medicine* 31, 651–65.

Mazzeo, R.S. and Tanaka, H. (2001). Exercise prescription for the elderly: current recommendations. *Sports Medicine* 31 (11), 809–18.

Messent, P.R., Cookes, C.B. and Long, J. (1998). Daily physical activity in adults with mild and moderate learning disabilities: is there enough? *Disability and Rehabilitation* 20, 424–7.

Morrison, J.A., Barton, B.A., Biro, F.M., Daniels, S.R. and Sprecher, D.L. (1999). Overweight, fat patterning, and cardiovascular disease risk factors in black and white boys. *Journal of Pediatrics* 135 (4), Oct. 451–7.

Mullis, R., Campbell, I.T., Wearden, A.J., Morriss, R.K. and Pearson, D.J. (1999). Prediction of peak oxygen uptake in chronic fatigue syndrome. *British Journal of Sports Medicine* 33, 352–6.

Nied, R.J. and Franklin, B. (2002). Promoting and prescribing exercise for the elderly. *American Family Physician* 65 (3), 419–26.

Nixon, S., O'Brien, K., Glazier, R.H. and Wilkins, A.L. (2001). Aerobic exercise interventions for people with HIV/AIDS. *Cochrane Database of Systematic Reviews* 1, CD001796.

Okura, T. and Tanaka, K. (2001). A unique method for predicting cardiorespiratory fitness using rating of perceived exertion. *Journal of Physiological Anthropology and Applied Human Science* 20 (5), 255–61.

Sallis, J.F. and Patrick, K. (1994). Physical activity guidelines for adolescents: consensus statement. *Pediatric Exercise Science* 6, 302–14.

Sculley, D., Kremer, J., Meade, M.M., Graham, R. and Dudgeon, K. (1998). Physical exercise and psychological well-being: a critical review. *British Journal of Sports Medicine*, 32, 111–20.

Telema, R., Leskinen, E. and Yang, X. (1996). Stability of habitual physical activity and sports participation: a longitudinal tracking study. *Scandinavian Journal of Medicine and Science in Sports* 6, 371–8.

Thompson, P.D., Buchner, D., Pina, I.L., Balady, G.J., Williams, M.A., Marcus, B.H., Berra, K., Blair, S.N., Costa, F., Franklin, B., Fletcher, G.F., Gordon, N.F., Pate, R.R., Rodriguez, B.L., Yancey, A.K. and Wenger, N.K. (2003). *Exercise and Physical Activity in the Prevention and Treatment of Atherosclerotic Cardiovascular Disease: A Statement from the Council on Clinical Cardiology (Subcommittee on Exercise, Rehabilitation and Prevention) and the Council on Nutrition, Physical Activity, and Metabolism (Subcommittee on Physical Activity).* Circulation, 107 (24), 24 June, 3109–16.

Tremblay, M.S. and Willms, J.D. (2000). Secular trends in the body mass index of Canadian Children. *Canadian Medical Association Journal* 163, 1429–33.

Weil, E., Wachterman, M., McCarthy, E.P., Davis, R.B., O'Day, B., Iezzoni, L.I. and Wee, C.C. (2002). Obesity among adults with disabling conditions. *Journal of American Medical Association* 288, 1265–8.

Bibliography

Colangelo, R.M., Stillman, M.J., Kessier-Fogil, D. and Kessler-Hartnett, D. (1997). The role of exercise in rehabilitation for patients with end-stage renal disease. *Rehabilitation Nursing* 22, 288–92.

O'Brien, C. (1996). Exercise prescription: lessening the risk of physical activity. *Journal of Cardiovascular Risk* 3, 141–7.

US Department of Health and Human Services (1996). *Physical Activity and Health: A Report of the Surgeon General.* US Department of Health and Human Services, Centres for Disease Control and Prevention, National Centre for Chronic Disease Prevention and Health Promotion, Atlanta.

Chapter 8

EXERCISE IN PREVENTION AND TREATMENT OF CARDIOVASCULAR DISEASE

John Gormley

Key words: cardiovascular disease, coronary heart disease, prevention, cardiac rehabilitation.

Introduction

In Chapter 2 the cardiovascular responses to exercise are described in detail. The following chapter examines the effect of exercise in diseases of the cardiovascular system. Cardiovascular diseases (CVD), (coronary heart disease (CHD), cerebrovascular disease and peripheral vascular disease) accounted for 41% of all deaths in the United Kingdom in 2001 (British Heart Foundation (BHF), 2003). Diseases of this nature are recognised as one of the major health challenges in the twenty-first century. It is only relatively recently that inactivity has been accepted as an independent risk factor for coronary heart disease.

There is no doubt that exercise is underutilised as an intervention for either the prevention or treatment of CVD. The utilisation of exercise in CVD with patients following myocardial infarction and cardiac artery bypass grafting (CABG) is widely accepted. These cardiac rehabilitation programmes, however, are not available to, or taken up by, many patients despite their well researched benefits. If many patients do not receive an exercise prescription following a myocardial infarction, it is not surprising that exercise is not widely used as a preventative measure in CVD. This situation may be due to many factors, including ignorance of health professionals, lack of resources and the problems associated with adherence discussed in Chapter 13.

The purpose of this chapter is therefore to provide the reader with an overview of the beneficial effects of exercise in CVD, concentrating mainly on coronary heart disease. Furthermore, it is the contention of this chapter that there is major potential for the use of exercise as both a treatment and a preventative measure in CVD.

The benefits of exercise in positively influencing CVD risk factors are discussed, along with the benefit of exercise in other CVD.

The problem of cardiovascular disease

CVD is a major health problem in developed countries especially in Western Europe and in America. Until recently CVD was regarded as a disease of the West, but now increasing rates of CVD are becoming evident in developing countries in Asia and Eastern Europe. In the ten years from 1988 the death rate from coronary heart disease in Croatia increased by 60% (BHF, 2003). It is estimated that one in four Americans (62 million people) have some form of CVD and one in every 2.5 deaths in the United States is as a result of CVD. In America CVD has been the major cause of death in every year except 1918 since 1900 and every year it accounts for almost as many deaths as the next seven leading causes of death (American Heart Association (AHA), 2002).

In the countries of the European Union (EU) a similar picture is apparent. CVD is the major cause of mortality, accounting for 42% of all deaths (1.5 million people). For deaths occurring before the age of 65 CVD is the second main cause in the EU leading to 170 000 deaths. In men under 65 years of age CVD is the main cause of death in six countries of the EU: Austria, Finland, Greece, Sweden, Ireland and the United Kingdom.

Coronary Heart Disease (CHD) is a major problem in both the United Kingdom and Ireland. Although death rates in the countries of central and Eastern Europe are higher, the United Kingdom and Ireland, along with Finland, all have the highest death rates from coronary heart disease in developed countries. In 2001 one in four men and one in six women died from coronary heart disease, accounting for 120 000 deaths, and this was the most common cause of death. The highest mortality rates are mainly found in urban areas and are highest in Scotland and the north of England (BHF, 2003).

There are also ethnic and social differences with CVD. In the United States of America it has been found that black Americans have a considerably higher death rate compared to males (AHA, 2002). In the United Kingdom people from an Indian, Bangladeshi, Pakistani, or Sri Lankan background have a higher premature death rate from coronary heart disease compared to the average (BHF, 2003). An examination of socio-economic groups reveals that the premature death rate among male manual workers is 58% higher than male non-manual workers. In female manual workers the premature death rate is twice that of female non-manual workers.

Cardiovascular diseases

Cardiovascular diseases can be divided into three broad groups: diseases of the heart, cerebrovascular disease and peripheral vascular disease, each of which will be discussed separately.

Diseases of the heart

Coronary artery disease

Coronary artery disease is caused by narrowing of the coronary arteries that supply the myocardium. The narrowing of coronary arteries is caused by the gradual progressive formation of fatty plaques along the inner lining (intima) of the artery, known as atherosclerosis. As the plaques become bigger the lumen of the artery becomes narrower, which can eventually lead to the situation that the blood flow in the artery becomes severely restricted. When this occurs the area of the heart supplied by the narrowed artery is therefore unable to adequately perfuse an area of the heart with blood. Lack of blood results in lack of oxygen in the myocardium, supplied by the coronary artery, so the area of myocardium becomes ischaemic. Ischaemia of the heart leads to tight central chest sensation or pain, which may radiate into the left arm or sometimes the right arm. This pain, which is called angina pectoris, can also radiate into the neck, jaw or back and can be accompanied by breathlessness. It is often brought about by exercise and ceases a few minutes after stopping exercise. 'Unstable angina' is pain of the same distribution that occurs at rest. When a patient presents with chest pain it can be difficult to diagnose whether the patient is having a myocardial infarction (see below) or the pain is due to unstable angina. As the presentations of both conditions are similar and the initial management is the same, patients presenting with such symptoms are considered to have what is known as 'acute coronary syndrome'.

If the coronary artery becomes completely blocked the myocardium loses all its oxygen supply and dies. This is referred to as a myocardial infarction (MI). The complete occlusion of an artery usually happens as a result of a plaque rupturing, and material entering the blood, with the formation of a clot at a narrowed area of a coronary artery. The pain produced by myocardial infarction is similar to angina, and other symptoms include dyspnoea, cold sweat, pallor and nausea and fainting. Sometimes, however, people can have a 'silent MI' when some of the symptoms, especially pain, are not present. An MI can lead to sudden death either as a result of the infarct or more commonly as a result of ventricular fibrillation. Most of these deaths occur outside hospital.

Congestive heart failure

If heart muscle becomes severely damaged, either as a result of coronary artery disease or structural defects, it may lose the ability to pump an adequate amount of blood to meet the body's oxygen demands. If the left ventricle is affected blood backs up in the pulmonary vein, leading to the build up of blood in the pulmonary circulation, which results in dyspnoea on mild exertion and the production of frothy sputum. If the right ventricle is unable to pump adequately, excess fluid accumulates in the legs and ankles. These conditions are known as left-sided heart failure or right-sided heart failure, respectively.

Valvular heart disease

Heart valves control the flow of blood in and out of the heart. Valvular heart diseases occur when there is a problem in the functioning of one or more of the four heart valves. Stenosis of a valve occurs when a valve will not fully open, which requires the heart to pump harder. Insufficiency of a valve is when it will not close properly and blood returns back into the chamber. In this case also, the heart must pump harder in order to maintain cardiac output. Valvular heart disease can also contribute to congestive heart failure.

Cerebrovascular disease

When the arteries of the brain are affected by disease similar to coronary artery disease, this is referred to as cerebrovascular disease. At its worst blockage of one of the cerebral arteries can lead to a stroke or cerebrovascular accident (CVA). In a stroke the area of brain tissue supplied by an artery that has become occluded develops ischaemia and dies. Depending on the severity and location of the infarct a stroke can lead to a loss of speech, loss of motor or sensory control on one side, and loss of memory. Sometimes a person may suffer some of the above symptoms and appear to have had a stroke, but they resolve within 48 hours. This is referred to as a transient ischaemic attack (TIA). Not all strokes are caused by blockage of an artery. A haemorrhage from a weakened artery, often as a result of an aneurysm, can put pressure on brain tissue causing some or all of the symptoms above. As with an ischaemic stroke the severity of the symptoms depends on the size and location of the haemorrhage.

Peripheral vascular disease

Peripheral vascular disease involves the systemic arteries and veins outside the heart and brain. The most serious form of peripheral vascular disease is atherosclerosis, where the arteries in the peripheries, usually the legs, become narrowed in a mechanism similar to coronary artery disease. Patients with atherosclerosis will complain of a severe pain in their legs during exercise, progressing to pain on minimal activity or rest. This is an ischaemic pain due to the narrowing of the arteries, which are unable to supply sufficient blood to the working muscles during exercise. When the exercise is terminated the pain subsides as the oxygen demands of the working muscles decrease. This pain is referred to as intermittent claudication. In its most severe form intermittent claudication will cause a patient to waken at night with pain, and the pain is relieved by sitting on the edge of the bed, which allows gravity to restore the circulation. If the artery in a leg becomes completely occluded, and this blockage cannot be reversed through angiography or bypass surgery, then amputation of the limb above the area of occlusion is necessary.

Risk factors for cardiovascular disease

Non-modifiable risk factors

Non-modifiable risk factors are factors such as age, sex and family history. Coronary heart disease increases with age in both males and females and is more prevalent in males before the age of 60. After 60 years of age the incidence of CHD increases in females and is similar to males by approximately the age of 75. Indeed, the mortality rate from CHD is greater in women than men in the over 75 age group. A positive family history of CHD, especially in a first degree relative, leads to a greater risk to the individual.

Modifiable risk factors

Smoking

Cigarette smoking is linked to all major cardiovascular diseases and is one of the major modifiable risk factors. Evidence from the Multiple Risk Factor Intervention Trial (MRFIT), carried out on over 300 000 men, identified a relationship between the number of cigarettes smoked and the risk of death from CHD (Neaton and Wentworth, 1992). Smoking is associated with sudden death in those who were previously thought to be risk free (Escobedo and Caspersen, 1997). Smokers who continue to smoke after a myocardial infarction have a higher mortality rate than those who give up (Hermanson et al., 1988). The mechanism by which smoking affects arteries is not yet totally understood, but the acute effects of smoking include vasoconstriction and alteration in clotting of blood. Smoking may have an effect on lipoproteins, as individuals that smoke have lower levels of HDL cholesterol. The level of smoking has dropped since 1978 in England, but this decline in the rate of smoking levelled off in the 1990s. In the United Kingdom in 2001, 29% of men and 25% of women smoked (BHF, 2003).

Hyperlipidaemia

A lipid is a substance that is insoluble in water but dissolves in solvents. The two most important lipids associated with risk of CVD are cholesterol and triglyceride. Cholesterol is only found in animal cells, as plants do not manufacture cholesterol. As these two lipids are not soluble in blood they are transported around the body in combination with a protein to form a lipoprotein. There are four main types of lipoproteins the most important of which in terms of CVD are the low density lipoproteins (LDL), the very low density lipoproteins (VLDL) and the high density lipoproteins (HDL). LDL and VLDL transport cholesterol and triglyceride, respectively, around the body to the various organs of the body including the walls of arteries. It is therefore accessible to form fatty plaques in the arteries. HDL, however, transports cholesterol from the organs of the body, including blood vessels, to the liver and after it is synthesised it is excreted from the body. It is therefore no surprise that a high level of LDL and VLDL are associated with an increased risk of CVD, whereas increased levels of HDL have a protective effect on risk of CVD. A low level of HDL is an increased risk for CVD. Guidelines recommend that total cholesterol should be below 5 millimoles per litre (mmol/l) and LDL below 3 mmol/l. In patients with CVD the recommended levels of total cholesterol is < 4.5 mmol/l and LDL < 2.5 mmol/l (De Backer et al., 2003). Cholesterol levels can be altered by dietary interventions and more recently major success has been achieved with lipid lowering drugs known as statins (Scandinavain Simvastatin Survival Study, 1994). Later in this chapter the role of exercise in reducing cholesterol is discussed.

Hypertension

The pressure of blood in the arterial system is known as blood pressure. It is measured as a combination of both systolic and diastolic pressures. The systolic pressure, which is the maximum pressure, occurs when the left ventricle expels blood into the aorta. The diastolic pressure is the pressure that occurs when the ventricle is filling. The normal blood pressure is usually 120 mmHg for the systolic and 80 mmHg for the diastolic pressure. Individuals with blood pressure above 140 mmHg systolic and 90 mmHg diastolic are considered to have elevated blood pressure, also known as hypertension. The European guidelines on cardiovascular disease state that individuals with a high cardiovascular disease profile accompanied by systolic blood pressures above 140 mmHg and/or diastolic blood pressure above 90 mmHg require therapy to lower their blood pressure (De Backer et al., 2003).

For much hypertension there is no known cause, but it is a risk factor for coronary heart disease and stroke (MacMahon et al., 1990). A reduction in blood pressure, through pharmaceutical means, can result in a reduced risk of stroke and myocardial infarction (Collins et al., 1990). Indeed a 6 mm reduction in diastolic blood pressure can result in a risk reduction of stroke of 42% (Collins et al., 1990).

Obesity and diabetes

Obesity and diabetes are covered in detail in Chapter 7. Obesity is associated with an increased risk of coronary heart disease and stroke and was designated by the American Heart Association as a major modifiable risk factor for CHD in 1998. Obesity as an adolescent leads to a greater risk of coronary artery disease in later life (Must et al., 1992). Obesity is linked to other risk factors, for example, hypertension, diabetes, hyperlipidaemia and inactivity. Loss of weight with reduction in percentage body fat can have positive effects on hypertension, lipid profile and diabetes.

Both type 1 and type 2 diabetes lead to an increased risk of all the main types of CVD. CHD and stroke are the major causes of death among patients with diabetes. Kannel and McGee (1979) found that diabetes doubled the risk of CVD in men and tripled the risk in women. The presence of one or more other risk factors in an individual with diabetes leads to a greater risk of CVD.

Inactivity

Lack of physical activity is now recognised as an independent risk factor for CVD. There is, however, a major problem, especially in developed countries, with the lack of physical activity in the population. In the USA only 15% of the population partake in vigorous activity for 20 minutes, three times per week and 25% reported no activity (US Surgeon General, 2002). In the UK only 37% of men and 25% of women exercise for 30 minutes five times per week (BHF 2003). The problem is not only confined to adults, but there is increasing alarm at the lack of physical activity in children. One of the earliest studies to identify a link between activity and risk of CHD was carried out on bus workers in London in 1966. It was found that bus conductors who had to walk up and down double-decker buses suffered less severe myocardial infarctions and had a lower risk of CHD than the bus drivers. (Morris et al., 1966). Studies carried out on other occupational groups have shown similar results.

Not surprisingly, physical fitness can have an effect on cardiovascular disease risk. An inverse relationship between physical fitness and risk of CVD was identified in 17 000 US college alumni who were followed for up to 16 years (Paffenbarger et al., 1978). A study by Blair et al. (1989) examined physical fitness in 13 000 males and females over an eight-year period. The results of the study demonstrated that a moderate amount of exercise reduced the risk of death from CVD. There was three-fold increase in the risk of death from CVD in middle-aged men who had a leisure time energy expenditure of 800 Kcal per week, compared to those who had a leisure time energy expenditure of 2100 Kcal per week. In a more recent study by Kavanagh et al. (2002) exercise capacity as measured by $\dot{V}O_2$peak was found to be a powerful predictor of cardiac and all-cause mortality in men.

Physical activity must be current, as the 'protective' effect of exercise on CVD disappears quickly if exercise is ceased. Previous activity does not confer protection from risk of CVD. Morris et al. (1980) found the risk of a fatal MI was three times higher among sedentary men compared to men participating in vigorous sports. Those men who had participated in vigorous exercise many years previously and had since ceased had the same levels of mortality from MIs as the sedentary men.

The mechanisms by which exercise can have a preventative effect on CVD risk are becoming clearer. Regular exercise can lead to an increased efficiency of muscle to extract oxygen from circulating blood leading to a decreased demand on the heart at any given workload. There are blood volume changes, changes in blood pressure and heart rate at rest and during exercise and changes in heart muscle and vasculature. The reader is referred to Chapter 2 for a detailed discussion of these mechanisms.

Exercise as a preventative measure for cardiovascular disease

The use of exercise as a preventative treatment in CVD was recognised as far back as 1768. The physician who first recognised angina, Heberden, noted that one of his patients received major relief of his symptoms by sawing wood for half an hour each day (Coats et al., 1995). It is, however, only in recent years that the use of exercise as a preventative measure for CVD has been recognised. Aerobic exercise has a positive influence on CVD risk factors. In this section of the chapter the preventative effects of exercise on hyperlipidaemia and hypertension are discussed. The beneficial effects of exercise in diabetes and obesity are presented in Chapter 5 and 11.

Hyperlipidaemia

Exercise can favourably alter blood lipid profiles. Cullinane et al. (1982) found an acute effect of exercise on triglyceride levels in both trained cyclists and sedentary men after exercise, which was maintained for 48 hours. The main effect on lipid profile is, however, an increase in HDL without necessarily altering LDL. A reduction in triglyceride concentrations is also found. The level of exercise necessary to achieve positive effects does not necessarily have to be high intensity, as moderate levels of exercise may be sufficient to bring about an increase in high density lipoproteins (Durstine et al., 2001). When exercise is combined with weight loss or dietary interventions, low density lipoproteins may also be affected (Tran et al., 1985; Stefanick et al., 1998; Lalonde et al., 2002).

Hypertension

There is strong evidence to suggest that regular exercise can lower blood pressure. Low levels of physical activity or fitness would appear to increase the risk of hypertension in the future (Paffenbarger et al., 1983; Blair et al., 1984). In a recent study in Japan, Hayashi et al. (1999) examined physical activity levels in over 6000 men aged between 35 to 60 years who had normal blood pressure. The men were followed up over ten years and cases of hypertension identified. It was found that activity, especially the duration of the walk to work, decreased the risk of hypertension. There have been numerous intervention studies examining the effect of exercise on blood pressure. These studies have varied in the duration, frequency and intensities of exercise and some have used resistance training as opposed to the majority that have examined aerobic training. A number of meta-analyses have been carried out to determine an overall effect. Fagard (1993) reviewed 36 trials and found a significant decrease of 5.3 mmHg and 4.8 mmHg in systolic and diastolic blood pressures, respectively. The greatest reductions were found in those with hypertension (> 140/90 mmHg) of −10 mmHg (systolic) and −8 mmHg (diastolic). Halbert et al. (1997) used stricter criteria and only examined randomised controlled trials. Aerobic exercise was found to reduce systolic pressure by 4.7 mmHg and diastolic pressure by 3.1 mmHg.

Exercise in the treatment of myocardial infarction (cardiac rehabilitation)

Cardiac rehabilitation has been defined as:

> 'the sum of activity required to ensure cardiac patients the best possible physical, mental and social conditions so that they may by their own efforts regain as normal as possible a place in community and lead a normal life.' (World Health Organization, 1993)

More recently the Scottish Intercollegiate Guidelines Network (SIGN) and the British Association of Cardiac Rehabilitation (BACR) defined cardiac rehabilitation as:

> 'the process by which patients with cardiac disease, in partnership with a multi-disciplinary team of health professionals, are encouraged and supported to achieve and maintain optimial physical and psychological health.' (SIGN/BACR, 2002)

Exercise is an integral part of most cardiac rehabilitation programmes and the aim is to promote the uptake and maintenance of exercise as part of a healthier lifestyle. For cardiac rehabilitation to be effective patients must continue to exercise after the organised 6–8 week outpatient programme is completed.

Exercise for the treatment of patients following an MI is relatively new and has only become accepted as an effective form of therapy in the last 25 years. Up to the 1960s the standard treatment for a patient following an MI was prolonged bed rest in order to allow the injured part of the myocardium to recover sufficiently. The length of time that a patient spent in bed could be up to four weeks, followed by a month of gradual and careful convalescence (Coats et al., 1995). Bed rest meant bed rest: patients were often fed and washed by nurses, and bedpans were used for toileting. This is despite the fact that using a bedpan required more energy expenditure than using a commode at the bedside. (Benton et al., 1950).

In the USA a move away from this strict regime was reported by Levine and Lown in 1952. They described the benefit of getting patients up out of bed and sitting in a chair within two days, walking at the end of the third week and sending patients home after four weeks. Some of the earliest rehabilitation programmes were commenced by Kellerman (1967) and Gottheiner (1968) in Israel, and in the US by Hellerstein and Ford in the 1950s. Early mobilisation of cardiac patients gradually became more accepted, leading to a much shorter stay in hospital for the patient. Aerobic exercises to improve cardiovascular fitness were offered to patients on an outpatient basis providing the genesis of today's cardiac rehabilitation.

Over the years cardiac rehabilitation programmes have expanded from pure exercise programmes to become multifaceted interventions aimed at educating the patient, modifying risk factors and stress management. In the UK there has been a gradual increase in the number of cardiac rehabilitation programmes from 9 in 1970 (Groden et al., 1971) to 90 in 1989 (Horgan et al., 1992). A programme multiplying initiative was launched by the British Heart Foundation in 1989 and was, in part at least, responsible for the increase in programmes to 186 in 1992. In 1997 a total of 273 programmes were identified (Lewin et al., 1998) rising to 300 programmes in 1998 (Bethell et al., 2001). In a meta-analysis of data of over 8000 patients, exercise-based cardiac rehabilitation programmes were found to reduce all cause mortality by 27% and mortality attributed to cardiac disease by 31% (Jolliffe et al., 2002). Cardiac rehabilitation programmes are nowadays recommended for the rehabilitation of patients following cardiac surgery and cardiac revascularisation, stable angina and stable chronic heart failure as well as patients post-MI (SIGN/BACR, 2002). For patients with these conditions, modifications to a programme may be necessary but the basic principles are the same. Cardiac rehabilitation can be divided into four distinct phases each of which have exercise as their core.

Phase I covers the period from admission to the hospital to their discharge from hospital. Depending on the severity of the MI the duration of phase I may vary from between five to seven days in the case of a small, uncomplicated MI to a number of weeks with a more complicated larger MI. Although the level of exercise that can be safely achieved by a patient is limited it is important that the exercise is gradually introduced to the patient during their inpatient stay, provided there are no contraindications to exercise, for example, unstable angina.

After the first 48 hours the patient will be sitting out of bed and exercise can commence, mainly based on walking short distances in the ward 2–3 times daily. As with all exercise prescription the progress should be gradual and the activity should be approximately 2–3 metabolic equivalents (METs) (see Chapter 7), which means the pace of walking is slow. In preparation for discharge stairs should be climbed towards the end of phase I. The patient is shown how to take their own pulse so that they can monitor their own heart rate during exercise. The heart rate during exercise should be about resting heart rate + 20 beats/minute (bpm) (Coats et al., 1995). A sub-maximal exercise test can also be performed at this stage, which is useful for prescribing exercise at home. If possible, the rating of perceived exertion (RPE) (Chapter 6) should be introduced to the patient at this point especially those who are on drugs that alter the heart rate response to exercise, for example, beta blockers.

Phase II is the period from discharge to the start of the formalised outpatient programme. This is usually a period of 4–6 weeks and during this time the patient may attend programmes which aim to educate the patient about coronary heart disease and to modify risk factors, for example, smoking, diet, etc. Prior to discharge the patient will have been given clear written instructions on exercise to be taken during this period at home. The mode of exercise prescribed is usually walking on level ground for short periods initially. The length of walk can be increased gradually up to approximately two miles by the end of phase II. The intensity of exercise will commence at a slow pace and be gradually increased to an intensity of 4 METs, which is equivalent to walking at a fast pace. The patient should not exceed 20 bpm above their resting heart rate or 11–12 on the RPE (Coats et al., 1995). If the exercise brings on symptoms or excessive fatigue the patient should slow down. At least two weeks after the MI the patient is usually requested to return to the hospital for a symptom limited exercise test.

Exercise test

The aim of this test is to assess the intensity of exercise that a patient can perform without symptoms. The test is used as a diagnostic and prognostic tool and therefore provides information that is essential for the accurate prescription of exercise. The test has traditionally been carried out either using either a treadmill or a cycle ergometer with monitoring of ECG, heart rate and blood pressure. Recently it has been recommended that for uncomplicated patients risk stratification by history, examination and resting ECG, in conjunction with a functional capacity test (for example, shuttle walking test or six-minute walking test), is sufficient assessment before exercise training (SIGN/BACR, 2002). Details of these tests are given in Chapter 9. As testing by the more traditional methods is still common and is indicated in more complicated patients the exercise testing will concentrate on these methods.

There are advantages and disadvantages in using treadmills and bicycle ergometers, so the choice may depend on individual preferences of the staff carrying out the test. Treadmills are noisy, therefore making blood pressure monitoring difficult and patients are sometimes fearful and therefore need to hold on to handrails, which means that estimation of exercise capacity may not be accurate (McConnell et al., 1996). However, they do mimic the exercise that patients are most familiar with, that is, walking. Cycle ergometers are quiet, patients may feel more secure as they can stop at any time, and allow the easy measurement of blood pressure. The main disadvantage is that the patient's body weight is supported and it may be more preferable to exercise test a patient in a situation that more closely resembles everyday life.

The exercise test is an incremental test, that is, the difficulty of the test is increased in steady stages until the patient reaches a maximum. Examples of different protocols for treadmill testing are given in Chapter 6. Measurements are taken of heart rate, blood pressure and maximal oxygen uptake (usually calculated by the increment reached on the test or infrequently by direct gas analysis). The rating of perceived exertion (RPE) (Borg, 1982) is also assessed as heart rate may not truly reflect the patient's exertions and because many patients may be on medication that lowers heart rate response to exercise.

Termination of the test may occur due to the achievement of physiological end points, for example, maximum heart rate (220 bpm − age in years for males, in the case of a maximal test, or more usually 85% of maximum heart rate for a submaximal test). If there is a drop of greater than 10 mmHg in systolic pressure accompanied by other signs of ischaemia the test should also be terminated (Gibbons et al., 1997). ECG evidence of ventricular tachycardia or other significant arrhythmias or an ST segment depression of 2 mm can also indicate termination of the test (Coats et al., 1995). Patient fatigue, or a desire on the part of the patient to stop the test are further indications for termination. If signs of cyanosis or pallor, or symptoms of moderate to severe angina, wheezing, leg cramps or claudication pain become apparent the test should be stopped (Gibbons et al., 1997). Other reasons for stopping the test include a blood pressure response exceeding 250 mmHg systolic and/or 115 mmHg diastolic.

The exercise test allows the prescribed intensity of exercise to be calculated. The $\dot{V}O_2$max can be used to prescribe exercise in terms of METs. At its simplest a patient could have achieved a $\dot{V}O_2$max of 10 METs so an exercise prescription of 60–80% $\dot{V}O_2$max would equate to activities in the 6–8 MET region. Heart rate is often used to prescribe exercise and is the more usual method with cardiac patients. There are three ways of using heart rate. First, heart rate can be plotted against $\dot{V}O_2$max and the appropriate training range between two levels of heart beat extrapolated. This is useful when the patient is taking medication that alters the exercise heart rate response (ACSM, 2000). The second method is based on the the fact that 60–75% of maximum heart rate equates to 40 to 60% of an individuals $\dot{V}O_2$max. The training heart rate is simply calculated by taking 60% and 75% of the maximum heart rate. The final method is to use the Heart Rate Reserve (Karvonen, 1957). Resting heart rate is subtracted from the maximal heart rate to give the heart rate reserve. If the required exercise intensity is 60 to 80% $\dot{V}O_2$max then 60% and 80% of the heart rate reserve are calculated. Resting heart rate is added to each of the values to give the training heart rates.

Phase III

Phase III is the period of exercise-based outpatient rehabilitation which lasts for 8–12 weeks. An educational programme is often carried out during this stage in conjunction with the exercise programme. The frequency of attendance usually varies between 2–3 times per week, but this can vary between programmes. The aims of this phase are for the patient to exercise safely and symptom free, to be aware of their own limitations and to understand the benefits of exercise in coronary heart disease (Coates et al., 1995). The training heart rate is set at 60–75% HRmax, which is 12–13 on the RPE scale (Taylor et al., 2002). An exercise class will usually consist of 8–10 patients of similar functional capacities, exercising together. The number of patients in a group can vary depending on the severity of their disease, the limitation of functional capacity and the number of trained staff available. Guidelines on the ratio of instructors to patients vary across countries. The Chartered Society of Physiotherapy recommends a ratio of not more than 1:5, whereas Australian guidelines recommend a ratio not greater than 1:10.

As with any exercise there is a warm up for 15 minutes at the start of the class. For patients with cardiac disease this is especially important as a gradual warm up prevents the development of cardiac ischaemia or arrhythmias. (Coats et al., 1995). It is recommended that the patient should be within 20 bpm of their prescribed heart rate at the end of the warm up (Taylor et al., 2002). Following a warm up the actual aerobic exercise regime commences. For many years this part of the class consisted almost exclusively of aerobic type activities, for example, step-ups, cycling or rowing. Although these type of activities are still used, resistance exercises are becoming more popular. Resistance training is only recommended for low to moderate risk cardiac patients and furthermore it is recommended that patients spend some time on aerobic exercises until they become used to monitoring their exercise intensity (SIGN/BACR, 2002). The class is usually organised as circuit training, where the patient exercises at one station, for example, treadmill and then moves on to the next, for example, bicycle. The number of stations used will depend on the availability of equipment and the number of patients in the class. The aerobic exercise programme lasts for approximately 20–30 minutes and resistance training can follow the aerobic programme if appropriate. When the exercise regime has been completed patients carry out a cool down. After the cool down 10–15 minutes should be allowed for relaxation. It is recommended that patients exercise to their prescribed exercise intensity on the days of the week that there is no formal exercise class.

Safety of the patients is of the utmost importance during the exercise class. Blood pressure should be monitored prior to commencing the warm up and again when the cool down is completed. Heart rate can be monitored in a number of ways. The patient can take their own pulse but this can be difficult while exercising, so it is more usual to wear a heart rate monitor. If necessary the heart rate monitor can be linked by telemetry to a central screen where staff can monitor the heart rate response of the patients. The need for heart rate monitors becomes less as the patients become used to the RPE scale. In terms of life support training for low to moderate risk patients staff should be able to determine when patients are in distress and all should be trained in basic life support and have the knowledge and the ability to use a defibrillator (SIGN/BACR, 2002). An onsite resuscitation team should be available.

Phase IV

The BACR recommends that for patients to be discharged to Phase IV they should be clinically stable, able to regulate their own exercise and have a minimum capacity of 5 METs (Coats et al., 1995). Phase IV of cardiac rehabilitation is when the patient leaves the structured programme and maintains exercise and lifestyle modifications indefinitely. Most of the emphasis in the last twenty years has been on promoting phase III programmes, probably to the detriment of phase IV. Despite the fact that there are some phase IV exercise programmes, secondary prevention clinics and self-help groups (SIGN/BACR, 2002) there is often little choice for the patient except to exercise alone. The maintenance of exercise beyond the supervised setting is one of the essential components of cardiac rehabilitation. It is therefore important that measures to support patients in phase IV are addressed.

Exercise in the treatment of other cardiovascular disease

In Chapter 12 the effect of exercise in cerobrovascular disease is discussed. In peripheral vascular disease intervention studies have found a significant benefit from exercise. Intermittent claudication is ischaemic pain in the legs and is common in patients with peripheral vascular disease. It will limit the distance that can be walked and can also cause pain in bed. The effect of exercise programmes on intermittent claudication has been investigated in many trials, but most were hampered by a limited number of results. A meta-analysis of ten randomised controlled trials found that programmes of at least twice weekly exercise intervention, for at least twelve weeks, significantly increased walking time compared to controls (Leng et al., 2004). The walking time was assessed by treadmill testing in all studies and was the time at which the onset of claudication appeared. The overall improvement in walking ability was 150%. The results of the meta-analysis demonstrates the positive effect of exercise in peripheral vascular disease.

Exercise has positive effects in CVD. It is now an integral part of the treatment of patients post-MI and is indicated in heart failure, revascularisation procedures and post-cardiac surgery. To be effective exercise has to be maintained over a lifetime. Adherence therefore becomes an issue and this is discussed in Chapter 13.

References

American Heart Association (2002). *Heart Disease and Stroke-2003 Update*. American Heart Association, Dallas, Texas.

Benton, J.G., Brown, H. and Rusk, H.A. (1950). Energy expended by patients on the bedpan and bedside commode. *Journal of American Medical Association* 44, 1443–7.

Bethell, H.J., Turner, S.C., Evans, J.A. and Rose, L. (2001). Cardiac rehabilitation in the United Kingdom. How complete is the provision? *Journal of Cardiopulmonary Rehabilitation* 21 (2), March–April, 111–5.

Blair, S.N., Goodyear, N.N., Gibbons, L.W. and Cooper, K.H. (1984). Physical fitness and incidence of hypertension in healthy normotensive men and women. *Journal of American Medical Association* 252 (4), 27 July, 487–90.

Blair, S.N., Kohl, H.W. 3rd, Paffenbarger, R.S. Jr., Clark, D.G., Cooper, K.H. and Gibbons, L.W. (1989). Physical fitness and all-cause mortality. A prospective study of healthy men and women. *Journal of American Medical Association* 262 (17), 3 Nov. 2395 401.

Borg, G. (1982). The psychophysical bases of perceived exertion. *Medicine and Science in Sports and Exercise* 14, 377–81.

British Heart Foundation (2003). *Coronary Heart Disease Statistics*. British Heart Foundation Health Promotion Research Group, University of Oxford, Oxford.

Chartered Society of Physiotherapy (CSP) (1999). *Standards for the Exercise Component of Phase III Cardiac Rehabilitation*. Chartered Society of Physiotherapy, London.

Coats, A., McGee, H. Stokes, H. and Thompson, D. (1995). BACR *Guidelines for Cardiac Rehabilitation*. Blackwell Science, Oxford.

Collins, R., Peto, R., MacMahon, S., Hebert, P., Fiebach, N.H., Eberlein, K.A., Godwin, J., Qizilbash, N., Taylor, J.O. and Hennekens, C.H. (1990). Blood pressure, stroke and coronary heart disease. Part 2, Short-term reductions in blood pressure: overview of randomised drug trials in their epidemiological context. *Lancet* 335 (8693), 7 April, 827–38.

Cullinane, E., Siconolfi, S., Saritelli, A. and Thompson, P.D. (1982). Acute decrease in serum triglycerides with exercise: is there a threshold for an exercise effect? *Metabolism* 31 (8), Aug., 844–7.

De Backer, G., Ambrosioni, E., Borch-Johnsen, K., Brotons. C., Cifkova, R., Dallongeville, J., Ebrahim, S., Faergeman, O., Graham, I., Mancia, G., Manger Cats, V., Orth-Gomer, K., Perk, J., Pyorala, K., Rodicio, J.L., Sans, S., Sansoy, V., Sechtem, U., Silber, S., Thomsen, T. and Wood, D. (2003). Third joint task force of European and other societies on cardiovascular disease prevention in clinical practice. European guidelines on cardiovascular disease prevention in clinical practice. *European Heart Journal* 24 (17), Sep., 1601–10.

Durstine, J.L., Grandjean, P.W., Davis, P.G., Ferguson, M.A., Alderson, N.L. and DuBose, K.D. (2001). Blood lipid and lipoprotein adaptations to exercise: a quantitative analysis. *Sports Medicine* 31 (15), 1033–62.

Escobedo, L.G. and Caspersen C.J. (1997). Risk factors for sudden coronary death in the United States. *Epidemiology.* **8** (2), March, 175–80.

Fagard, R.H. (1993). Physical fitness and blood pressure. *Journal of Hypertension* **11**, (Suppl. 5), Dec., S47–52.

Gibbons, R.J., Balady, G.J., Beasley, J.W., Bricker, J.T., Duvernoy, W.F., Froelicher, V.F., Mark, D.B., Marwick, T.H., McCallister, B.D., Thompson, P.D., Winters, W.L. Jr., Yanowitz, F.G., Ritchie, J.L., Cheitlin, M.D., Eagle, K.A., Gardner, T.J., Garson, A. Jr., Lewis, R.P., O'Rourke, R.A. and Ryan, T.J. (1997) *ACC/AHA Guidelines for Exercise Testing: Executive Summary. A report of the American College of Cardiology/American Heart Association Task Force on Practice Guidelines (Committee on Exercise Testing).* Circulation **96** (1), 1 July, 345–54.

Gottheiner, V. (1968). Long-range strenuous sports training for cardiac reconditioning and rehabilitation. *American Journal Cardiology* **22** (3), Sep., 426–35.

Groden, B.M., Semple, T. and Shaw, G.B. (1971). Cardiac rehabilitation in Britain (1970). *British Heart Journal* **33** (5), Sep., 756–8.

Hayashi, T., Tsumura, K., Suematsu, C., Okada, K., Fujii, S. and Endo, G. (1999). Walking to work and the risk for hypertension in men: the Osaka Health Survey. *Annals of Internal Medicine* **131** (1), 6 July, 21–6.

Hellerstein, H.K. and Ford, A.B. (1957). Rehabilitation of the cardiac patient. *Journal of American Medical Association* **164** (3), 18 May, 225–31.

Hermanson, B., Omenn, G.S., Kronmal, R.A. and Gersh, B.J. (1988). Beneficial six-year outcome of smoking cessation in older men and women with coronary artery disease. Results from the CASS registry. *New England Journal of Medicine* **319** (21), 24 Nov., 1365–9.

Horgan, J., Bethell, H., Carson, P., Davidson, C., Julian, D., Mayou, R.A. and Nagle, R. (1992). Working party report on cardiac rehabilitation. *British Heart Journal* **67** (5), May, 412–8.

Jolliffe, J.A., Rees, K., Taylor, R.S., Thompson, D., Oldridge, N. and Ebrahim, S. (2002). Exercise-based rehabilitation for coronary heart disease (Cochrane Review). In: *The Cochrane Library*, **1**. John Wiley and Sons, Ltd, Chichester.

Kannel, W.B. and McGee, D.L. (1979). Diabetes and cardiovascular disease. The Framingham study. *Journal of American Medical Association* **241** (19), 11 May, 2035–8.

Karvonen, M.J., Kentala, E. and Mustala, O. (1957). The effects of training on heart rate; a longitudinal study. *Annales Medicinale Experimentalis et Biologiale Fenniale* **35** (3), 307–15.

Kavanagh, T., Mertens, D.J., Hamm, L.F., Beyene, J., Kennedy, J., Corey, P. and Shephard, R.J. (2002). Prediction of long-term prognosis in 12 169 men referred for cardiac rehabilitation. *Circulation* **106** (6), 6 Aug., 666–71.

Kellermann, J.J., Levy, M., Feldman, S. and Kariv, I. (1967). Rehabilitation of coronary patients. *Journal of Chronic Diseases* **20** (10), Oct. 815–21.

Lalonde, L., Gray-Donald, K., Lowensteyn, I., Marchand, S., Dorais, M., Michaels, G., Llewellyn-Thomas, H.A., O'Connor, A. and Grover, S.A. (2002). Canadian Collaborative Cardiac Assessment Group. Comparing the benefits of diet and exercise in the treatment of dyslipidemia. *Preventive Medicine* **35** (1), July, 16–24.

Leng, G.C., Fowler, B. and Ernst, E. (2004). Exercise for intermittent claudication (Cochrane Review). In: *The Cochrane Library*, **1**. John Wiley and Sons, Ltd Chichester.

Levine, S.A. and Lown, B. (1952). 'Armchair' treatment of acute coronary thrombosis. *Journal of American Medical Association* **148** (16), 19 April, 1365–9.

Lewin, R.J., Ingleton, R., Newens, A.J. and Thompson, D.R. (1998). Adherence to cardiac rehabilitation guidelines: a survey of rehabilitation programmes in the United Kingdom. *British Medical Journal* 316 (7141), 2 May, 1354–5.

McConnell, T.R. and Clarke P.A. (1996). Exercise prescription: when the guidelines do not work. *Journal of Cardiopulmonary Rehabilitation* 16 (1), 34–37.

MacMahon, S., Peto, R., Cutler, J., Collins, R., Sorlie, P., Neaton, J., Abbott, R., Godwin, J., Dyer, A. and Stamler, J. (1990). Blood pressure, stroke and coronary heart disease. Part 1, Prolonged differences in blood pressure: prospective observational studies corrected for the regression dilution bias. *Lancet* 335 (8692), 31 March, 765–74.

Morris, J.N., Kagan, A., Pattison, D.C. and Gardner, M.J. (1966). Incidence and prediction of ischaemic heart disease in London busmen. *Lancet* 2 (7463), 10 Sep., 553–9.

Morris, J.N., Everitt. M.G., Pollard, R., Chave, S.P. and Semmence, A.M. (1980). Vigorous exercise in leisure-time: protection against coronary heart disease. *Lancet* 2 (8206), 6 Dec., 1207–10.

Must, A., Jacques, P.F., Dallal, G.E., Bajema, C.J. and Dietz, W.H. (1992). Long-term morbidity and mortality of overweight adolescents. A follow-up of the Harvard Growth Study of 1922 to 1935. *New England Journal of Medicine* 327 (19), 5 Nov., 1350–5.

Neaton, J.D. and Wentworth, D. (1992). Serum cholesterol, blood pressure, cigarette smoking, and death from coronary heart disease. Overall findings and differences by age for 316 099 white men. Multiple Risk Factor Intervention Trial Research Group. *Archives of Internal Medicine* 152 (1), Jan., 56–64.

Paffenbarger, R.S. Jr., Wing, A.L. and Hyde, R.T. (1978). Physical activity as an index of heart attack risk in college alumni. *American Journal Epidemiology* 108 (3), Sep., 161–75.

Paffenbarger, R.S. Jr., Wing, A.L., Hyde, R.T. and Jung, D.L. (1983). Physical activity and incidence of hypertension in college alumni. *American Journal Epidemiology* 117 (3), March, 245–57.

Scandinavain Simvastatin Survival Study 1994 (1994). Randomised trial of cholesterol lowering in 4444 patients with coronary heart disease: the Scandinavian Simvastatin Survival Study (4S) *Lancet* 344 (8934), 19 Nov., 1383–9.

Scottish Intercollegiate Guidelines Network (SIGN) (2002). *Cardiac Rehabilitation: A National Clinical Guideline*. Scottish Intercollegiate Guidelines Network Edinburgh. Endorsed by the British Association for Cardiac Rehabilitation (BACR).

Stefanick, M.L., Mackey, S., Sheehan, M., Ellsworth, N., Haskell, W.L. and Wood, P.D. (1998). Effects of diet and exercise in men and post-menopausal women with low levels of HDL cholesterol and high levels of LDL cholesterol. *New England Journal of Medicine* 339 (1), 2 July, 12–20.

Taylor, A., Bell, J., Lough, F. (2002). Cardiac rehabilitation. In: *Physiotherapy for Respiratory and Cardiac Problems* (Pryor, J.A. and Prasad, S.M. eds), 3rd edn. Churchill Livingstone, Edinburgh.

Tran, Z.V. and Weltman, A. (1985). Differential effects of exercise on serum lipid and lipoprotein levels seen with changes in body weight. A meta-analysis. *Journal of American Medical Association* 254 (7), 16 Aug. 919–24.

World Health Organization Expert Committee (1993). *Rehabilitation after Cardiovascular Disease with Special Emphasis on Developing Countries*. Technical report series 831. World Health Organization, Geneva.

Bibliography

American College of Sports Medicine (2000). *Guidelines for Exercise Testing and Prescription*, 6th ed. Lippincott Willaims and Wilkins, Baltimore.

Goble, A.J. and Worcester, M.U.C. (1999). *Best Practice Guidelines for Cardiac Rehabilitation and Secondary Prevention*. Heart Research Centre. Melbourne (on behalf of Department of Human Services Victoria).

Halbert, J.A., Silagy, C.A., Finucane, P., Withers, R.T., Hamdorf, P.A. and Andrews, G.R. (1997). The effectiveness of exercise training in lowering blood pressure: a meta-analysis of randomised controlled trials of four weeks or longer. *Journal of Human Hypertension* **11** (10), Oct., 641–9.

US Surgeon General (1996). *Physical Activity and Health: A Report of the Surgeon General*. Department of Health and Human Services, Centers for Disease Control and Prevention, National Center for Chronic Disease Prevention and Health Promotion, and The President's Council on Physical Fitness and Sports Atlanta, Ga.

Chapter 9

EXERCISE IN THE TREATMENT OF RESPIRATORY DISEASE

Brenda O'Neill, Judy M. Bradley and Fidelma Moran

Key words: respiratory disease, exercise testing and training, exercise prescription.

Introduction

This chapter concentrates on exercise in the treatment of patients with respiratory disease. The first part provides a descriptive overview of the abnormal responses to exercise in patients with respiratory disease. The second part summarises the results of Cochrane reviews undertaken to evaluate the evidence for exercise training in respiratory conditions. The third part describes exercise testing in respiratory disease and briefly summarises other outcome measures used in the evaluation of exercise training for respiratory conditions. The final section considers the general principles of exercise training and prescription in respiratory disease.

The most common respiratory diseases are summarised in Box 9.1 and the pathophysiological processes involved in these diseases are detailed in other texts. The clinical symptoms of these respiratory diseases are outlined in Box 9.2.

The abnormal responses to exercise in patients with respiratory disease

Often patients with respiratory disease do not achieve their $\dot{V}O_2max$; consequently the term $\dot{V}O_2peak$ may be preferred to $\dot{V}O_2max$ for this group of patients. $\dot{V}O_2peak$ is the highest level attained by a patient in the absence of fulfilling the criteria for $\dot{V}O_2max$ (McArdle et al., 2001). $\dot{V}O_2max$ or $\dot{V}O_2peak$ can be expressed as an absolute value (litres/min), or a relative value (ml/kg/min) where it is referenced to body weight.

In patients with respiratory disease the factors that limit $\dot{V}O_2max$ (or $\dot{V}O_2peak$) are complex, and include pulmonary factors such as abnormal ventilatory mechanics, abnormal rib cage mechanics and impaired gas exchange. These are complicated by psychosocial issues, abnormal symptom perception, general deconditioning,

Box 9.1 Six common respiratory disorders.

Chronic obstructive pulmonary disease (COPD) (Global Obstructive Lung Disease (GOLD), 2001)

- *Definition*: a disease characterised by airflow limitation that is not fully reversible. Airflow limitation is usually progressive and associated with an abnormal inflammatory response of the lungs to noxious particles and gases.
- *Diagnosis*: cough, sputum production or abnormal shortness of breath and history of exposure to risk factors. Diagnosis is confirmed by spirometry.
- *Classification*:
  Stage 0, At Risk: normal spirometry, chronic symptoms (cough, sputum production)
  Stage I, Mild: $FEV_1/FVC < 70\%$, $FEV_1 \geq 80\%$ predicted with or without chronic symptoms (cough, sputum production)
  Stage II, Moderate: $FEV_1/FVC < 70\%$, $30\% \leq FEV_1 < 80\%$ predicted (IIA $50\% \leq FEV_1 < 80\%$ predicted; IIB $30\% \leq FEV_1 < 50\%$ predicted with or without chronic symptoms (cough, sputum production, dyspnoea)
  Stage III, Severe: $FEV_1/FVC < 70\%$, $FEV_1 < 30\%$ predicted or $FEV_1 < 50\%$ predicted and respiratory failure or clinical signs of right heart failure.
  NB: FEV_1 values refer to post bronchodilator FEV_1.

Asthma (British Thoracic Society and Scottish Intercollegiate Guidelines Network, 2003)

- *Definition*: there is no agreed definition. Chronic inflammatory disorder of the airways. In susceptible individuals, inflammatory symptoms are usually associated with widespread but variable airflow obstruction and an increase in airway response to a variety of stimuli. Obstruction is often reversible either spontaneously or with treatment.
- *Diagnosis*: there is no diagnostic blood test, radiograph or histopathological investigation. Therefore asthma is diagnosed clinically. In some patients the diagnosis can be corroborated by changes in lung function tests. Symptoms are wheeze, shortness of breath, chest tightness and cough. These are variable, intermittent, worse at night, and provoked by triggers including exercise.

Lung function:

- 20% diurnal variation on ≥ three days in a week for 2 weeks on Peak Expiratory Flow (PEF) diary; or $FEV_1 \geq 15\%$ (and 200 ml) increase after short acting β 2 agonist; or $FEV_1 \geq 15\%$ (and 200 ml) increase after trial of steroid tablets; or $FEV_1 \geq 15\%$ (and 100 ml) decrease after six minutes of exercise (running). Histamine or methacholine challenge is necessary in difficult cases.
- Using Peak Expiratory Flow (PEF) in adults: Amplitude % best = (highest PEF-lowest PEF)/highest PEF x100 = X%. A 20% greater variation in amplitude % best with a minimal change of at least 60 litres/min, ideally for three days in a week for two weeks seen over a period of time is highly suggestive of asthma.
- *Classification*: childhood: wheeze heard on auscultation. Family history of atopy. Adult: persistent wheeze with few known precipitants except infection.

Cystic fibrosis (CF) (CF Trust, 2001)

- *Definition*: CF is a generalised disease caused by dysfunction in the exocrine glands and characterised by accumulation of mucus in the respiratory and gastrointestinal tracts and a high concentration of electrolytes in the sweat.
- *Diagnosis*: sweat test, nasal potential difference test, immunoreactive trypsin test, genotyping to identify mutations. Diagnosis of intestinal malabsorption and of a pancreatic abnormality supports the diagnosis.
- *Classification:* mild disease $FEV_1 < 30\%$; moderate FEV_1 30–70%; severe $FEV_1 > 70\%$.

Box 9.1 *Continued.*

Bronchiectasis (Mysliwiec and Pina 1999; Barker, 2002)

- *Definition*: bronchiectasis is defined as irreversible dilation of one or more bronchi. It is associated with various lung conditions and commonly accompanied by chronic infection. The disease may be congenital, for example, Kartagener's syndrome or acquired, for example, post-infection, post-obstruction, aspiration, inhalation, immuncompromised.
- *Diagnosis*: high resolution computerised tomography. Sputum bacteriology. Chest x-ray will show loss of lung volume locally and clinical symptoms are cough with purulent sputum.
- *Classification*: localised resulting from a focal insult, for example, severe lobar pneumonia; generalised/diffuse, that is, resulting from a global disorder predisposing to chronic inflammation.

Pneumonia (BTS, 2001a)

- *Definition*: a bacterial or viral infection that causes an inflammatory process in the lung spread by droplet infection.
- *Diagnosis*: patient history, chest x-ray and sputum bacteriology.
- *Classification*: community acquired, that is, due to organisms of high virulence. Nosocomial, that is, hospital acquired due to impaired defence mechanisms of the respiratory tract either mechanical or immunological. Clinical classification based on appearances, that is, lobar, bronchopneumonia or interstitial pneumonia.

Diffuse parenchymal lung disease (DPLD) (BTS, 1999)

- *Definition*: DPLD is a generic term for a large group of disorders that affect the lung parenchyma resulting in restrictive lung abnormatilies with loss of lung volume and increasing shortness of breath. There are over 200 entities previously labelled interstitial lung disease or diffuse lung disease. Examples are cryptogenic fibrosing alveolitis, pulmonary fibrosis and sarcoidosis.
- *Diagnosis*: patient history, past medical history, occupations, medications, hobbies, pets, travel, immunosuppression, systemic drugs, smoking. Investigations include chest x-ray, urine, erythrocyte sedimentation rate, lung function, liver function, bronchoscopy, electrocardiograph, bronchioalveolar lavage, video assisted thoracoscopy surgery, open lung biopsy.
- *Classification*: acute, episodic (which may present acutely), chronic due to occupational or environmental aspects or drugs, chronic with evidence of systemic disease, chronic with no evidence of systemic disease.

Box 9.2 Common signs and symptoms of respiratory disease.

Signs	Symptoms
- Tachypnoea	- Chest tightness
- Accessory muscle use	- Dyspnoea
- Cyanosis	- Wheeze
- Finger clubbing	- Sputum production
- Hyperinflation	- Orthopnoea
- Peripheral oedema	- Reduced exercise tolerance
- Neck vein distention	

peripheral muscle dysfunction, cardiovascular abnormalities and nutritional status (Kealy et al., 2003). Factors such as age, gender, environment and mode of exercise will also influence $\dot{V}O_2$peak in patients with respiratory disease, but the remainder of the discussion will relate to the pathophysiological factors. All these have important implications for exercise prescription in respiratory disease (see section on general principles of exercise training, p. 151).

Patients with mild disease may have a $\dot{V}O_2$peak which is within normal range but exhibit abnormal cardiorespiratory responses. Patients with moderate or severe disease usually exhibit a reduced $\dot{V}O_2$peak and abnormal cardiorespiratory responses to exercise.

Abnormal ventilatory mechanics

Most patients with respiratory disease have reduced maximum voluntary ventilation (MVV) compared to healthy individuals at rest. The MVV evaluates ventilatory capacity and can be determined by measuring the volume during rapid and deep breathing for 15 seconds, and this 15-second volume is extrapolated to the volume if breathing was continued for 1 minute (McArdle et al., 2001). Alternatively the MVV can be estimated by multiplying the FEV_1 by 35 to 40 (ATS/ACCP, 2003). The MVV is a good marker of the overall function of the ventilatory apparatus, including muscle strength, endurance, airway function, and lung compliance. Breathing reserve, defined as the difference in MVV and maximum ventilation ($\dot{V}_E$max), enables determination of the ventilatory contribution to exercise limitation. The pathophysiology of respiratory diseases result in a reduced MVV. Reduced expiratory airflow prevents the lungs from emptying on expiration. There is a progressive increase in end expiratory lung volume (EELV) and physiological dead space (V_D). Hyperinflation, as a result of increased EELV and V_D, limits the change in tidal volume (V_T), increases the V_D/V_T ratio and also reduces inspiratory capacity (IC). To compensate patients breathe at shallow rapid (increased respiratory rate) tidal volumes and recruit abdominal and accessory muscles during respiration. Consequently ventilation ($\dot{V}_E$) for a given exercise intensity in respiratory disease is higher than for a healthy individual. As a result of reduced MVV and increased $\dot{V}_E$ there is less breathing reserve (MVV–$\dot{V}_E$max) available for exercise. At maximal exercise patients with respiratory disease have low or no breathing reserve, but a high heart rate reserve, so patients stop exercising, usually because of severe dyspnoea and not because of cardiac limitations. Studies of patients with moderate and severe disease have shown that as disease severity progresses $\dot{V}O_2$peak and breathing reserve decrease and heart rate reserve increases (ATS/ACCP, 2003).

Abnormal ribcage mechanics

In chronic respiratory disease there are a number of mechanical changes of the thorax and ribcage that may contribute to the altered cardiorespiratory responses and limitations to exercise. These include thoracic kyphosis, use of accessory muscles, respiratory muscle wasting, fatigue and altered elastic properties, rib and thoracic pain, and inflammation. The contribution of these changes may differ for individual patients but they have the potential to increase EELV, increase respiratory rate, reduce IC, and ultimately reduce breathing reserve. This increases the oxygen cost of breathing and symptoms such as breathlessness and fatigue.

Impaired gas exchange

The abnormal ventilatory mechanics described above contribute to impaired gas exchange during exercise. This can be evidenced by changes in PaO_2 and $P(A-a)O_2$ and $PaCO_2$ with exercise, particularly in patients with severe disease. The causes of impaired gas exchange during exercise in respiratory disease are multifactorial and include impaired V_A/Q, intrapulmonary shunting (increased perfusion of underventilated airways) and diffusion abnormalities (Dantzker et al., 1982). These impairments occur primarily as a result of formation of scar tissue, alveolar hypoventilation in some lung regions and hyperventilation in others. The hypoventilation contributes to increased physiological dead space (V_D) and a greater than normal V_D/V_T ratio and an increased $\dot{V}_E/\dot{V}CO_2$ and $\dot{V}_E/\dot{V}O_2$ ratios. Impaired gas exchange further contributes to the higher $\dot{V}_E$ for a given exercise intensity and reduced breathing reserve and reduced $\dot{V}O_2$peak.

Anaerobic threshold

Anaerobic threshold (AT) is considered an estimation of the onset of metabolic acidosis, caused predominantly by an increase in cellular lactate acid during exercise (ATS/ACCP, 2003). This occurs at approximately 50–60% of $\dot{V}O_2$max in healthy untrained individuals with a wide range of normal values extending from 35–80% (European Respiratory Society, 1997; Roca and Whipp, 1997). In patients with mild respiratory disease AT usually occurs within the normal range. As disease severity progresses it may be low or undeterminable. Low breathing reserves and severe breathlessness mean that patients are often unable to exercise to a level which produces anaerobic metabolism. A low AT may also reflect deconditioning due to physical inactivity or skeletal muscle dysfunction.

Restrictive versus obstructive components

The relative contribution of abnormal ventilatory mechanics and gas exchange may be different in lung diseases with obstructive and/or restrictive components. With primarily airflow obstruction (for example, COPD), destruction of the alveolar wall and increased airflow resistance causes increased dead space and inefficient ventilation during exercise. These abnormal ventilatory mechanics result in a reduced ability to eliminate CO_2 relative to the ability to make oxygen available at cellular level (Wasserman et al., 1994). The AT is often normal until disease becomes very severe.

With primarily restrictive components (for example, DPLD) the loss of capillary vascular bed due to inflammatory scar tissue or thickening of the membrane causes low V_A/Q and right-to-left shunting of blood, which limits the diffusing capacity of gases, decreases PaO_2 and lowers the AT. Lung compliance is reduced and formation of scar tissue limits ability to increase V_T and the patient must increase their breathing frequency to achieve the necessary increases in $\dot{V}_E$ (Durstine and

Moore, 2003). Patients with restrictive diseases often increase their breathing frequency at maximal exercise to greater than 50 breaths per minute (Wasserman et al., 1994).

In summary, hypercapnia, as a result of impaired ventilatory mechanics, may be the more predominant factor in exercise limitation in patients with severe obstructive components. Hypoxaemia, as a result of impaired gas exchange, may be the more predominant factor in reduced exercise capacity in patients with primarily restrictive components.

Physical deconditioning

The impact of physical deconditioning on exercise capacity has been detailed in Chapter 4. Physical deconditioning as a consequence of the disease process may be an important additional factor, which contributes to the reduced exercise response in respiratory patients. In these patients respiratory muscle and skeletal muscle may compete for the limited pool of available oxygen. In respiratory disease the resultant dyspnoea that arises leads to a downward spiral of inactivity as the patient tries to avoid symptoms. This in turn leads to a lack of confidence, fear and anxiety and further inactivity, deconditioning and reduced function.

Evidence of benefit of exercise in respiratory disease

The importance of exercise within the care package of patients with respiratory disease has been the focus of research for many years. A plethora of research has resulted in some evidence for the proposed benefits of exercise in respiratory disease (Box 9.3) (ACCP/AACVPR, 1997; AACVPR, 1998; ACSM, 2003). A number of Cochrane reviews have been undertaken in an attempt to systematically review the evidence from existing randomised controlled trials designed to investigate the efficacy of exercise in respiratory disease. Where relevant, these Cochrane reviews have undertaken meta-analyses but in some reviews meta-analyses were not possible due to difficulties pooling data from the original trials.

Box 9.3 Proposed benefits of exercise in respiratory disease.

- Increased exercise capacity
- Increased muscle strength and endurance
- Decreased breathlessness
- Improved body image
- Enhanced body composition
- Enhanced sputum clearance
- Improved morale and health related quality of life (HRQoL)
- Increased lung function
- Increased activities of daily living (ADL)
- Increased coping skills
- Decreased health care utilisation

Box 9.4 Summary of Cochrane reviews assessing efficacy of exercise training in respiratory disease.

Cochrane review	Benefits
Physical training in CF (Bradley and Moran, 2003)	1a (meta-analysis) none 1b (non-pooled data) • increased peak exercise capacity • increased muscle strength • improved lung function • improved quality of life • slower decline in lung function
Pulmonary rehabilitation in COPD (Lacasse et al., 2003)	1a (meta-analysis) • decreased breathlessness • increased peak exercise capacity • improved quality of life 1b (non-pooled data) none
Physical training in asthma (Ram et al., 2003)	1a (meta-analysis) • increased $\dot{V}O_2$max 1b (non-pooled data) • increased work capacity
Physical training in bronchiectasis (Bradley et al., 2003)	1a (meta-analysis) none 1b (non-pooled data) • increased endurance exercise capacity • increased quality of life • increased lung function
Physical training in diffuse parenchymal lung disease (DPLD)	No Cochrane review to date
Physical training in pneumonia	No Cochrane review to date

Box 9.5 Levels of evidence (reprinted with permission from Agency for Health Care Policy and Research, 1992).

Level	Type of evidence
Ia	Evidence obtained from meta-analysis of randomised controlled trials
Ib	Evidence obtained from at least one randomised controlled trial
IIa	Evidence obtained from at least one well designed controlled study without randomisation
IIb	Evidence obtained from at least one other type of well designed quasi-experimental study
III	Evidence obtained from well designed non-experimental descriptive studies, such as comparative studies, correlation studies and case control studies
IV	Evidence obtained from expert committee reports or opinions and/or clinical experience of respected authorities

Box 9.4 provides a summary of Cochrane reviews (levels 1a and 1b evidence) assessing the efficacy of exercise training in respiratory disease. Box 9.5 identifies the criteria used to determine the levels of evidence. The Cochrane reviews highlight the need for further adequately powered, well designed long-term randomised controlled trials using appropriate outcome measures to quantify fully the role of exercise training within the already demanding care package of many respiratory diseases.

In summary, there is evidence to support the inclusion of exercise in the management of patients with respiratory disease. The benefit of exercise is dependent on multiple factors such as disease pathology, disease severity, baseline exercise capacity, intensity, type, frequency and duration of exercise training programmes. Not all exercise training programmes will achieve the same benefits, and it is important that exercise prescription and training are targeted towards individual treatment goals.

Exercise testing and assessment of outcome in respiratory disease

Exercise tests (maximal, sub-maximal, clinical laboratory and field tests) are important in the evaluation of patients with respiratory disease, as resting parameters, such as lung function, cannot reliably predict exercise performance. Additionally, functional capacity and health status correlate better with exercise tolerance than lung function.

Exercise tests are used for:

- The evaluation of functional or exercise capacity
- Determining the origin of exercise limitations
- Individualised safe and effective exercise prescription
- Determination of disease progression
- Prognosis
- Evaluation of efficacy of interventions
- Assessment of hypoxaemia
- Assessment of impairment/disability for applications for state benefits
- Pre-surgical evaluation and evaluation for transplantation

Maximal versus sub-maximal exercise tests

Maximal and sub-maximal tests are used in clinical practice and the choice of test depends on the information required, the facilities available, staff availability and expertise and the patient's clinical condition.

There is some debate regarding the comparative clinical utility of maximal versus sub-maximal exercise tests. Maximal exercise tests are most commonly performed in a clinical laboratory where equipment facilitates the collection of accurate metabolic ventilatory and circulatory data. This is resource intensive and consequently clinical laboratory exercise tests are used when the determination of $\dot{V}O_2$peak is necessary or when an in-depth understanding of cardiopulmonary responses to exercise are required, such as determining the origin of exercise limitations and clarifying change in respiratory disease progression or response to treatment.

For patients with respiratory disease sub-maximal exercise tests provide an alternative to maximal exercise testing. Some sub-maximal exercise tests provide an opportunity to predict $\dot{V}O_2$peak.

Clinical laboratory testing in respiratory disease

Clinical laboratory based tests may use a treadmill or cycle ergometer, although there is some argument that cycle ergometry is more useful (Box 9.6). The principal advantages of cycle ergometry over the treadmill is that the work performed is more easily quantified. This is because cycle ergometry is less prone to the introduction of artefacts such as the impact of arm and torso movement on ventilatory and ECG measurements (Wasserman et al., 1994). Also the work rate of the subject is less affected by the weight of the subject, the pacing strategy used and whether the patient holds on to the handlebars (Wasserman et al., 1994).

There are several protocols that can be used with either a cycle ergometer or a treadmill (ATS/ACCP, 2003). Some of the protocols have been developed for assessing maximal (or peak) exercise capacity while others have been developed to assess sub-maximal exercise capacity. Maximal exercise testing protocols can increase the intensity by a uniform amount each time increment or can be increased on a more continuous basis. Maximal exercise testing protocols, where the intensity increases on a more continuous basis, are often preferred for patients with respiratory disease as they are associated with a steadier rise in cardiopulmonary responses. It has been suggested that the length of the incremental phase of the maximal exercise test is between 8–12 minutes (ATS/ACCP, 2003).

Box 9.6 Practical comparisons, when measuring exercise responses, of cycle ergometry versus treadmill testing.

	Cycle versus treadmill
$\dot{V}O_2$peak	Lower
Work rate measurement	More quantifiable
Blood gas collection	Easier
Noise and artefacts	Less
Safety	More
Degree of leg muscle involvement	More
Cost	Less
Space	Less
Related to activities daily living	Less
Patient anxiety	Less

Sub-maximal protocols can apply the intensity at a percentage of the $\dot{V}O_2$max, for example, 70% $\dot{V}O_2$max (or $\dot{V}O_2$peak). Alternatively an intensity can be used which relates to the patient's usual activities of daily living (ADL), for example, three miles per hour treadmill walk, 50 watts on the cycle ergometer. Patients are asked to work at this rate for a set time, for example, six minutes (ATS/ACCP, 2003).

Field exercise tests in respiratory disease

Field exercise tests are an alternative to clinical laboratory exercise tests. Field tests do not provide in-depth information on the systems involved in exercise limitation, yet they have many advantages over laboratory testing and probably have greater applicability to health care professionals in their role as clinical exercise specialists.

For this reason this section will review the merits of field exercise tests in terms of their psychometric properties (validity, reliability, repeatability and responsiveness) and clinical utility. These properties ensure that the test can accurately measure exercise capacity at a single point in time and measure changes over time. There are different statistical methods for assessing the psychometric properties of a test. A valid test should exhibit a strong relationship and good agreement with a recognised gold standard. In a reliable and repeatable test there should be a strong relationship and good agreement between two tests performed within a period of clinical stability (Bland and Altman, 1986; Nevill and Atkinson, 1997). It is also important to note that evidence for the usefulness of a test in one population does not mean it is applicable or transferable to other populations.

Peak tests

The incremental shuttle walk test (ISWT) by Singh and colleagues is an externally paced test and the protocol and equipment for this test is readily available (Singh et al., 1992). Bradley and colleagues modified the original ISWT test by the addition of three levels and by permitting the patients to run (Bradley et al., 1999a). This has facilitated the use of a single test to assess exercise capacity in patients with minimal disability, as well as those with more severe disability, and has enabled a single test to be used to monitor changes in exercise capacity from childhood through to adulthood and through the course of the disease from mild disease through to severe disease (Bradley et al., 1999a). Validation studies have demonstrated good agreement between distance covered on ISWT (or modified shuttle test, MST) and $\dot{V}O_2$peak during treadmill testing in COPD and CF (Singh et al., 1994; Bradley et al., 1999a). Consequently $\dot{V}O_2$peak can be estimated using the results of the ISWT (or MST) (Singh et al., 1994; Bradley et al., 1999a). Studies have also shown that this test has good reliability and repeatability following familiarisation in COPD and CF (Singh et al., 1992; Bradley et al., 2000). This test has been shown to be sensitive to treatment induced changes in exercise capacity and a study in COPD has shown that a change of 48 metres represents a clinically important difference in exercise capacity (Singh et al., 1998; Bradley et al., 2000; Dyer et al., 2002; Singh et al., 2002). There are no reference ranges for respiratory populations. In clinical practice the ISWT (and where applicable the MST) can be used to establish the extent of exercise-induced desaturation, discriminate between different levels of exercise capacity, assess efficacy of interventions and assess for lung transplantation. It can also be used to establish a training zone. Exercise training can be prescribed at a speed equivalent to, for example, 70% maximum speed attained at the end of the exercise test. Alternatively, a percentage of peak HR can be used to prescribe a training zone.

Sub-maximal tests

Self-paced test

A number of self-paced tests (12, 6, 2-minute walk tests) have been developed and have been used to assess exercise capacity in respiratory disease (Butland et al., 1982). The most common self-paced test is the six-minute walk test (6 MWT) (ATS, 2002). The procedures for the 6 MWT are detailed in the ATS statement on the 6 MWT (ATS, 2002). There are many sources of variability when conducting the 6 MWT, including practical aspects, equipment required and patient preparation (Solway et al., 2001; ATS, 2002).

A comprehensive summary of the studies which have investigated the psychometric properties of this test in a variety of populations is provided by Solway and colleagues (Solway et al., 2001). The majority of studies in this review focused on validating the 6 MWT by correlating distance walked to several other reference criteria such as $\dot{V}O_2$peak, lung function, measures of function and dyspnoea. In brief, these studies show that the 6 MWT has a moderate to strong relationship with $\dot{V}O_2$peak, although correlation with lung function or dyspnoea is less consistent. Actual agreement between the 6 MWT and $\dot{V}O_2$peak is less clear (ATS, 2002). Investigation of the reliability of the 6 MWT has shown fairly consistent results in a variety of respiratory populations, with variability in the total distance between the first and second tests, and establishing consistency with the third test. Consequently the ATS have highlighted that one practice test is necessary (ATS, 2002). There is evidence that the 6 MWT is sensitive to change in exercise capacity, and studies in COPD have shown that a change of 54 metres represents a clinically important difference in exercise capacity (Redelmeir et al., 1997). There are some reference values available for the 6 MWT for healthy individuals but no reference ranges for respiratory populations (Enright and Sherrill, 1998; Gibbons et al., 2001; Enright et al., 2003). In clinical practice the 6 MWT can be used to establish the extent of exercise-induced desaturation, discriminate between different levels of exercise capacity, assessment efficacy of interventions and assessment for transplantation. It can also be used to establish a training zone. Speed during the 6 MWT (km/h) can be calculated using the distance (metres) and time walked, and exercise training can be prescribed at a speed equivalent to, for example, 70% of this. Alternatively, a percentage of peak HR (highest HR during test) can be used to prescribe a training zone.

Endurance shuttle walk test

The endurance shuttle walk test (ESWT) has been developed to compliment the ISWT (Revill et al., 1999). The protocol and equipment for this test is readily available (Revill et al., 1999). The ESWT facilitates assessment of endurance capacity using constant walking speeds and external regulation of pace at an intensity that is predetermined from the individual's peak performance on the ISWT. There is some evidence of the validity, reliability, repeatability (after familiarisation) and responsiveness of this test in COPD (Revill et al., 1999). There is no data on what represents a clinically significant improvement in endurance exercise capacity. There are no reference ranges for respiratory populations. The clinical utility of the ESWT likely rests in its usefulness to discriminate between different levels of endurance exercise capacity, assessment efficacy of interventions and assessment for transplantation.

Step test

The original step test was developed by Master and Oppenheimer, although a number of different step test protocols are now used (Master and Oppenheimer., 1929; Swinburn et al., 1985; Balfour-Lyn et al., 1998). Differences in protocols are mainly related to step height and stepping frequency, and whether or not these are fixed or graded. A standardised procedure has been described for step testing in respiratory disease, where patients are required to step up and down a six inch step at a rate of 30 steps per minute for three minutes; time is kept by a metronome and encouragement is standardised (Balfour-Lyn et al., 1998). The validity of this test in respiratory disease is unclear. Reproducibility of step testing suggests that there is a large learning effect with this type of exercise testing. The interpretation of step test results is more difficult than other tests and there are no reference ranges for respiratory populations. The clinical utility of this test has not been fully investigated and there is no data on what represents a clinically significant improvement in exercise capacity. The step test may be used in clinical practice to establish the extent of exercise-induced desaturation.

Stair climbing

Stair climbing has been used in some cases as a guide to general fitness and in determining fitness for surgery in patients with chronic respiratory disease. Patients are either asked to gauge how many flights of stairs they can climb or they are asked to perform stair climbing to assess their response. There is no standard protocol and data on the psychometric properties of this method of exercise testing is limited. However, a relationship has been demonstrated between performance on stair climbing and $\dot{V}O_2$peak, and stair climbing has some predictive ability in determining post-operative complications (Holden et al., 1992; Pollock et al., 1993; Girsh et al., 2001).

The timed up and go

The timed up and go, modified from the get up and go is an exercise test which was originally developed to assess balance and basic mobility skills in the frail elderly patient (Mathias et al., 1986; Podsiadlo and Richardson, 1991). It requires the patient to stand up from a chair, walk a short distance (three metres), turn around, return, and sit down again. This assessment of functional ability may be useful in patients with very severe disease who are unable to perform other tests. The clinical utility of this test is probably limited to gaining some estimate of functional ability in patients with very severe lung disease.

Metabolic equivalents (METs) and exercise testing

The energy cost of exercise can be expressed in terms of the metabolic equivalent (MET). The concept of the MET is based on the assumption that the resting $\dot{V}O_2$ is approximately 3.5 ml/kg/min. The energy cost of activities can be described in multiples of resting $\dot{V}O_2$ or METS (Durstine and Moore, 2003). The MET value associated with performance on exercise tests can be calculated, provided the speed is available (AACVPR, 1998). This information is useful in formulating an exercise prescription focused on activities of daily living (Box 9.10 on p. 153).

General principles for exercise testing in respiratory disease

Regardless of which test is used it is important to standardise the test procedure to ensure the accuracy of the results. The purpose and type of test should be explained to the patient. Information should be given to the patients regarding preparation for the test (clothing/footwear, avoid strenuous activity for 24 hours prior to test and avoid a heavy meal, caffeine or nicotine within two hours of testing, timing of medication). Patients should be familiarised with the equipment and test procedures and the appropriate number of practice tests should be performed with adequate rest periods between each practice. Other important factors include the calibration of equipment, time of day, expertise of the assessor and standardisation of instruction and encouragement (Noonan and Dean, 2000; ATS/ACCP, 2003). Consideration should also be given to current medications and coexisting diseases, as these may have implications for exercise testing and prescription (ACSM, 2003).

In clinical practice an exercise test may be useful if:

- It provides an estimate of exercise and/or functional capacity
- It can be used to prescribe an individualised exercise programme
- It can reliably detect a change in exercise capacity
- It gives the patient a clear understanding of their capabilities
- Perceived and physiological measures (for example, heart rate, SpO_2, and perceived breathlessness) can be easily recorded at appropriate intervals throughout the test
- It can predict $\dot{V}O_2$peak or $\dot{V}O_2$max

Training required

There are clear guidelines for the qualifications and training of personnel required to run and work in a formal exercise testing laboratory (ATS/ACCP, 2003). There is less information available regarding the qualifications and training of personnel

Box 9.7 Contraindications to exercise testing in respiratory disease (reproduced from ATS, 2001, with permission of the ATS/ACCP).

Absolute

- Acute myocardial infarction (3–5 days)
- Unstable angina
- Uncontrolled arrhythmias causing symptoms or haemodynamic compromise
- Syncope
- Active endocarditis
- Acute myocarditis or pericarditis
- Symptomatic severe aortic stenosis
- Uncontrolled heart failure
- Acute pulmonary embolus or pulmonary infarction
- Thrombosis of lower extremities
- Suspected dissecting aneurysm
- Uncontrolled asthma
- Pulmonary oedema
- Room air desaturation at rest ≤ 85%
- Respiratory failure
- Acute non-cardiopulmonary disorder that may affect exercise performance or be aggravated by exercise (that is, infection, renal failure, thyrotoxicosis)
- Mental impairment leading to inability to cooperate

Relative

- Left main coronary stenosis or its equivalent
- Moderate stenotic valvular heart disease
- Severe untreated arterial hypertension at rest (> 200 mmHg systolic, > 120 mmHg diastolic)
- Tachyarrhythmias or bradyarrhythmias
- High degree atrioventricular block
- Significant pulmonary hypertension
- Advanced or complicated pregnancy
- Electrolyte abnormalities
- Orthopaedic impairment that compromises exercise performance

required to perform field exercise tests. However, it is proposed that these tests should only be carried out under the direction of a physician, although physicians do not always need to be present during testing (ATS/ACCP, 2003). The health care professional carrying out the test is responsible for the type of test chosen, well-being and safety of the patient, monitoring of the patient, interpretation of results. Testing should be in a location that has access to oxygen, a cardiac arrest trolley, and adequate telephone and emergency services. The health care professional should have gained expertise in the field of exercise physiology in respiratory patients. Absolute and relative contraindications for exercise testing are outlined in Box 9.7.

Indications for stopping an exercise test

In general, patients should be encouraged to give a maximal effort during a test. The general indications for stopping any exercise test before the symptom limited maximum is reached apply to patients with respiratory disease (Box 9.8). When extensive cardiac and pulmonary monitoring is not being carried out during the exercise test, for example during field exercise testing, particular attention should be given to the following criteria: chest pain, SpO_2 levels, heart rate,

Box 9.8 Indications for exercise termination (reproduced with permission of ATS/ACCP, 2003).

- Chest pain suggestive of ischaemia
- Ischaemic electrocardiogram changes
- Complex ectopy
- Second or third degree heart block
- Fall in systolic pressure > 20 mmHg from the highest value during the test
- Hypertension (> 250 mmHg systolic; > 120 mmHg diastolic)
- Severe desaturation: arterial oxygen saturation as indicated by pulse oximetry ($SpO_2 \leq 80\%$ when accompanied by symptoms and signs of severe hypoxemia)
- Sudden pallor
- Loss of coordination
- Mental confusion
- Dizziness or faintness
- Signs of respiratory failure

sudden pallor, severe breathlessness, loss of coordination, confusion, dizziness or faintness.

It is unclear at what level of SpO_2 an exercise test should be stopped. However, as oxygen desaturation is not always related to the onset of symptoms inclusion of a lower limit may mean that the patient does not perform a true symptom limited exercise test. Pulse oximetry also becomes less accurate at lower readings. A parameter for stopping informal exercise testing used in some clinical settings and research trials is 75%, although it has been argued that in some populations in the absence of symptoms SpO_2 should not be included as a criteria to indicate the end of the test (Balfour-Lyn et al., 1998; Bradley et al., 1999a).

Other outcome measures used in the evaluation of exercise training for respiratory conditions

The use of other outcome measures is important, with the realisation that exercise capacity alone cannot always assess the health related benefits of exercise. These other outcome measures often complement the usual measurements of respiratory impairment, such as lung function and exercise tolerance, in order to more fully reflect the net benefit (positive and negative effects) on disability, function and health. Although Box 9.9 is not meant to be exhaustive it provides some examples of other outcome measures that can be used in the evaluation of exercise training for respiratory conditions. The choice of outcome measure(s) is dependent on the purpose and context for which it is being used, the ease of use, the rigor with which it has been developed and the psychometric properties in the population of study. It is fundamental that the outcome measures chosen reflect the goals of exercise training and that they are used to assess effectiveness of the exercise training programme, for example, if improved quality of life is a goal of exercise training then a disease

Box 9.9 Examples of other outcomes which are used to monitor/measure training in respiratory disease.

Breathlessness scales	Borg breathlessness scale (Borg, 1982) Visual Analogue Scale (VAS) (Gift, 1989; Wilson and Jones, 1989) Medical Research Council (MRC) breathlessness scale (MRC, 1966) Chronic Respiratory Disease Questionnaire (CRDQ) Dyspnoea component (Guyatt et al., 1987)
Generic quality of life health scales	Nottingham Health Profile (Hunt et al., 1985) Quality of Well Being (Kaplan et al., 1984) Short Form 36 (SF 36) (Ware and Sherbourne, 1992)
Disease specific quality of life questionnaires (QoL)	St Georges Respiratory Disease Questionnaire (Jones et al., 1992) Chronic Respiratory Disease Questionnaire (CRDQ) (Guyatt et al., 1987; Bradley et al., 1999b) Breathing Problems Questionnaire (BPQ) (Hyland et al., 1994) The Cystic Fibrosis Questionnaire (CFQ) (Quittner et al., 2000) The Cystic Fibrosis QoL Questionnaire (CFQoL) (Gee et al., 2000) Asthma QoL questionnaire (Juniper et al., 1992)
Activities of daily living (ADL)	Pulmonary Functional Status and Dyspnoea Questionnaire (Lareau et al., 1994) London Chest Activity of Daily Living scale (LCADL) (Garrod et al., 2000a) Manchester Respiratory ADL Questionnaire (Yohannes et al., 2000) Activity monitors (Singh and Morgan, 2001) Life Shirt (Rosso et al., 2002)
Psychosocial	Hospital Anxiety and Depression Questionnaire (Zigmond and Snaith, 1983) The Manchester Cystic Fibrosis Coping Scale (Abbott et al., 1997)
Health care utilisation	The Manchester Cystic Fibrosis Compliance Questionnaire (Abbott et al., 1994) Evaluation of service costs, frequency of exacerbation and antibiotic use, number of GP visits and hospitalisations
Respiratory muscle strength	Test of incremental respiratory muscle endurance (TIRE) (Chatham et al., 1996) PiMax and Pemax (Ng and Stokes, 1991)
Strength tests	Isokinetic strength tests (Lands et al., 1994) Isometric strength (Farrell and Richards, 1986)

specific Quality of Life (QoL) questionnaire may be an appropriate outcome measure. This should be administered at the start and end of the training programme to enable changes in QoL to be ascertained. Outside the context of the research environment outcome measures should only be used if they provide useful information of clinical value and the technology, personnel, expertise to analyse and interpret and use the result is available.

General principles of exercise training and prescription in respiratory disease

There is a growing body of evidence that patients with respiratory disease should be advised to adhere to an exercise programme appropriate to their disease severity and/or level of disability. The format in which this is delivered to patients with respiratory disease varies considerably at local, regional and international level. It is dependent as much on local resources, funding, expertise and focus of the multidisciplinary team involved in the management of the patient population, as on disease severity and disability.

When patients have mild disease or minimal disability the primary aim of exercise training is to initiate and maintain adherence to an exercise training programme and incorporate this training programme into their lifestyle. In this group of patients the role of the health professional should focus on advice, such as type of exercise, importance of warm up and cool down, education, such as control of breathlessness, use of inhaled medication and monitoring of exercise capacity. As disease severity and disability progress patients may require a more individualised exercise programme, and more regular monitoring and reassessment. Regardless of whether the patient performs exercise training at hospital or at home, in a group or an individualised format the general principles of exercise training should be followed and patients assessed for possible contraindications to exercise (Chapter 7). Training should include a warm up to ensure a gradual increase in, for example, heart rate and ventilation, and a cool down to reduce the risk of, for example, arrhythmias and bronchospasm. Exercise should be of sufficient intensity, frequency, duration, type and length to improve cardiopulmonary fitness and muscle conditioning.

Intensity

The intensity of training should be based on individual patient assessment and results of exercise testing. Due to training specificity it is important that the exercise testing protocol selected is relevant to the proposed training programme, for example, if the proposed training programme involves cycling, a cycle ergometer should be used to determine training intensity. Guidelines for training intensity for COPD suggest a workload/speed equivalent to 60–70% of $\dot{V}O_2$peak and for CF 50–60% $\dot{V}O_2$max (BTS, 2001b; CF Trust, 2001). In patients with mild respiratory disease who achieve an AT during maximal/peak exercise testing a training intensity could be set at or above the AT, (AACVPR, 1998). Alternatively, and for patients who do not achieve AT, lower intensity training may be beneficial, as they often improve their exercise tolerance despite training at lower work rates (ACSM, 1995). Patients with severe disease may benefit from general whole body exercise. Training intensity may be set using peak heart rate during an appropriate exercise test. Equations for calculating peak heart rate in healthy individuals are not suitable for patients with respiratory disease because they exhibit a ventilatory limitation to exercise. It is also possible to guide intensity by symptoms and advise patients to work at an intensity that induces dyspnoea, for example, a Borg breathlessness score of 3 equates to an intensity of 50% $\dot{V}O_2$peak (ACSM, 1995). This is particularly useful for unsupervised exercise and patients can be set a target level of breathlessness.

Frequency and duration of exercise sessions

In respiratory disease it is not known what duration or frequency of training is required. A pragmatic approach has been used and most exercise programmes follow the American College of Sports Medicine (ACSM) guidelines for healthy individuals, such as, exercising for a tolerable time and aiming to progress to at least 20–30 minutes exercise for 3–5 days a week (ACSM, 1998). Patients with severe disease and/or deconditioning may need to undertake multiple short bouts of exercise in order to achieve this volume.

Type of exercise

An exercise programme should include endurance and strength training for the upper and lower body (ACCP/AACVPR, 1997). Endurance type exercise (continuous or interval training) aims to increase capacity and improve ability to perform more activities with fewer symptoms. This can involve periods of continuous training for a length of time at a target intensity. Interval training entails bouts of relatively intense work separated by periods of rest or low intensity training. Interval training is advantageous as it enables the patient to carry out a greater volume of exercise than they could achieve by continuous training. In addition, interval training resembles the bouts of work required in activities of daily living (Coppoolse et al., 1999). The energy costs of various daily activities have been extensively studied. Box 9.10 lists a variety of activities and equivalent MET and these may be useful when prescribing individualised exercise which relates to functional activity and activities of daily living.

Patients with mild disease should be encouraged to participate in sporting activities of their choice, for example, football, swimming and walking. For younger patients the development of skill and an interest in exercise in youth often means that patients will continue exercise/playing sport into adulthood. For these patients, liaison with local leisure centres may be appropriate to ensure access to adequate facilities and supervision. As disease severity and disability progress exercise training may need to be individualised and it may be better to have a more structured format. In those who are more disabled, training should focus on interval training in order to increase the total amount of exercise completed per session.

Strength training may lead to improved muscle strength and ability to perform activities of daily living (Simpson et al., 1992; ACCP/AACVPR, 1997). The effects are specific to the muscle group being trained, for example, training the arms will have little effect on the strength of the legs. Muscle strength is best increased by

Box 9.10 METS values for some activities of daily living and exercise in healthy individuals (AACVPR, 1998; ACSM, 1995).

1.5–2 METS
Walking 1 mph
Sitting at desk

2–3 METS
Bathing
Dressing
Walking 2.5–3 mph
Dusting
Preparing meal
Bowling

3–4 METS
Sweeping
Vacuuming
Food shopping with trolley
Walking 3 mph
Golfing

4–5 METS
Mowing lawn
Golfing, carrying clubs
Mopping
Washing windows
Cycling 6 mph

5–6 METS
Skiing downhill
Swimming
Walking 4 mph
Digging

> 6 METS
Cycling vigorously
Running

using a high resistance and low number of repetitions, and muscle endurance is best increased by using a low resistance and a high number of repetitions; although both of these will generally add to increased strength and endurance.

Although patients with respiratory disease may have respiratory muscle weakness, the role of respiratory muscle strength training remains controversial (ACCP/AACVPR, 1997; ACPCF, 2002). The effects of strength training are specific to the muscle group being trained and this is likely to be the case with the respiratory muscles (ACCP/AACVPR, 1997). A number of new respiratory muscle trainers have been manufactured and these overcome many of the problems with early muscle trainers in that they allow the training programme to be individualised. Research is ongoing to establish the role of these respiratory muscle trainers in the management of patients with respiratory disease.

Duration of exercise programmes

The length of training required to obtain physiological benefits in respiratory disease is unclear, yet general studies show that benefits from exercise will be attained after 4–12 weeks (ACSM, 1998; Green et al., 2001). It is also unclear how long after cessation of training that the benefits are maintained. However, a general guide is that benefits of training will be lost after 3–4 weeks of cessation of exercise (ACSM, 1998). Although there are no longitudinal studies in respiratory disease similar work in healthy individuals supports the need for lifelong training in order to maintain the initial benefits gained, promote long-term health benefits and prevent the onset of other co-morbidities.

Precautions to exercise in respiratory disease

There are no absolute contraindications to exercise in respiratory disease, but careful consideration should be given in some circumstances. Webb and Dodd (1999) have indicated that the sports that carry a medical risk for patients include parachute jumping, skiing and scuba diving. Skiing, for patients who are already hypoxic, is not advised and episodes of acute right heart failure brought on by a combination of altitude and unaccustomed fierce aerobic and anaerobic exercise are well documented (Webb and Dodd, 1999). Scuba diving is contraindicated for patients with lung disease if there is evidence of air trapping. Patients with coexisting cardiac status should be carefully assessed prior to exercise training to ensure that their cardiac status is stable and to facilitate stratification according to any possible risk. Careful consideration should be given to patients with acute exacerbations and although some studies have demonstrated benefits of training most guidelines state that exercise should be of lower intensity and for shorter periods of time, taking into account patients' increased respiratory symptoms. All patients should be well hydrated, and, in groups at risk of salt depletion, oral electrolyte replacement therapy should be considered. Patients with low bone density should avoid contact sport or high impact sports.

Precautions should be taken with patients who are at risk of pneumothorax, severe haemoptysis, exercise induced asthma and severe breathlessness or hypoxia. Patients with multi-system disease, for example, portal hypertension in CF with significant enlargement of spleen and liver, should probably be advised against contact sports (Webb and Dodd, 1999). Consideration should also be given to the microbiological status of the patient in view of infection control policies, for example, patients with methicillin-resistant *Staphylococcus aureus* (MRSA) are trained separately. Patients with CF are advised to exercise independently from other patients with CF.

Monitoring during exercise in respiratory patients

Patients can be monitored during exercise for several reasons: to ensure that they are meeting the predetermined target levels to achieve a training effect, to facilitate progression of the intensity of the exercise programme, to ensure that patients are exercising within safe parameters and to assess compliance with the training programme. When relevant, patients with mild disease or minimal disability can self monitor, for example, using heart rate and perceived breathlessness to ensure that they are training at sufficient intensity to achieve the intended benefit.

As disease progresses more in-depth monitoring during exercise may be required, such as level of breathlessness, heart rate, respiratory rate and oxygen saturation. Patients and health care professionals should be educated regarding when to stop exercise (Box 9.8). Special consideration should be give to specific populations, for example, patients using non-invasive ventilation (NIV), patients on long-term oxygen therapy (see section on special populations on pages 158–62). Patients with exercise induced asthma should take their prescribed inhaled short acting β_2 agonists prior to exercise (BTS and SIGN, 2003).

Pulmonary rehabilitation

Exercise training can be delivered in the context of a pulmonary rehabilitation (PR) programme. The American Thoracic Society states that 'Pulmonary rehabilitation is a multidisciplinary programme of care for patients with chronic respiratory impairment that is individually tailored and designed to optimise physical and social performance and autonomy' (ATS, 1999).

Pulmonary rehabilitation aims to reduce the disability and loss of health associated with chronic respiratory disease, and to improve functional ability and quality of life while reducing health care utilisation. There is evidence to support the use of pulmonary rehabilitation in patients with chronic lung disease, and the following benefits have been observed.

- Improved quality of life
- Improved exercise capacity
- Reduced dyspnoea
- Reduced health care utilisation
- Improved coping skills

These benefits have been demonstrated in patients with mild as well as more severe disease (BTS, 2001b). Most of this evidence is from studies in patients with COPD (ACCP/AACVPR, 1997; Lacasse et al., 2003). It has been suggested that other respiratory patient populations, for example, DPLD, bronchiectasis and asthma will achieve benefit from PR (ACCP/AACVPR, 1997). Documents summarising the evidence for PR and guidelines for practice are available (ACCP/AACVPR, 1997; AACVPR, 1998; ATS, 1999; BTS, 2001b; Garrod, 2003).

Pulmonary rehabilitation format

Pulmonary rehabilitation comprises a programme of exercise training and educational sessions on a range of topics delivered by a multidisciplinary team. PR may be conducted in any setting: hospital inpatient, hospital outpatient, community and at home. The level of supervision for PR is dependent on the setting, number of patients, and disease severity. Patients should be assessed at the start and end of PR and this should include exercise testing, health related quality of life, functional status and psychosocial status (Box 9.4). A pragmatic approach to outpatient PR is 6–8 weeks of exercise training three to five times per week, and an education session delivered once per week (BTS, 2001b). Studies investigating the role of prolonged maintenance programmes are controversial (Vale et al., 1993). However, patients are advised to continue with an individualised home exercise programme and attend support groups for patients with respiratory disease. Follow-up is suggested at 6–12 months and this enables the health care practitioner to modify the patient's exercise programme and/or assess the need for re-entry into PR.

Exercise component

Exercise training should generally follow the principles outlined above for exercise in respiratory patients. Training components may vary and should be based

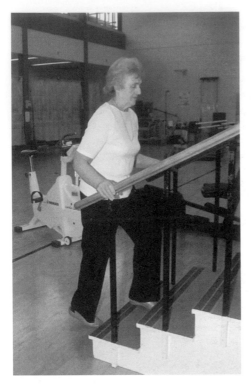

Figure 9.1 Patient performing step-ups on stairs.

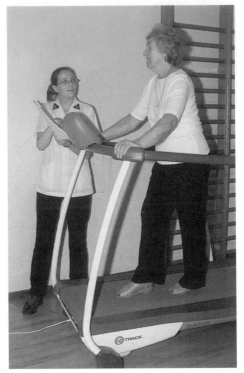

Figure 9.2 Patient walking on treadmill.

on individual patient assessment and the results of exercise testing. At all stages of disease severity an aerobic exercise component (either continuous or interval training) should be included, particularly using the lower extremities, for example, walking and cycling. Lower extremity exercises involve muscle groups and improve performance of activities of daily living, for example, walking or stairs (Figures 9.1, 9.2). Upper extremity training should also be included, for example, functional activities or arm exercises (Figures 9.3a–c). Upper extremity training improves performance for task specific activities, for example, shaving. Interval training is advantageous for patients who have severe respiratory disease or who are deconditioned, as it enables the patient to carry out a greater volume of exercise than they could achieve by continuous training. Disease severity does not always relate well to exercise capacity; therefore training programmes for any particular patient are often based on the baseline assessment of symptoms and exercise capacity. Programmes that are specifically designed for the individual are superior to those with a standard protocol (Vallet et al., 1997).

Guidelines have been developed at the Belfast City Hospital for the prescription of exercise training based on initial Incremental Shuttle Walk Test (ISWT) results (Boxes 9.11, 9.12). Training can be progressed by increasing the intensity of exercise to a higher level (for example, level 1 to level 3) and/or increasing the duration of

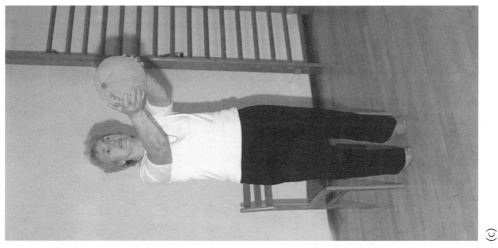

(a)

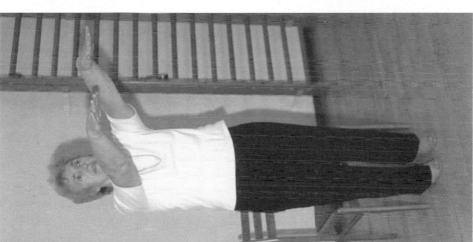

(b)

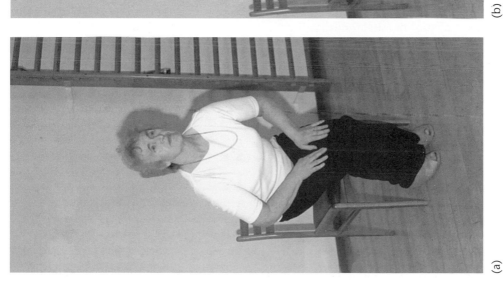

(c)

Figure 9.3 (a) Patient performing stand-up sit-down exercise. (b) Patient performing stand-up sit-down with arms at shoulder height. (c) Patient performing stand-up sit-down with ball.

Box 9.11 Belfast City Hospital guidelines for prescription of exercise training based on initial Incremental Shuttle Walk Test (ISWT).

Exercise tolerance ISWT < 50 m Interval training = Level 1	Exercise tolerance ISWT ≥ 50 m to < 100 m Interval training = Level 2	Exercise tolerance ISWT ≥ 100 m Interval training = Level 3
Exercise alternative(s) or progression: • Repeat level 1 • Increase level 1 exercise time • Move to level 2 • Strength training and functional activities • Walking at 50% $\dot{V}O_2$peak for 10–20 minutes	Exercise alternative(s) or progression: • Repeat level 2 • Increase level 2 exercise time • Move to level 3 • Strength training • Walking or cycling at 60% $\dot{V}O_2$peak for 10–20 minutes	Exercise alternative(s) or progression: • Repeat level 3 • Increase level 3 exercise time • Strength training • Walking or cycling at 60–70% $\dot{V}O_2$peak for 10–20 minutes

* Patients with higher exercise capacity may participate in, for example, sport multi-gym activities and/or exercise up to 70% $\dot{V}O_2$peak

each exercise (for example, 30 seconds each, progressing to 120 seconds each) and/or the addition of weights to incorporate some strength training (Box 9.12).

Educational component

It is agreed that education is a central component of pulmonary rehabilitation, but there is no consensus regarding which sessions are essential or which should be included (BTS, 2001b; ATS, 1999). Sessions cover a variety of topics and are usually delivered by the multidisciplinary team (Box 9.13). Consideration should be given to the diagnosis and level of disability of the patient group attending. Patients who require additional individual education sessions for, for example, airway clearance, change of inhaler device, flight assessment, should be identified. Written and audiovisual material (for example, video, CD ROMs) may be advantageous in improving patient knowledge and compliance with the information provided. It may also be helpful for patient's carers or family members to attend the educational sessions in order to better assist patients in the management of their respiratory condition.

Special considerations for exercise in respiratory disease

Patients using oxygen

Patients who are hypoxaemic at rest and require long-term oxygen therapy (LTOT) should exercise with supplementary oxygen. The level of oxygen required in this case may need to be increased/titrated for the duration of the exercise training to maintain oxygen saturations at an acceptable level ($SpO_2 > 90\%$) (GOLD, 2001; BTS, 2001b). The level of oxygen required for exercise can be confirmed by

Box 9.12 Exercise circuit for interval training at Belfast City Hospital.

	Exercise Level 1	Exercise Level 2	Exercise Level 3
(1)	Sitting down, shoulder circles in one direction then the other.	Standing up, shoulder/elbow circles with right hand placed on right shoulder, repeat with left arm.	Keep feet moving during this shoulder exercise, shoulder/elbow circles with right hand placed on right shoulder, repeat with left arm.
(2)	Trunk rotation. Sitting down, hold a stick out at shoulder height, turn all the way round to one side, return to starting position. Repeat to opposite side.	Trunk rotation. Sitting down, hold a stick out at shoulder height, turn all the way round to one side, return to starting position. Repeat to opposite side.	Trunk rotation. Sitting down, hold a stick out at shoulder height, turn all the way round to one side, return to starting position. Repeat to opposite side.
(3)	Step up and down from a step, hold railing(s) as necessary.	Step up and down from a step without holding railings.	Step up and down on two alternate steps without holding railings.
(4)	Standing, single alternate arm forward flexion to shoulder height.	Standing, keep feet moving during this shoulder exercise. Single alternate arm forward flexion to shoulder height.	Keep feet moving during this shoulder exercise, bilateral arm overhead flexion circles (front crawl swimming motion).
(5)	Standing holding onto a secure surface, lunge alternate foot backwards.	Standing, lunge alternate foot backwards while raising alternate arms to shoulder height in front.	Standing, raise one heel towards buttock and touch heel with opposite hand, then alternate with opposite side.
(6)	Bicycle/cycle ergometry with no resistance, or alternatively patient seated marching feet on the spot	Bicycle/cycle ergometry with increased resistance/time.	Bicycle/cycle ergometry with increased resistance/time.
(7)	Push-ups. Stand with hands on wall at shoulder height, allow elbows to bend then push out straight.	Push-ups. Stand with hands on wall at shoulder height, allow elbows to bend then push out straight.	Push-ups. Stand with hands on wall at shoulder height, allow elbows to bend then push out straight.
(8)	Stand up, sit down.	Stand up, sit down with arms held at shoulder height when standing and by the sides when sitting.	Stand up, sit down, with arms holding ball at shoulder height when standing and by the sides when sitting.
(9)	Trunk flexion. Sitting down, back straight, hold a stick tucked under the chin, bend trunk slowly to alternate sides.	Trunk flexion. Sitting down, back straight, hold a stick tucked under the chin, bend trunk slowly to alternate sides.	Trunk flexion. Sitting down, back straight, hold a stick tucked under the chin, bend trunk slowly to alternate sides.
(10)	Standing holding onto secure surface, alternate knee lifts to hip height.	Standing with arms at shoulder height, alternate knee lifts to hip height touching opposite knee to opposite hand.	Marching on the spot, lifting knees to hip height, elbows bent and moving elbows in a circular motion in time to leg movements.

Box 9.13 Suggested educational topics for pulmonary rehabilitation.

Educational topic	Suggestions for content of session
Disease process	Pathophysiology of respiratory disease Self-assessment of symptoms and recognition of infection and exacerbation Description and interpretation of medical tests Infection control
Medication	Rationale for use of respiratory medications, inhalers and nebulisers Care of equipment Correction of inhaler technique
Psychosocial and coping skills	Support systems and support groups Goal setting, desensitisation Anxiety management, relaxation
Airway clearance	Active cycle of breathing technique, positive expiratory pressure, flutter. Correction of forced expiration technique
Nutrition	Advice on healthy eating for patients with respiratory disease Advice on healthy eating for patients who are exercising Advice for patients with malnutrition or obesity
Smoking cessation	Advice regarding smoking cessation Information about local programmes/referral to smoking cessation clinic
Benefits of exercise	Principles of exercise and exercise activity General health related and disease specific benefits
Management of breathlessness	Positions of ease Pursed lip breathing and breathing control Pacing techniques for exercise and activities of daily living
Travel with respiratory disease	Effects of air travel on the respiratory system Preparation for travel abroad for patients with respiratory disease Appropriate referral for flight assessment, oxygen use while flying
Oxygen therapy	Long term oxygen therapy and ambulatory oxygen Oxygen use during acute exacerbation in hospital or at home
Energy conservation	Home adaptations Mobility aids Energy conservation for activities of daily living

assessment for ambulatory oxygen, and in liaison with the patient's consultant as there is a need to ensure patients do not retain carbon dioxide (RCP, 1999).

Many patients who are not hypoxaemic at rest demonstrate significant desaturation ($SpO_2 < 90\%$) (BTS, 1997; RCP, 1999). At present there is no consensus regarding the use of supplemental oxygen during exercise training in these patients. Recent studies (Rooyackers et al., 1997; Garrod et al., 2000c) have shown no additional benefit from oxygen administered during PR. Patients should be assessed if they desaturate significantly and those who meet the criteria for ambulatory oxygen should wear their oxygen during exercise and activities of daily living (RCP, 1999). Alternatively, in either case (chronic or transient hypoxaemia) patients can be taught to pace themselves and modify exercise regimes to avoid significant levels of desaturation during exercise and activities of daily living.

Lung surgery

Exercise prior to lung surgery (lung volume reduction surgery and lung transplant) can maximise pre-operative exercise and functional capacity, and manage breathlessness. Where appropriate this may be delivered within the context of a PR programme. As disease progresses patients on the waiting list for lung surgery may require frequent assessment and modification of exercise/activity programmes. Patients following lung volume reduction surgery have improved exercise performance as a direct result of the surgical procedure (Criner et al., 1999; BTS, 2001b). As these patients still have chronic lung disease the goals of exercise training may need to be readdressed post-surgery (AACVPR, 1998). Multiple factors contribute to reduced exercise capacity in patients following lung transplantation. Patients need to be reassessed post-transplant and the goals of exercise training readdressed. There is evidence that adherence to a long-term exercise training programme increases strength and endurance in these patients (Steibellebner et al., 1998).

Non-invasive ventilation (NIV)

Non-invasive ventilation (NIV) is the provision of mechanical ventilatory assistance without the need for an invasive airway and can be used during exercise training (Figure 9.4). In patients with severe COPD there is some evidence that the use of NIV during exercise training may enable patients to train at a higher exercise intensity (Kielty et al., 1994; Hawkins et al., 2002; Van't Hull et al., 2002). Alteration of the NIV settings and oxygen entrainment should be considered, to meet the increased demands during exercise (AACVPR, 1998). The use of nocturnal ventilation in patients with severe COPD has been shown to have a positive impact on exercise performance and dyspnoea (Garrod et al., 2000b). Therefore NIV used for a period prior to an exercise training session could enhance patients' exercise performance.

Smokers

Currently, there is no evidence that smokers should be excluded from exercise programmes or pulmonary rehabilitation. There is no evidence that smokers achieve any more or any less benefit from exercise training and in some cases opportunity exists for referral to smoking cessation programmes (ATS, 1999).

Patients with acute exacerbations

Patients with respiratory disease often have unstable pathophysiology and may develop acute exacerbations and/or infection which can increase oxygen consumption (Stiller and Phillips, 2003). There is controversy regarding the efficacy of exercise training during an acute exacerbation/infection. However, a significant increase in exercise capacity and lung function has been reported (Kirsten et al., 1998; Bradley et al., 2003). It is important that exercise is modified and individually tailored according to the patient's symptoms at the time of the exacerbation.

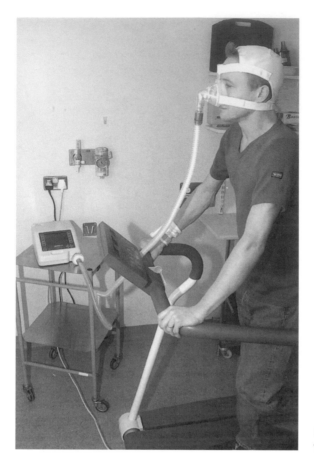

Figure 9.4 Patient exercising with non-invasive ventilation.

Patients in intensive care unit (ICU)

The deleterious effects of immobilisation in patients is documented (Sciaky, 1994) and there is evidence that exercise activity is of benefit to patients with respiratory compromise in ICU (Nava, 1998). Exercise is included in the rehabilitation of patients in ICU, and for those with existing respiratory disease or those who develop respiratory disease the underlying disease pathology needs to be considered as well as their critical status (Smith and Ball, 1998; Lewis, 2003; Stiller and Phillips, 2003). In ventilated patients requiring high levels of oxygen, positive end expiratory pressure and inotropic support, active or repetitive exercise is less appropriate and functional assisted movement is advised. Once the patient is cooperative with a stable cardiovascular status, a decreased dependence on inotropic support and is able to increase their minute ventilation by taking spontaneous breaths, then active exercise using the major muscle groups can begin.

Nutritional status

Patients with chronic respiratory disease have an altered nutritional status which may have an impact on their exercise performance (Kealy et al., 2003; Lewis and

Bellman, 1987). Respiratory diseases are associated with increased energy expenditure, which contributes to poor nutritional status. Assessment and modification of nutritional intake is important prior to commencing an exercise programme (AAVCPR, 1998). Weight gain may be indicated for malnourished patients and a weight loss programme may be required for obese patients.

Conclusion

This chapter has provided rationale for including exercise training and/or PR in the management of patients with respiratory disease. The use of exercise testing in assessment and prescription is also detailed.

References

American College of Chest Physicians/American Association of Cardiovascular and Pulmonary Rehabilitation (ACCP/AACVPR) Pulmonary Rehabilitation Guidelines Panel (1997). Pulmonary Rehabilitation. Joint ACCP/AACVPR evidence-based guidelines. *Chest* 112, 1363–96.

American Association of Cardiovascular and Pulmonary Rehabilitation (AACVPR) (1998). *Guidelines for Pulmonary Rehabilitation Programes*, 2nd edn. Human Kinetics, Champaign, Ill.

Abbott, J., Dodd, M., Bilton, D. and Webb, A.K. (1994). Treatment compliance in adults with cystic fibrosis. *Thorax* 49, 115–20.

Abbott, J., Dodd, M., Gilling, S. and Webb, K. (1997). 'Coping styles and treatment adherence in adults with cystic fibrosis'. Proceedings of the 21st European Cystic Fibrosis Conference, European Working Group in Cystic Fibrosis. Davos, Switzerland.

American College of Sports Medicine (ACSM) (1995). *ACSM's Guidelines for Exercise Testing and Prescription*, 5th edn. Williams and Wilkins, Philadelphia.

American College of Sports Medicine (ACSM) (1998). The recommended quantity and quality of exercise for developing and maintaining cardiorespiratory and muscular fitness, and flexibility in healthy adults. *Medicine and Science in Sports and Exercise* 30, 975–1001.

American College of Sports Medicine (ACSM) (2003). *ACSM's Exercise Management for Persons with Chronic Diseases and Disabilities* (Durstine, S.L. and Mocre, G.F. eds), 2nd edn. Human Kinetics, Champaign, Ill.

American Thoracic Society (ATS) (1999). Pulmonary Rehabilitation. *American Journal of Respiratory and Critical Care Medicine* 159, 1666–82.

American Thoracic Society (ATS) (2002). ATS Statement: guidelines for the 6-minute walk test. *American Journal of Respiratory and Critical Care Medicine* 166, 111–7.

American Thoracic Society/American College of Chest Physicians (ATS/ACCP) (2003). ATS/ACCP Statement on Cardiopulmonary Exercise Testing. *American Journal of Respiratory and Critical Care Medicine* 167, 211–77.

Balfour-Lyn, I.M., Prasad, S.A., Laverty, A., Whitehead, B.F. and Dinwiddie, R. (1998). A step in the right direction: assessing exercise tolerance in cystic fibrosis. *Pediatric Pulmonology* 225, 278–84.

Barker, A.D. (2002). Bronchiectasis. *New England Journal of Medicine* 346, 1383–93.

Bland, J.M. and Altman, O.J. (1986). Statistical methods for assessing agreement between two methods of clinical measurement. *Lancet* i, 307–10.

Borg, G. (1982). Psychophysical basis of perceived exertion. *Medicine and Science in Sport and Exercise* 14, 377–81.

Bradley, J.M., Howard, J., Wallace, E. and Elborn, S. (1999a). Validity of the modified shuttle test in adult cystic fibrosis. *Thorax* 54, 437–9.

Bradley, J.M., Dempster, M.T., Wallace, E.S. and Elborn, J.S. (1999b). The adaptations of a quality of life questionnaire for routine use in clinical practice: the chronic respiratory disease questionnaire in cystic fibrosis. *Quality of Life Research* 8, 65–71.

Bradley, J.M., Howard, J., Wallace, E. and Elborn, S. (2000). Reliability, repeatability and sensitivity of the modified shuttle test in adult cystic fibrosis. *Chest* 117, 1666–71.

Bradley, J.M. and Moran, F. (2003). Physical training in cystic fibrosis (Cochrane Review). In *The Cochrane Library* 2, Oxford Update Software (Accessed 23 June 2003).

Bradley, J.M., Moran, F. and Greenstone, M. (2003). Physical training in bronchiectasis (Cochrane Review). In *The Cochrane Library* 2, Oxford Update Software (Accessed 23 June 2003).

British Thoracic Society (BTS) (1997). Guidelines for the Management of Chronic Obstructive Pulmonary Disease. *Thorax* 52 (S5), S1–S28.

British Thoracic Society (BTS) (1999). Standards of Care Committee. The diagnosis, assessment and treatment of diffuse parenchymal lung disease in adults. *Thorax* 54 (Suppl 1), S1–S28(April).

British Thoracic Society (BTS) (2001a). Guidelines for the management of community acquired pneumonia in adults. *Thorax* 56 (Suppl 4), iv1–64(December).

British Thoracic Society (BTS) (2001b). Standards of Care Subcommittee for Pulmonary Rehabilitation. BTS Statement: pulmonary rehabilitation. *Thorax* 56, 827–834.

British Thoracic Society (BTS) and Scottish Intercollegiate Guidelines Network (SIGN) (2003). Guidelines for asthma. *Thorax* 58 (Suppl 1), i1–i83.

Butland, R.J.A., Pang, J., Gross, E.R., Woodcock, A.A. and Geddes, D.M. (1982). 2, 6, and 12-minute walking tests in respiratory disease. *British Medical Journal* 284, 1607–8.

Chatham, K., Baldwin, J., Olwen, W., Summer, L. and Griffiths, H. (1996). Fixed load incremental respiratory muscle training: a pilot study. *Physiotherapy* 82, 422–6.

CF Trust (2001). *Clinical Guidelines for Cystic Fibrosis Care*. Cystic Fibrosis Trust, Bromley, Kent.

Coppoolse, R., Schols, A.M.W.J., Baarendss, E.M., Mostert, R., Akkermans, M.A., Janssen, P.P. and Wouters, E.F.M. (1999). Interval versus continuous training in patients with severe COPD: a randomised clinical trial. *European Respiratory Journal* 14, 258–63.

Criner, G.J., Cordova, F.C., Furukawa, S., Kuzma, A.M., Travaline, J.M., Leyenson, V. and O'Brien, G.M. (1999). Prospective randomised trial comparing bilateral lung volume reduction surgery to pulmonary rehabilitation in severe COPD. *American Journal of Respiratory and Critical Care Medicine* 160, 2018–27.

Dantzker, D.R., Patten, G.A. and Bower, J.S. (1982). Gas exchange at rest and during exercise in adults with cystic fibrosis. *American Review Respiratory Disease* 125, 400–405.

Durstine, S.L. and Moore, G.E. (2003). *ACSM Exercise Management for Persons with Chronic Diseases and Disabilities*. Human Kinetics, Champaign, Ill.

Dyer, C.A.E., Singh, S.J., Stockley, R.A., Sinclair, A.J. and Hill, S.L. (2002). The incremental shuttle walking test in elderly people with chronic airflow limitation. *Thorax* 57, 34–8.

Enright, P.L. and Sherrill, D.L. (1998). Reference equations for the six-minute walk in healthy adults. *American Journal of Respiratory and Critical Care Medicine* 158 (5 Pt 1), 1384–7.

Enright, P.L., McBurnie, A., Bittner, V., Tracey, R.P., McNamara, R., Arnold, A. and Newman, A.B. (2003). The 6-minute walk test – a quick measure of functional status in elderly adults. *Chest* **123** (2), 387–98.

European Respiratory Society (ERS) (1997). Clinical testing with reference to lung diseases: indications, standardisation and interpretation strategies. ERS task force on standardisation of clinical exercise testing. *European Respiratory Journal* **10**, 2662–89.

Farrell, M. and Richards, J. (1986). Analysis of the reliability and validity of the kinetic communicator exercise device. *Medicine and Science in Sports and Exercise* **18**, 44–9.

Garrod, R. (2003). *The Effectiveness of Pulmonary Rehabilitation: Evidence and Implications for Health Care Practitioners.* Chartered Society of Physiotherapy, London.

Garrod, R., Bestall, J.C., Paul, E., Wedzicha, J.A. and Jones, P.W. (2000a). Development and validation of a standardised measure of activity of daily living in patients with severe COPD: the London Chest Activity of Daily Living Scale (LCADL). *Respiratory Medicine* **94**, 589–96.

Garrod, R., Mickelsons, C., Paul, E. and Wedzicha, J.A. (2000b). Randomised controlled trial of domicillary positive pressure ventilation and physical training in severe chronic obstructive pulmonary disease. *American Journal of Respiratory and Critical Care Medicine* **162** (4), 1335.

Garrod, R., Paul, E.A. and Wedzicha, J.A. (2000c). Supplemental oxygen during pulmonary rehabilitation in patients with COPD with exercise hypoxaemia. *Thorax* **55**, 539–43.

Gee, L., Abbott, J., Conway, S.P., Etherington, C. and Webb, A.K. (2000). Development of a disease specific health related quality of life measure for adults with cystic fibrosis. *Thorax* **55**, 946–54.

Gibbons, W.J., Fruchter, N., Sloan, S. and Levy, R.D. (2001). Reference values for a multiple repetition six-minute walk test in healthy adults older than 20 years. *Journal of Cardiopulmonary Rehabilitation* **21** (2), 87–93.

Gift, A.G. (1989). Validation of a vertical visual analogue scale as a measure of clinical dyspnoea. *Rehabilitation Nursing* **14**, 323–325.

Girsh, M., Trayner, E., Dammann, O., Pinto-Plata, V. and Celli, B. (2001). Symptom-limited stair climbing as a predictor of post-operative cardiopulmonary complications after high-risk surgery. *Chest* **120**, 1147–51.

Global Initiative for Chronic Obstructive Lung Disease (GOLD) NHLBI/WHO Workshop Summary (2001). Report on the global strategy for the diagnosis, management and prevention of COPD. *American Journal of Respiratory and Critical Care Medicine* **163**, 1256–76.

Green, R.H., Singh, S.J., Williams, J. and Morgan, M.D. (2001). A randomised controlled trial of four weeks versus seven weeks of pulmonary rehabilitation in chronic obstructive pulmonary disease. *Thorax* **56**, 143–5.

Guyatt, G.H., Berman, L.B., Townsend, M., Pugsley, S.O. and Chambers, L.W. (1987). A measure of quality of life for clinical trials in chronic respiratory disease. *Thorax* **42**, 733–88.

Hawkins, P., Johnson, L.C., Nikoletou, D., Hamnegard, C.H., Sherwood, R., Polkey, M.I. and Moxham, J. (2002). Proportional assist ventilation as an aid to exercise training in severe chronic obstructive pulmonary disease. *Thorax* **57**, 853–9.

Holden, D.A., Rice, T.W., Stelmach, K. and Meeker, D.P. (1992). Exercise testing, 6 minute walk and stair climb in the evaluation of patients at high risk for pulmonary resection. *Chest* **102**, 1774–79.

Hunt, S.M., McEwan, J. and McKenna, S.P. (1985). Measuring health status: a new tool for clinicians and epidemiologists. *Journal of the Royal College of Practitioners* **35**, 185–88.

Hyland, M.E., Bott, J., Singh, S. and Kenyon, C.A. (1994). Domains, constructs and the development of the breathing problems questionnaire. *Quality of Life Research* 3, 245–56.

Jones, P.W., Quirk, F.H., Baveystock, C.M. and Littlejohns, P. (1992). A self complete measure of health status for chronic airflow limitation: the St George's respiratory questionnaire. *American Review of Respiratory Disease* 145, 1321–7.

Juniper, E.F., Guyatt, G.H., Epstein, R.S., Ferrie, P.J., Jaesche, R. and Hiller, J.K. (1992). Evaluation of impairment of health related quality of life in asthma: development of a questionnaire for use in clinical trials. *Thorax* 47, 76–83.

Kaplan, R.M., Atkins, C.J. and Timms, R. (1984). Validity of a quality of well-being scale as an outcome measure in chronic obstructive pulmonary disease. *Journal of Chronic Diseases* 37, 85–95.

Kealy, S., Hussey, J. and Lane, S.J. (2003). Reasons for exercise intolerance in patients with COPD. *Physical Therapy Reviews* 8, 17–26.

Kielty, S.E.J., Ponte, J., Fleming. T.A. and Moxham, J. (1994). Effect of inspiratory pressure support on exercise tolerance and breathlessness in patients with severe stable chronic obstructive pulmonary disease. *Thorax* 49, 990–4.

Kirsten, D.K., Taube, C., Lehnigk, B., Jorres, A. and Magunssen, H. (1998). Exercise training improves recovery in patients with COPD after an acute exacerbation. *Respiratory Medicine* 92, 1191–8.

Lacasse, Y., Brosscan, L., Milnes, S., Martins, S., Wong, E., Buyatt, G.H., Goldstein, R.J. and White, J. (2003). Pulmonary rehabilitation for COPD (Cochrane Review). In *The Cochrance Library*, 2. John Wiley and Sons, Chichester.

Lands, L.C., Hornby, L., Desrochers, G., Iler, T. and Heigenhauser, G.J. (1994). A simple isokinetic cycle for measurement of leg muscle function. *Journal of Applied Physiology* 77, 2506–10.

Lareau, S.C., Carrieri-Kohlman, V., Janson-Bjerklie, S. and Roos, P.J. (1994). Development and testing of the pulmonary function status and dyspnoea questionnaire (PFSGQ). *Heart and Lung* 23, 242–50.

Lewis, M. (2003). Intensive care unit rehabilitation within the United Kingdom: Review. *Physiotherapy* 89, 531–8.

Lewis, M.I. and Belman, M.J. (1987). Nutritional supplementation in ambulatory patients with chronic obstructive pulmonary disease. *American Review Respiratory Disease* 135, 1062–7.

McArdle, W.D., Katch, F. and Katch, V. (2001). *Exercise Physiology, Energy Nutrition and Human Performance*. Lippincott Williams and Wilkins, Baltimore.

Master, A.M. and Oppenheimer, E.T. (1929). A simple exercise tolerance test for circulatory efficiency with standard tables for normal individuals. *American Journal of Medical Science* 177, 223–43.

Mathias, S., Nayak, U.S.L. and Isaacs, B. (1986). Balance in elderly patients: the 'get-up and go' test. *Archives of Physical Medicine and Rehabilitation* 67, 387–9.

Medical Research Council (1966). *Committee on Research into Chronic Bronchitis: Instructions for Use on the Questionnaire on Respiratory Symptoms*. W.J. Holman, Devon.

Mysliwiec, V. and Pina, S.E. (1999). Bronchiectasis; the 'other' obstructive lung disease. *Postgraduate Medicine* 106 (1), 123–31.

Nava, S. (1998). Rehabilitation of patients admitted to a respiratory intensive care unit. *Archives of Physical Medicine and Rehabilitation* 79, 849–54.

Nevill, A.M. and Atkinson, G. (1997). Assessing agreement between measurements recorded on a ratio scale in sports medicine and sports science. *British Journal Sports Medicine* 31, 314–8.

Ng, G.Y. and Stokes, M.J. (1991). Maximal inspiratory and expiratory mouth pressures in sitting and half lying positions in normal subjects. *Respiratory Medicine* 3, 209–11.

Noonan, V. and Dean, E. (2000) Sub-maximal exercise testing: clinical application and interpretation. *Physical Therapy* 80, 782–807.

Podsiadlo, D. and Richardson, S. (1991). The timed 'up and go': a test of basic functional mobility for frail elderly persons. *Journal of the American Geriatric Society* 39, 142–8.

Pollock, M., Roa, J., Benditt, J. and Celli, B. (1993). Estimation of ventilatory reserve by stair climbing: a study in patients with chronic airflow obstruction. *Chest*, 104, 1378–83.

Quittner, A.L., Sweeny, S., Watrous, M., Munzberger, P., Bearss, K., Gibson, N.A., Fisher, L. and Henry, B. (2000). Translation and linguistic validation of a disease-specific quality of life measure for cystic fibrosis. *Journal of Pediatric Psychology* 25, 403–14 .

Ram, F.S.F., Robinson, S.M. and Black, P.N. (2003). Physical training in asthma. (Cochrane Review). In *The Cochrane Library*, 2. Oxford: update software. (Accessed 25 June 2003).

Redelmeir, D.A., Bayoumi, A.M., Goldstein, R.S. and Guyatt, G.H. (1997). Interpreting small differences in functional status: the six-minute walk test in chronic lung disease patients. *American Journal of Respiratory and Critical Care Medicine* 155, 1278–82.

Revill, S.M., Morgan, M.D.L., Singh, S.J., Williams, J. and Hardman, A.E. (1999). The endurance shuttle walk: a new field test for the assessment of endurance capacity in chronic obstructive pulmonary disease. *Thorax* 54, 213–22.

Roca, J. and Whipp, B.J. (eds). (1997). *European Respiratory Society Monograph 6: Clinical Exercise Testing*. European Respiratory Society, Lausanne.

Rooyackers, J.M., Dekhuijzen, P.N., Van Herwaarden, C.L. and Folgering, H.T. (1997). Training with supplemental oxygen in patients with COPD and hypoxaemia at peak exercise. *European Respiratory Journal* 10, 1278–84.

Rosso, V., Passino, C., Assunta, A., Bonaguidi, F., Bramanti, F., Bruno, F., Mariari, L. and Emdin, M. (2002). Cardiopulmonary monitoring of patients with chronic heart failure: use of a new system for ambulatory monitoring. In: X11 National Meeting of the Italian Association of Sleep Medicine, Pemgia. Institute of Clinical Physiology CNR National Research Council, Pisa.

Royal College of Physicians (RCP). (1999). *Domiciliary Oxygen Therapy Services. Clinical Guidelines and Advice for Prescribers*. A Report of the Royal College of Physicians, London.

Sciaky, A.J. (1994). Mobilising the intensive care patient: pathophysiology and treatment. *Physical Therapy Practice* 3, 69–80.

Simpson, K., Killian, K., McCartney, N., Stubbing, D.G. and Jones, N.L. (1992). Randomised controlled trial of weightlifting exercise in patients with chronic airflow limitation. *Thorax* 47, 70–5.

Singh, S.J. and Morgan, M.D. (2001). Activity monitors can detect brisk walking in patients with chronic obstructive pulmonary disease. *Journal of Cardiopulmonary Rehabilitation* 21 (3), 143–8.

Singh, S.J., Morgan, M.D.L., Scott, S., Walters, D. and Hardman, A.E. (1992). Development of a shuttle walking test of disability in patients with chronic airways obstruction. *Thorax* 47, 1019–25.

Singh, S.J., Morgan, M.D.L., Hardman, A.E., Rowe, C. and Bardsley, P.A. (1994). Comparison of oxygen uptake during a conventional treadmill test and the shuttle walking test in chronic airflow limitation. *European Respiratory Journal* 7, 2016–20.

Singh, S.J., Smith, D.L., Hyland, M.E. and Morgan, D.L. (1998). A short outpatient pulmonary rehabilitation programme: immediate and longer term effects on exercise performance and quality of life. *Respiratory Medicine* 92, 1146–54.

Singh, S.J., Jones, P.J., Sewell, L., Williams, J.E. and Morgan, M.D. (2002). What is the minimum clinically important difference in the incremental shuttle walking test (ISWT) observed in pulmonary rehabilitation. *European Respiratory Society* 120 (S38), 520.

Smith, M. and Ball, V. (1998). *Cardiovascular/Respiratory Physiotherapy*. Mosby, London.

Solway, S., Brooks, D., Lacasse, Y. and Thomas, S.A. (2001). Qualitative systematic overview of the measurement properties of functional walk tests used in the cardiorespiratory domain. *Chest* 119, 256–70.

Steibellebner, L., Quittan, M., End, A., Wieselthaler, G., Klepekto, W., Haber, P. and Burghuber, O.C. (1998). Aerobic endurance training program improves exercise performance in lung transplant recipients. *Chest* 113, 906–12.

Stiller, K. and Phillips, A. (2003). Safety aspects of mobilising acutely ill patients. *Physiotherapy Therapy and Practice* 19, 239–57.

Swinburn, C.R., Wakefield, J.M. and Jones, P.W. (1985). Performance, ventilation and oxygen consumption in three different types of exercise test in patients with chronic obstructive lung disease. *Thorax* 40, 581–6.

Vale, F., Reardon, J.Z. and ZuWallack, R.L. (1993). The long-term benefits of outpatient pulmonary rehabilitation on exercise endurance and quality of life. *Chest* 103, 42–5.

Vallet, G., Ahmaidi, S., Serres, I., Fabre, C., Bourgouin, D., Desplan, J., Varray, A. and Prefaut, C. (1997). Comparison of two training programmes in chronic airway limitation patients: standardised versus individualised protocols. *European Respiratory Journal* 10, 114–22.

Van't Hull, A., Kwakkel, G. and Gosselink, R. (2002). The acute effects of non-invasive ventilatory support during exercise on exercise endurance and dyspnoea in patients with chronic obstructive pulmonary disease: a systematic review. *Journal of Cardiopulmonary Rehabilitation* 22 (4), 290–7.

Ware, J.E. and Sherbourne, C.D. (1992). The MOS 36-item short form health survey (SF–36). 1: Conceptual framework and item selection. *Medical Care* 30, 473–83.

Wasserman, K., Hansen, J.E., Sue, D.Y., Whipp, B.J. and Casaburi, R. (1994). *Principles of Exercise Testing and Interpretation*, 2nd edn. Lea and Febiger, Philadelphia.

Webb, A.K. and Dodd, M.E. (1999). Exercise and sport in cystic fibrosis: benefits and risks. *British Journal of Sports Medicine* 33, 77–8.

Wilson, R.C. and Jones, P.W. (1989). A comparison of the visual analogue scale and modified Borg scale for the measurement of dyspnoea during exercise. *Clinical Science* 76, 277–83.

Yohannes, A.M., Roomi, J., Winn, S. and Connolly, M.J. (2000). The Manchester Activities of Daily Living questionnaire: development, reliability, validity, and responsiveness to pulmonary rehabilitation. *Journal of the American Geriatrics Society* 48, 1496–500.

Zigmond, A. and Snaith, R.P. (1983). The Hospital Anxiety and Depression Score. *Acta Psychiatrica Scandinavia* 67, 361–70.

Bibliography

Agency for Health Care Policy and Research (1992). *Acute Pain Management, Operative or Medical Procedures and Trauma*. (Clinical Practice Guideline). Publication No. AHCPR 92–0032. Agency for Health Care Policy and Research, Public Health Service, US, Department of Health and Human Services, Rockville, Md.

Association of Chartered Health Care Practitioners in Cystic Fibrosis (ACPCF) (2002). *Clinical Guidelines for the Physiotherapy Management of Cystic Fibrosis*. Cystic Fibrosis Trust, Bromley, Kent.

Chapter 10
EXERCISE IN THE TREATMENT OF MUSCULOSKELETAL DISEASE

Fiona Wilson-O'Toole

Key words: aerobic exercise, flexibility and range of movement exercises, osteoporosis, back pain, resistance.

Introduction

Traditionally, exercise therapy was the mainstay of treatment for musculoskeletal dysfunction for many physiotherapists. Work by clinicians such as Cyriax, and later Grieve and Maitland, popularised the use of manipulation/mobilisation therapy from the 1950s onwards. This, along with the increased availability and use of modern electrotherapy equipment, lead to a decrease in exercise being the primary treatment of choice. Research by authors such as Comerford, Jull, Richardson and Sahrmann (to name only a few) not only provided an evidence base for the use of exercise in the treatment of musculoskeletal disease, but also caused a renewed interest in the early 1990s.

The purpose of this chapter is to outline the use of exercise as therapy in the treatment of musculoskeletal disease. In particular, inflammatory arthropathies, osteoporosis, osteoarthritis and low back pain will be examined. The types of exercise employed will be discussed and evidence for its use investigated. The foundations of therapeutic exercise in musculoskeletal disease will be applied in each case. Shankar (1998) describes these as:

- Stretching
- Range of movement exercises
- Strengthening exercises
- Proprioceptive or balance training

In addition, the use of aerobic training and its benefits will be investigated. An understanding of the physiological effects of exercise on musculoskeletal tissues as discussed in previous chapters is required.

Exercise in the management of inflammatory arthropathies

Inflammatory arthropathies may be simply classified as pathologies which cause inflammation of varying numbers of joints. Examples include rheumatoid arthritis (RA), ankylosing spondylitis and juvenile rheumatoid arthritis (JRA). All are characterised by symptoms of:

- Pain
- Fatigue
- Joint stiffness

McMeeken et al. (1999) also described symptoms of progressive symmetrical joint destruction, muscle atrophy, loss of strength and increasing functional impairment in RA. Such symptoms may be used as objective markers when using exercise therapy, thus allowing its efficacy to be monitored. An objective marker is a sign or symptom that may demonstrate changes following the use of a treatment modality. For example: pain may be assessed using the visual analogue scale; fatigue or fitness levels may be measured using tests described in previous chapters; and changes in joint stiffness may be measured with goniometry. The management option of choice, which in this case is exercise therapy, is aimed at causing positive changes in the objective markers.

Aerobic training

Traditionally, the most important objectives of exercise therapy in RA were to maintain joint range of movement (ROM) and improve muscle strength. The exercise forms of choice tended to be those which put little stress on the joints. Historically, dynamic exercises which were of sufficient intensity to improve aerobic fitness and enhance muscle strength were avoided as they were presumed to provoke joint damage. During the last twenty years dynamic exercise has been recommended more, particularly in patients with active disease (Van Den Ende et al., 1998). A large evidence base supports this approach. Van Den Ende et al. performed a systematic review of six randomised studies on the effect of dynamic exercise in RA. The findings suggest that dynamic exercise therapy is effective in improving aerobic capacity, muscle strength and joint mobility with no evidence of negative side effects on joint inflammation or disease activity.

The type of exercise recommended is summarised well in an earlier study by Van Den Ende et al. (1996). Patients were randomly divided into a high and a low intensity exercise group. The high intensity group met for one hour three times a week and followed a programme of twelve exercises, which included twenty minutes cycling at a heart rate of 70–85% of the age predicted maximum. The group also performed dynamic weight-bearing exercises which included knee bending, step-ups, walking at fast speed, alternating with muscle strengthening exercises for the trunk and upper extremities. All exercises were performed at high pace and every four weeks a new programme with a higher exercise load was offered. The patients in this group displayed a greater improvement in joint mobility, aerobic capacity and muscle strength than a group who performed low intensity, non-weight-bearing ROM and isometric strengthening exercises.

Klepper (1999) investigated use of a similar management approach in JRA. Children and adolescents performed a sixty-minute conditioning programme which consisted of a ten-minute warm up, ten minutes of low impact aerobics, fifteen minutes of strengthening exercises and ten minutes of cool down and flexibility exercises. Fitness levels improved, as in the study described previously, and there was a decrease in mean VAS scores, which suggested that the programme had an effect on decreasing symptoms of pain. Thus, research suggests that provided that the inflammatory disease is under control, an exercise programme very similar to that given to any other non-rheumatoid patient to improve their fitness levels may be prescribed. Dosage of exercises may be progressed according to improvement, that is, positive changes in objective markers.

It must be noted at this point that none of the evidence discussed suggests that exercises described have any true effect on disease activity as measured by markers such as ESR levels and radiological changes. However, a significant change in signs and/or symptoms is demonstrated. This will be a recurring theme when applying exercise in the management of much other pathology.

Range of movement exercises

The evidence discussed to this point suggests that ROM exercises in isolation will have a limited effect on signs and symptoms. However, aerobic exercise, practised to the levels described, requires that the disease is well controlled, which may exclude patients in a distinct inflammatory phase. Of course, patients with well controlled symptoms will perform ROM exercises in conjunction with aerobic exercise as described above.

When a patient has a very painful joint, ROM exercises may improve blood flow and joint metabolism, reducing oedema and thus improving symptoms (David and Lloyd, 1999). During normal daily activity few joints are put through their full ROM. In a healthy joint this is not a problem, but in one with inflammatory disease, progressive loss of joint range will occur. It is essential to put all affected joints through their full ROM every day. This may be done actively or passively, which may be more appropriate if a joint is very painful. With active ROM assisted movements may be chosen when active movements require some assistance to reach the end of range. An important factor which must be remembered when performing ROM exercises, particularly passive, is that instability of joints is a common progression of inflammatory arthropathies, both as a result of classic pathological changes and as a side effect of drug therapy. Therefore care must always be exercised.

A simple approach to management would be to select affected joints and move each joint daily through full range of movement a specific number of times. This may be done following aerobic exercise when appropriate. No research could be identified to stipulate optimum repetition of ROM exercise, but at least ten repetitions of a movement would be a good starting point.

Strengthening exercises

The physiological effects of strengthening exercises and their importance in the treatment of disease have been discussed in previous chapters and should be considered at this point. In particular, when considering inflammatory arthropathies, joint effusions inhibit contraction of surrounding muscle groups and if a joint contracts while misaligned it will not be able to generate its peak force (Hakkinen et al., 2001). Again, the use of strengthening exercises within a programme that includes aerobic exercise has already been described, but it must be remembered that the strengthening programme must be designed to suit the individual's signs and symptoms.

In a two-year study, Hakkinen et al. (2001) examined the effects of dynamic strength training on muscle strength, disease activity, functional capacity and bone mineral density in early RA. One group of patients performed exercises for the upper and lower extremities using elastic bands for resistance, as well as abdominal and back muscle exercises using dumb-bells. Subjects exercised twice a week with loads at 50–70% of the repetition maximum, two sets per exercise and 8–12 repetitions per set. The programme took approximately 45 minutes and was combined with 30 minutes of aerobic exercise twice a week. Patients in a control group performed ROM and stretching exercises twice a week without additional resistance. Results showed that dynamic strength training showed greater improvement in outcome measures than pure static strength training. This theory was reinforced by research by Bostrom et al. (1998), which demonstrated that patients who performed dynamic shoulder rotator exercises showed greater improvements in outcome measures in RA than a group performing static exercises.

Although there is a lack of clarity in research as to how great the contribution of aerobic exercise in such programmes is on symptom reduction, the evidence appears to suggest that dynamic, rather than static or isometric strength training, should be the management of choice when disease activity permits. Resistance may be provided by elastic bands, loaded pullies, dumb-bells or water, which will be briefly described later. All these modalities will allow loading through the joint range of motion as recommended. When joints are acutely inflamed and dynamic exercise may not be appropriate, rhythmic stabilisations may be used to exercise the joint with minimal movement. As the inflammation settles, slow reversals, hold relax and repeated contractions may be used to improve muscle power.

Flexibility

Maintenance of flexibility in the patient with inflammatory arthropathies is perhaps better considered within ROM exercises. However, as with all exercises, it must be remembered that in most inflammatory arthropathies the viability of different tissues is compromised by the disease and as a result of drug therapy. The resulting instability of joints is a factor, which must be considered when designing a flexibility programme as aggressive stretching may lead to damage, producing further instability.

Along with ROM exercises, flexibility programmes may help temper progression of deformities associated with such diseases as ankylosing spondylitis.

Exercise in water

Hydrotherapy has been widely used for many years in the management of rheumatological conditions. A warm pool (traditionally maintained at 36°C) assists the patient by providing buoyancy as well as the palliative effect of heat on the tissues. A patient who may otherwise have difficulty mobilising and weight bearing through stiff and painful joints can follow a programme of exercises in the water, based on the principles described previously. The water may be used to assist and then resist movement and exercises may be graded without stressing joints.

Exercise in the management of osteoporosis

Osteoporosis may be defined as a metabolic disorder characterised by low bone mass and micro-architectural deterioration, leading to skeletal fragility and increased fracture risk. One of the major problems associated with the development of osteoporosis is an increased risk of fractures, which, at best, may be disabling for the individual and, at worst, poses a risk to life. The costs associated with such fractures are not only to the health of the individual but also to the health care budget. It is a major public health problem and one expected to increase with the significant ageing of the population (Kannus et al., 1999).

Exercise in osteoporosis is focused on bone loading, with its consequences on bone mineral density. The management approach should be towards prevention of development of osteoporosis as well as prevention of falls in those with well-established disease. The mechanical stresses that are put through bone during weight-bearing exercises are thought to directly affect the structure and geometrical characteristics of bone. As well as changes in bone density, improvements in aerobic fitness, muscle strength and balance, as a result of exercise, may help prevent falls and thus fracture rates (Mitchell et al., 1998).

There are many risk factors for osteoporosis, one of which is a sedentary lifestyle. Of all factors, this is one which may obviously be changed by participation in an exercise programme.

Signs and symptoms of osteoporosis

The signs and symptoms in osteoporosis are vague, in that an individual may be developing osteoporosis (osteopenia), or may have early or well-established osteoporosis and be unaware until they sustain a fracture. Measurement of bone mineral density by dual energy X-ray absorptiometry is currently the definitive way to diagnose the condition. Thus, a good knowledge of risk factors in a patient may allow a preventative programme to be developed.

The major osteoporotic fracture sites are the vertebrae, hip and radius (Rutherford, 1999). Pain is obviously associated with such fractures and so may be regarded as a symptom of the disease, although the presence of osteoporosis in itself should not be a cause of pain. This may be one of the reasons why many patients may be ignorant of the condition until a fracture is sustained. Postural changes are frequently associated with well established osteoporosis. One such change is the increasing development of a thoracic kyphosis, which may be due to anterior wedge fractures in the thoracic vertebrae. This will obviously cause pain at the time of the fracture, but the associated change in thoracic biomechanics may lead to dysfunction and pain in thoracic joints. The decreased mobility in the thorax may lead to associated pulmonary consequences.

Assessment of an osteoporotic patient prior to provision of an exercise programme would include measurement of those principles discussed previously such as, aerobic capacity, ROM, strength and balance, as well as a review of investigations such as BMD levels (bone mineral density). As with inflammatory arthropathies, the programme must not be generic but should be prescribed precisely for the patient according to levels of pathology.

Aerobic training

There are a number of epidemiological studies as well as controlled trials to suggest that weight-bearing, aerobic exercise has beneficial effects on bone (Baumann et al., 1999; Rutherford, 1999; Khan et al., 2001; Zhao, 2001). Current recommendations are that high impact exercise which produces ground reaction forces greater than two times the body weight is required for optimum benefit (Heinonen et al., 1998). The type of exercise that would be suitable could include power walking, running, stair climbing and dancing at moderate intensity, such as 70–80% of $\dot{V}O_2$max. Khan et al. (2001) recommend that such exercise should be undertaken for one hour at least three times a week for at least eight to nine months, but preferably indefinitely. Activities such as cycling and swimming, which are non-weightbearing, have not been proven to have any beneficial effects and therefore should not be prescribed.

In older age groups at risk, such as post-menopausal females, high impact exercise may not be appropriate because of risk of injury. In these cases, the beneficial effects of strengthening exercises may be utilised as an alternative form of bone loading.

Strengthening exercises

A number of recent studies have demonstrated that resistance training has a positive effect on bone mineral density (Swezey et al., 2000; Taaffe and Marcus, 2000; Kelley et al., 2001). A review of such literature suggests that mechanical strains of resisted muscle contraction stimulates an osteogenic response in the spine in particular, but also in the femur and radius, particularly in post-menopausal women.

Strength training at 70% 1 RM is recommended as safe and effective at maintaining bone mass (Hartard et al., 1996). A programme of approximately ten exercises covering the major muscle groups should be designed. Each exercise should be repeated eight to twelve times with the set repeated twice. Swezey et al. (2000) recommend resisted isometric exercises for ten minutes daily as being adequate to strengthen muscles and enhance bone formation. A typical programme could include the following exercises:

- Biceps curl
- Triceps extension
- Bench press
- Overhead pull-downs
- Wrist extension
- Leg press
- Hamstring curls
- Hip abduction/adduction
- Hip flexion/extension
- Toe raises

Pulleys, fixed or free weights, or elastic bands of differing resistance may provide resistance.

Flexibility and range of movement exercises

Maintenance of normal range of movement of joints is a challenge presented by ageing. However, specific postural changes that occur in osteoporosis may lead to joint dysfunction in associated joints. Also, following a fracture, ROM exercises are essential to achieve good return to normal movement in joints. One of the areas presenting the greatest problem is the thorax. Flexion loading increases the chance of vertebral wedge fractures (Khan et al., 2001). Flexibility exercises, which encourage thoracic extension, may provide a preventative role. For the same reason, patients with osteoporosis should avoid exercises which train trunk flexion. This particularly applies when the exercise involves loading, such as sit-ups.

General range of movement exercises of the thoracic spine may also have a beneficial effect on pulmonary function, which can be affected in developing kyphotic posture.

General posture should be observed and imbalance in muscle groups corrected in as early a stage as possible in the disease. Exercise classes which include yoga or Pilates may be useful, providing the instructor has a good understanding of the level of disease pathology and exercises are adapted accordingly. The usual rules of warm up and stretching prior to an exercise programme apply in osteoporosis management.

Proprioceptive and balance training

A major consequence of osteoporosis is that a sufferer is at a higher risk of sustaining a fracture from what might otherwise be an innocuous fall. Although

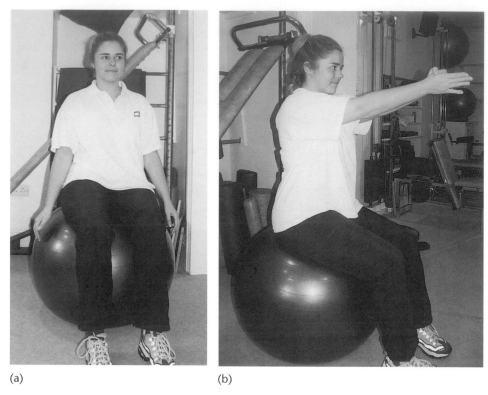

(a)   (b)

Figure 10.1 Using a Swiss ball for proprioceptive training.

evidence to support it is scant, it would make sense that balance training and correction of proprioceptive deficits may help prevent falls. Such training may be included in the programmes of exercise described previously and may include activity such as walking along a narrow line, using a Swiss ball (Figure 10.1a,b) or balancing on a wobble board. For further information in this area, the reader should refer to the work of Skelton and McLoughlin (1996).

It must be remembered that much of the research has been done on post-menopausal women and exercises designed with this group in mind. However, with the knowledge available regarding the influence of exercise on bone health, these principles should be applied early in life. The aim should be to maximise peak bone mass in children and adolescents by encouraging regular participation in high impact weight-bearing activity. In the older population, where signs of osteopenia or established osteoporosis are present, the aim is to preserve mass with activities described above.

Exercise in the management of osteoarthritis

Osteoarthritis (OA) is the most common form of arthritis and has been identified as affecting millions of people in the USA (Felson et al., 2000). It is a degenerative process acquired because of metabolic, mechanical, genetic and other influences. It is characterised by progressive loss of cartilage and bony overgrowth (Oddis, 1996). In the US, symptomatic disease in the knee occurs in approximately 6% and symptomatic hip OA in roughly 3% of the population. As OA prevalence increases with age, it is estimated to become more prevalent in the future (Felson et al., 2000). Symptoms can be disabling and treatment of a disease with such high incidence in the population has considerable socio-economic costs.

The management of OA has shown progressions in recent years, with more sophisticated drug and surgical treatment being offered. However, exercise therapy remains one of the main treatment options of choice for physiotherapists.

Signs and symptoms of osteoarthritis

The diagnosis of OA is made primarily radiographically and from analysis of presenting clinical features. A patient may present with advanced radiographic evidence of OA, which may not necessarily be married with clinical signs and symptoms of parity. Because cartilage is not innervated, it is thought that the pain of OA arises from secondary effects such as joint capsule distension, stretching of periosteal nerve endings and synovial inflammation (Oddis, 1996). Symptoms include pain in affected joints, which may be aggravated by both prolonged movement and rest. Decreased ROM is frequently seen in joints, which may be a result of protective splinting or pathology of disease on tissues such as the joint capsule. Localised oedema and other signs of inflammatory processes, such as increased temperature, are also seen, particularly in the acute phase. Some joint enlargements such as Heberden's nodes, along with joint tenderness, are classic clinical features of OA. Considering the signs and symptoms of OA, it is not surprising that it is frequently associated with loss of function and consequently varying levels of disability.

Aerobic training

When considering the role of aerobic training in the management of OA it is worth initially reviewing the established risk factors. Felson et al. (2000) cite obesity as a major risk factor, stating that for every one pound increase in weight, the over-all force across the knee in a single leg stance increases two to three pounds. A study showed that women who lost an average of eleven pounds decreased their risk for knee OA by 50% (Felson et al., 1992). The role of aerobic exercise in management of obesity has been discussed in Chapter 5 and 10.

Anecdotal evidence suggests that repeated loading of a joint may lead to destructive changes. Epidemiological studies support this, to an extent, when reviewing the particular cases of former athletes (Kujala et al., 1994; Spector et al., 1996). This volume of loading should therefore be avoided when prescribing a programme of aerobic exercise. A number of studies have highlighted the benefits of aerobic activity in the osteoarthritic patient and cite inactivity as a negative factor. Manninen et al. (2001) state that exercise, when it is moderate and recreational, is associated with a decrease in the risk of knee OA.

Oddis (1996), Rogind et al. (1998), Deyle et al. (2000), Felson et al. (2000), March et al. (2001) and Fransen et al. (2002) all studied the effect of a conditioning, that is, an aerobic exercise programme, on the signs and symptoms of osteoarthritis. None showed any deleterious effects and all showed varying levels of improvement of some outcome measures such as pain and disability. All the studies included strength training within the programme so it is difficult to assess if aerobic exercise alone is sufficient. However, exercise such as swimming, walking and cycling may be recommended, all of which will also strengthen muscles, as there is some form of loading. The type of exercise recommended included cycling for twenty minutes at 50–60% of the maximum heart rate (Fransen et al., 2002). However, no dose response relationship in aerobic exercise in osteoarthritis management has been established (Petrella et al., 2000).

In conclusion, aerobic exercise at levels normally recommended for maintenance of cardiovascular health is deemed suitable for patients suffering from OA. However, when there is advanced disease in a weight-bearing joint, exercise could be adapted to be non-weightbearing, such as cycling or swimming. There is some evidence that some forms of exercise that induce repeated very high level loading should be minimised to maintain long-term joint health.

Strengthening exercises

As well as a reduction in aerobic capacity, inactivity as a result of the symptoms of OA also results in a decrease in muscle strength. Well conditioned muscle and muscular balance are needed to attenuate impact loads and provide joint stability (Felson et al., 2000). Research has shown that good muscle function around a joint may not only have a stabilising effect but may also reduce pain. Baker et al. (2002) held a randomised controlled trial which examined the effect of home-based progressive strength training in OA. Their findings demonstrated an improvement in strength, pain, physical function and psychosocial well-being in an exercising group compared to controls. The type of exercise recommended based on such a programme could include:

- Squats and step-ups using body weight for resistance.
- Knee extension in sitting, with an ankle weight.
- Knee flexion in standing, with an ankle weight.
- Hip adduction and abduction in standing, with an ankle weight.

The intensity of the exercise set is based on difficulty perception using a modified Borg scale. Patients should perform two sets of twelve repetitions three times a week for each exercise. Figure 10.2 demonstrates the use of a pulley system to strengthen muscles around the hip (10.2a) and shoulder (10.2b).

This type of programme could be combined well with an aerobic training programme already described. It is notable that many of the studies have concentrated on knee OA; however, this is one of the most common disease sites. Slemenda et al. (1997) suggested that quadriceps weakness is a risk factor for OA, which

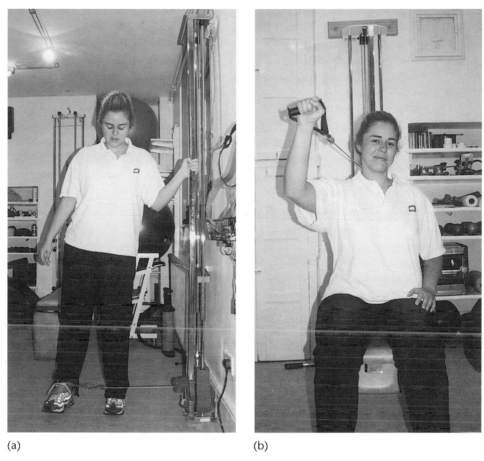

(a)   (b)

Figure 10.2 (a) Use of a pulley system to strengthen muscles around the hip. (b) Use of a pulley system to strengthen muscles around the shoulder.

would be a strong argument to include quadriceps-strengthening exercise in any fitness programme aimed at the older population. Recently, a hypothesis has been proposed that maintenance of well-conditioned muscles may result in a delay in development of OA, as pathogenesis of motor and sensory dysfunction of muscle may be important factors of pathogenesis of articular damage. (Hurley, 1999).

In conclusion, there is no doubt that strength training appears to play an important part in the management of OA, with pain reduction, functional and psychosocial well-being the improvements demonstrated (Oddis, 1996; Rogind et al., 1998; Van Baar et al., 1998; Felson et al., 2000; Penninx et al., 2001; Fransen et al., 2001). There is no clear evidence for the optimum dose response relations in strength training in OA (Vuori, 2001), so a programme must be designed with the individual symptoms and exercise response in mind.

Flexibility and range of movement exercises

As a result of pain and joint surface changes, a decrease in joint range of movement is common in OA. However, this does not appear to be an inevitable change. The author's own experience of treating elderly Muslim patients who had advanced OA changes in the knee suggests that taking the joint through the full range of movement a number of times a day, appears to help maintain joint range. Such patients prayed a number of times a day, involving a full kneeling position, taking the knee into full flexion. Such exercise appeared to help maintain full knee flexion. As mentioned previously, flexibility exercises should be routinely carried out before all the exercise programmes described above. Affected joints may then be taken through full active and passive ranges of movement. Some of the reasoning behind this has already been explained when discussing inflammatory arthropathies.

Proprioceptive and balance training

As a result of altered joint biomechanics, normal joint proprioception and balance may be altered in the OA patient. This occasionally may necessitate the use of walking aids. However, the continued use of a walking aid for pain relief may have the effect of altering normal balance reactions when the stick is removed. Both scenarios would benefit from balance exercises incorporated into a programme. The types of exercises which are suitable are included in the above discussion of osteoporosis.

Exercise in the treatment of low back pain

Back pain is a major health problem in Western society. Tulder et al. (1995) calculated that in the Netherlands in 1991, the cost of back pain to society was 1.7% of the GNP. They also showed that musculoskeletal disease was the fifth most expensive regarding hospital care and the most expensive regarding work absenteeism and disablement. Epidemiological studies by the same authors demonstrated a lifetime prevalence of low back pain (LBP) of 51% for men and 58% for women. Similar studies carried out in the USA and Scandinavia showed comparable results. Although research into causes and management of low back pain features heavily in physiotherapy and orthopaedic based journals, a definitive method of treatment remains elusive. Inevitably, management methods change over years in response to research. Following years of a manipulation based approach, clinicians are returning to exercise as a primary treatment of choice. This is mainly as a response to published evidence from clinical trials.

Koes et al. (2001) compared national clinical guidelines on low back pain around the world. Consistent features advised early and gradual activation of patients and the discouragement of prescribed bed rest. Most countries advise those with an acute back pain episode to 'stay active', while back specific exercises are not recommended at this stage. However, in the USA, low-stress aerobic exercises are recommended as a therapeutic option at this stage. Beyond the acute stage, all countries advised exercise therapy as a treatment option of choice.

Aerobic training

The benefit of aerobic exercise in the management of low back pain is not clear. A number of studies appear to produce conflicting evidence. Aerobic exercise is frequently incorporated into rehabilitation programmes on the assumption that relative disability due to LBP leads to low levels of fitness. However, the literature in this area is inconclusive. Hurri et al. (1991) analysed aerobic capacity in chronic low back pain patients as 'average' while McQuade et al. (1988) described similar patients as having 'very low' aerobic fitness. This is in conflict with a study by Wittink et al. (2000), which analysed the aerobic fitness of 50 chronic low back pain patients in comparison to normative data. Levels of fitness in such patients were found to be comparable to healthy subjects. A controlled trial by Mannion et al. (2001a) compared the efficacy of active physiotherapy, muscle reconditioning on training devices and low impact aerobics on patients with low back pain. The patients in the aerobics group took part in low impact aerobics classes lasting one hour. The class included warm up, stretching, low impact aerobic exercises and 20 to 30 minutes of specific trunk and leg muscle exercises. The three active treatments were equally efficacious in improving outcome measures. The aerobics classes were found to be the most cost efficient as 12 patients could be treated at one time. This presents a strong economic argument for the use of aerobic exercise as a management tool.

In the absence of a definitive answer, clinical guidelines, which suggest a return to normal activity (including exercise) following an incident of acute LBP, should be followed (Underwood, 2000). McGill (1998) suggests that not only does aerobic exercise have a function in the treatment of LBP but also that it may have a preventative role. He cites Videman et al. (1995), who examined age-related changes in the spines of elderly people as a function of lifelong activity level. They found that those who were involved in aerobic exercise as opposed to power sports showed less age-related changes in lumbar tissues. It would therefore seem that aerobic exercise, such as walking or cycling, has a role both in management and prevention of LBP. Normal guidelines for improvement of cardiovascular function should be followed when selecting heart rates and duration of exercise. However, the pathology of the disease must be taken into account when positioning the patient. For example, the flexed position of the lumbar spine may aggravate a lumbar disc problem and in this case, swimming may be a more suitable exercise.

Strengthening exercises

When many clinicians describe exercise therapy in LBP patients, they probably frequently mean strength training of lumbar and abdominal musculature. There has been a large amount of research performed in this area in recent years with many schools of thought providing different approaches. Many of these studies have documented an association between LBP and sub-optimal back muscle function and reduced muscle strength (Cassisi et al., 1993), increased muscle fatigueabilty (Latimer et al., 1999) and alterations in muscles' internal size and structure (Kaser et al., 2001). Although some of these factors may have lead to a development of LBP, the consensus is that these factors arise as a consequence of the pain, associated inactivity and the subsequent onset of the disease process (Mannion et al., 2001b). Although the research is not clear it would appear to be logical to try and reverse this deconditioning in rehabilitation. Hence the role of exercise.

To understand the physiological effects that strengthening exercises have on tissues, the chapter discussing this must be reviewed. When considering the case of LBP, the role that muscles play in stabilising a joint has been given particular importance in recent years. Hides et al. (1994, 1996) suggest that certain muscle groups, in particular multifidus, show evidence of wasting following an episode of low back pain. It appears that recovery of this muscle is not automatic following injury and that this may predispose the patient to further injury. Biomechanical studies have shown that the lumbar multifidus is an important muscle for lumbar segmental instability. It is able to provide segmental stiffness and control motion in the neutral zone (Panjabi, 1989). The role of transversus abdominus in spinal stabilisation has also been highlighted and comprehensively researched in recent years. It is thought that this muscle also has a significant role in the generation of spinal stiffness and hence a stabilising function (Hodges and Richardson, 1996). Such muscles should be retrained to stabilise the joint in the neutral zone before moving into more dynamic positions. The aim should be to sustain a consistent low force hold, typically a 10×10 second hold in a neutral position. Aids, such as biofeedback, may be useful to help the patient isolate multifidus and transversus (Comerford and Mottram, 2001). It is believed that control of a joint is attained when the local stabilisers, global stabilisers and global mobilisers are rehabilitated. The work of Comerford and Mottram referenced above and Hides et al. (2001) should be read to glean a more comprehensive overview of this approach of management. Research is very much ongoing and there is insufficient room in this text to expand further. This type of approach is very specific and, as well as demonstrating improvements in outcome measures when used in isolation, it is frequently combined with a more dynamic approach such as medical exercise therapy. The basis of training therapies such as Pilates, which has seen a surge in popularity, bases much of its evidence on the work of the above authors.

Strength training may take a more dynamic approach using weights, pulleys, elastic bands or specific rehabilitation equipment such as the Swiss ball. Medical exercise therapy is another management approach which is becoming more popular. It is a system of progressively graded exercises designed by Norwegian physiotherapist, Oddvar Holten. The exercises aim to normalise function by mobilising hypomoblie areas and stabilising exercises for other parts. Patients are given individual programmes and exercise for up to one hour under the supervision of a therapist. The type of equipment that is used includes wall pulleys, lateral pulleys, angle bench dumb-bells and bar bells (Figure 10.3). Patients are given around nine exercises which they repeat 20 to 30 times in three sets with a

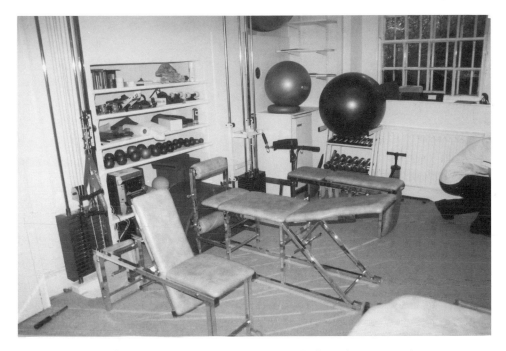

Figure 10.3 MET equipment set up for use in a small physiotherapy practice.

30 second rest between sets. By performing this number of repetitions, per set, a treatment will involve approximately 1000 repetitions, with theorised influences on circulation, endurance and coordination. Exercises are graded so that they are done free of pain, and work trunk flexion, extension and rotations exercising the abdominal and back muscles as well as the lower extremities (Torstensen et al., 1998). In a trial, Torstensen et al. demonstrated the efficacy of medical exercise therapy in improving pain, activities of daily living and patient satisfaction. They also demonstrated that such an approach might be more cost effective than conventional physiotherapy.

Flexibility and range of movement exercises

Following injury, splinting of joints or antalgic postures as a result of pain may lead to shortening of soft tissues. This may lead to altered joint biomechanics and further injury. The decision to include specific exercises in a flexibility programme must be made following examination of the patient and consideration of pathologies involved. The McKenzie method of management includes extension exercises of the lumbar spine with specific consideration of disc pathologies. However, extension exercises may be aggravating where there is a condition involving abnormality of the facet joint. Thus ROM exercises are designed following a good clinical reasoning process and according to the requirements of the patient. Shortened tissues, which may have lead to injury in the first place, should be mobilised

(Sahrmann, 2002). The type of flexibility and ROM exercises which are often included in a LBP rehabilitation programme often may include:

- Lumbar flexion in supine lying
- Lumbar extension in prone lying
- Hamstring stretches
- Hip extensor stretches
- Hip flexor stretches
- Postural correction
- Thoracic extension in sitting

These are very general examples and are not a list of generic exercises for all back pain patients.

Proprioceptive and balance training

Although there is a paucity of research in this area, there is some evidence that patients with low back pain have a less refined position sense than healthy subjects. This may be because of altered paraspinal muscle afference and central processing of this sensory input (Brumagne et al., 2000). In clinical trials Gill and Callaghan (1998) found that differences in proprioception do exist between individuals with back pain and those free from back pain. While the contribution that this deficit makes is still poorly understood, inclusion of balance training in a rehabilitation programme for LBP may have benefits.

It is important to note that there appears to be little evidence for the efficacy of exercise therapy in the treatment of low back pain in the acute stage (Frank et al., 1996; Tulder et al., 2000). In fact there is very little evidence for the efficacy of any management approach at this point. There is increasing evidence that exercise therapy may prove useful in the chronic stage (12 weeks and longer) although there seems to be no agreement on what exercises are the most effective (Faas, 1996). Most of the evidence discussed above refers to trials carried out on patients suffering from chronic back pain. The reader is encouraged to read the work of the various referenced authors to glean a more comprehensive understanding of this topic.

References

Baker, K.R., Nelson, M.E., Felson, J.E., Layne, R.S. and Roubenoff, R. (2001). The efficacy of home-based progressive strength training in older adults with knee osteoarthritis: a randomised controlled trial. *Journal of Rheumatology* **28**, 1655–65.

Bauman, W.A., Spungen, A.M., Wang, J., Pierson, R.N. and Schwartz, E. (1999). Continuous bone loss during chronic immobilisation: a monozygotic twin study. *Osteoporosis International* **10**, 123–7.

Bostrom, C., Harms-Ringdal, K., Karreskog, H. and Nordemar, R. (1998). Effect of static and dynamic shoulder rotator exercises in women with rheumatoid arthritis: a randomised comparison of impairment, disability, handicap and health. *Scandinavian Journal of Rheumatology* 27 (4), 281–90.

Brumagne, S., Cordo, P., Lysens, R., Verschueren, S. and Swinnen, S. (2000). The role of paraspinal muscle spindles in lumbo-sacral position sense in individuals with and without low back pain. *Spine* 25 (8), 989–94.

Cassisi, J.E., Robinson, M.E. and O'Connor, P. (1993). Trunk strength and lumbar paraspinal muscle activity during isometric exercise in chronic low back pain patients and controls. *Spine* 18, 245–51.

Comerford, M.J. and Mottram, S.L. (2001). Functional stability retraining: principles and strategies for managing mechanical dysfunction. *Manual Therapy* 6 (1), 3–14.

David, C. and Lloyd, J. (1999). *Rheumatological Physiotherapy*. Mosby International Limited, London.

Deyle, G.D., Henderson, N.E., Matekel, R.L., Ryder, M.G., Garber, M.B. and Allison, S.C. (2000). Effectiveness of manual physical therapy and exercise in osteoarthritis of the knee: a randomised clinical trial. *Annals of Internal Medicine* 132 (3), 173–81.

Faas, A. (1996). Exercises: which ones are worth trying, for which patients and when? *Spine* 21 (24), 2874–8.

Felson, D.T. (2000). Osteoarthritis: new insights. Part 1: The disease and its risk factors. *Annals of Internal Medicine* 133, 637–9.

Felson, D.T. (2000). Osteoarthritis: new insights. Part 2: Treatment approaches. *Annals of Internal Medicine* 133, 726–9.

Felson, D.T., Zhang, Y., Anthony, J.M., Naimark, A. and Anderson, J.J. (1992). Weight loss reduces the risk for symptomatic knee osteoarthritis in women. The Framingham study. *Annals of Internal Medicine* 116, 535–9.

Frank, J.W., Brooker, A., DeMaio, S.E., Kerr, M.S., Maetzel, A., Shannon, H.S., Sullivan, T.J., Norman, R.W. and Wells, R.P. (1996). Disability resulting from occupational low back pain. *Spine* 21 (24), 2918–29.

Fransen, M., Crosbie, J. and Edmonds, J. (2001). Physical therapy is effective for patients with osteoarthritis of the knee: a randomised controlled clinical trial. *Journal of Rheumatology* 28, 156–64.

Gill, K.P. and Callaghan, M.J. (1998). The measurement of lumbar proprioception in individuals with and without low back pain. *Spine* 23, 371–7.

Hakkinen, A., Sokka, T., Kotaniemi, A. and Hannonen, P. (2001). A randomised two-year study of the effects of dynamic strength training on muscle strength, disease activity, functional capacity and bone mineral density in early rheumatoid arthritis. *Arthritis and Rheumatism* 44 (3), 515–22.

Hartard, M., Haber, P., Ilieva, D., Preisinger, E., Seidl, G. and Huber, J. (1996). Systematic strength training as a model of therapeutic intervention. *American Journal of Physical Medicine and Rehabilitation* 75, 21–8.

Heinonen, A., Oja, P., Sievanen, H., Pasenen, M. and Vuori, I. (1998). Effect of two training regimes on bone mineral density in healthy peri-menopausal women: a randomised controlled trial. *Journal of Bone and Mineral Research* 13, 483–90.

Hides, J., Stokes, M., Saide, M., Jull, G. and Cooper, D.H. (1994). Evidence of lumbar multifidus muscle wasting ipsilateral to symptoms in patients with acute/subacute low back pain. *Spine* 19 (2), 165–72.

Hides, J., Richardson, C. and Jull, G. (1996). Multifidus recovery is not automatic after resolution of acute, first episode low back pain. *Spine* 21 (23), 2763–9.

Hides, J., Jull, G. and Richardson, C. (2001). Long-term effects of specific stabilising exercises for first episode low back pain. *Spine* 26 (11), e243–e248.

Hodges, P.W. and Richardson, C.A. (1996). Inefficient muscular stabilisation of the lumbar spine associated with low back pain. *Spine* 21 (22), 2640–50.

Hurley, M. (1999). The role of muscle weakness in the pathogenesis of osteoarthritis. *Rheumatic Disease Clinics of North America* 25 (2), 283–98.

Hurri, H., Mellin, G., Korhonen, O., Harjula, R. Harkapaa, K. and Luoma, J. (1991). Aerobic capacity among chronic back pain patients. *Journal of Spinal Disorders* 4, 34–8.

Kannus, P., Niemi, S., Parkkari, J., Palvenen, M., Vuori, I. and Jarvinen, M. (1999). Hip fractures in Finland between 1970 and 1997 and predictions for the future. *Lancet* 353, 802–5.

Kaser, L., Mannion, A.F., Rhyner, A., Weber, E., Dvorak, J. and Muntener, M. (2001). Active therapy for chronic low back pain. Part 2: Effects on paraspinal muscle cross sectional area, fibre type size and distribution. *Spine* 26 (8), 909–19.

Kelley, G.A., Kelley, K.S. and Tran, Z.V. (2001). Resistance training and bone mineral density in women. A meta-analysis of controlled trials. *American Journal of Physical Medicine and Rehabilitation* 80, 65–77.

Khan, K., Mckay, H., Kannus, P., Bailey, D., Wark, J. and Bennell, K. (2001). *Physical Activity and Bone Health*. Human Kinetics, Champaign, Ill.

Klepper, S.E. (1999). Effects of an eight-week physical conditing program an disease signs and symptoms in children with chronic arthritis. *Arthritis Care and Research* 12 (1), Feb., 52–60.

Koes, B.W., Van Tulder, M., Ostelo, R., Burton, A.K. and Waddell, G. (2001). Clinical guidelines for the management of low back pain in primary care. *Spine* 26, 2504–13.

Kujala, U.M., Kaprio, J. and Sarna, S. (1994). Osteoarthritis of the weight-bearing joints of lower limbs in former elite male athletes. *British Medical Journal* 308, 231–4.

Latimer, J., Maher, C.G., Refshauge, K. and Colaco, I. (1999). The reliability and validity of the Biering-Sorensen test in asymptomatic subjects and subjects reporting current or previous non-specific low back pain. *Spine* 24 (20), 2085–90.

McGill, S.M. (1998). Low back exercises: evidence for improving exercise regimes. *Physical Therapy* 78 (7), 754–65.

McMeeken, J., Stillman, B., Story, I., Kent, P. and Smith, J. (1999). The effects of knee extensor and flexor muscle training on the timed up and go test in individuals with rheumatoid arthritis. *Physiotherapy Research International* 4 (1), 55–67.

McQuade, K., Turner, J. and Buchner, D.M. (1988). Physical fitness and chronic low back pain: an analysis of the relationship between fitness, functional limitations and depression. *Clinical Orthopaedics and Related Research* 233, 198–204.

Manninen, P., Riihimaki, H., Heliovaara, M. and Suomalainen, O. (2001). Physical exercise and risk of severe knee osteoarthritis requiring arthroplasty. *Rheumatology* 40 (4), 432–7.

Mannion, A.F., Muntener, M., Taimela, S. and Dvorak, J. (2001a). Comparison of three active therapies for chronic low back pain: results of a randomised clinical trial with one year follow-up. *Rheumatology* 40 (7), 772–8.

Mannion, A.F., Taimela, S., Muntener, M. and Dvorak, J. (2001b). Active therapy for low back pain. Part 1: Effects on back muscle activation, fatigability and strength. *Spine* 26 (8), 897–908.

March, L.M. and Stenmark, J. (2001). Non-pharmacological approaches to managing arthritis. *Medical Journal of Australia* 175, s102–s107.

Mitchell, S.L., Grant, S. and Aitchison, T. (1998). Physiological effects of exercise on post-menopausal osteoporotic women. *Physiotherapy* 84 (4), 157–63.

Oddis, C.V. (1996). New perspectives on osteoarthritis. *American Journal of Medicine* **100** (2A), 10s–15s.

Panjabi, M., Abumi, K., Duranceau, J. and Oxland, T. (1989). Spinal stability and intersegmental muscle forces: a biomechanical model. *Spine* **14**, 194–200.

Penninx, B.W., Mesoier, S.P., Rejeski, W.J., Williamson, J.D., DiBari, M., Cavazzini, C., Applegare, W.B. and Pahor, M. (2001). Physical exercise and the prevention of disability in activities of daily living in older persons with osteoarthritis. *Archives of Internal Medical* **161** (19), Oct., 2309–16.

Petrella, R.J. (2001). Is exercise effective treatment for osteoarthritis of the knee? *British Journal of Sports Medicine* **34**, 326–31.

Rogind, H., Bibow-Nielson, B., Jensen, B., Moller, H.C., Frimodt-Moller, H. and Bliddal, H. (1998). The effects of a physical training programme on patients with osteoarthritis of the knees. *Archives of Physical Medicine and Rehabilitation* **79** (11), 1421–7.

Rutherford, O.L. (1999). Is there a role for exercise in the prevention of osteoporotic fractures? *British Journal of Sports Medicine* **33**, 378–86.

Sahrmann, S.A. (2002). *Diagnosis and Treatment of Movement Impairment Syndromes.* Mosby, St Louis, MO.

Shankar, K. (1998). *Exercise Prescription.* pp. 33–40. Hanley and Belfus Inc., Philadelphia.

Skelton, D.A. and McLoughlin, A.W. (1996). Training functional ability in old age. *Physiotherapy* **82** (3), 159 67.

Slemenda, C., Brandt, K.D., Heilman, D.K., Mazzuca, S., Braunstein, E.M., Katz, B.P. and Wolinskey, F.D. (1997). Quadriceps weakness and osteoarthritis of the knee. *Annals of Internal Medicine* **127**, 97–104.

Specter, T.D., Harris, P.A., Mart, D.J., Cicultini, F.M., Nandra, D., Ethemington, J., Wolman, R.L. and Doyle, D.V. (1996). Risk of osteoarthritis associated with long-term weight-bearing sports: a radiologic survey of the hips and knees in female ex-athletes and population controls. *Arthritis and Rheumatism* **39** (6), June, 988–95.

Swezey, R.L., Swezey, A. and Adams, J. (2000). Isometric progressive resistive exercise for osteoporosis. *Journal of Rheumatology* **27** (5), 1260–4.

Taaffe, D.R. and Marcus, R. (2000). Musculoskeletal health and the older adult. *Journal of Rehabilitation Research and Development* **37** (2), 245–54.

Torstensen, T.A., Ljunggren, A.E., Meen, H.D., Odland, E., Mowinckel, P. and Geijerstam, S. (1998). Efficiency and costs of medical exercise therapy, conventional physiotherapy and self-exercise in patients with chronic low back pain. *Spine* **23**, 2616–24.

Tulder, M., Koes, B.W. and Bouter, L.M. (1995). A cost of illness study of back pain in the Netherlands. *Pain* **62**, 233–40.

Tulder, M., Malmivaara, A., Esmail, R. and Koes, B. (2000). Exercise therapy for low back pain. A systematic review within the framework of the Cochrane back review group. *Spine* **25** (21), 2784–96.

Underwood, M.R. (2000). Exercise and the prevention of back pain disability. *British Journal of Sports Medicine* **34**, 5.

Van Baar, M.E., Dekker, J., Oostendorp, R.A., Bijl, Voorn, T.B., Lernmens, J.A. and Bijlsma, J.W. (1998). The effectiveness of exercise therapy in patients with osteoarthritis of the hip or knee: a randomised clinical trial. *Journal of Rheumatology* **25** (12), Dec., 2432–9.

Van Den Ende, C.H.M., Hazes, J.M.W., le Cassie, S., Mluder, W.J., Belfor, D.G., Breedveld, F.C. and Dijkmans, B.A. (1996). Comparison of high and low intensity training in well controlled rheumatoid arthritis. Results of a randomised clinical trial. *Annals of Rheumatic Diseases* **55** (11), Nov., 798–805.

Van Den Ende, C.H.M., Vlieland, T.P.M., Munneke, M. and Hazes, J.M.W. (1998). Dynamic exercise therapy in rheumatoid arthritis. A systematic review. *British Journal of Rheumatology* 37, 677–87.

Videman, T., Sarna, S. and Battie, M.C. (1995). The long-term effects of physical loading and exercise lifestyles on back-related symptoms, disability and spinal pathology among men. *Spine* 20, 696–709.

Vuori, I.M. (2001). Dose response of physical activity and low back pain, osteoarthritis and osteoporosis. *Medicine and Science in Sports and Exercise* 33 (6 suppl.), 609–10.

Wittink, H., Michel, T.H., Wagner, A., Sukiennik, A. and Rogers, W. (2000). Deconditioning in patients with chronic low back pain. Fact or fiction? *Spine* 25 (17), 2221–8.

Zhao, J. (2001). Effects of exercise modes on peak bone mineral density in human subjects. *Hong Kong Journal of Sports Medicine and Sports Science* 12, 54–72.

Chapter 11

EXERCISE AS PART OF THE MULTIDISCIPLINARY MANAGEMENT OF ADULTS AND CHILDREN WITH OBESITY

Alison Quinn and Juliette Hussey

Key words: obesity, multidisplinary team, prevention, diabetes.

Introduction

'Physical activity is an important determinant of body weight. In addition, physical activity and physical fitness (which relates to the ability to perform physical activity) are important modifiers of mortality and morbidity related to overweight and obesity.' (WHO, 2003)

As discussed in Chapter 5 there is a strong theoretical basis for exercise in the management of patients with obesity and diabetes. In this chapter the place of exercise therapy within the multidisciplinary management of these patients is described. Patients with obesity and diabetes frequently present with co-morbidities and these need to be considered when prescribing an exercise programme.

Understanding obesity

There are many factors thought to contribute to obesity:

- *Physical inactivity*: modern lifestyles are becoming more sedentary as advances in technology reduce the need for physical activity.
- *Dietary*: levels of energy consumption have increased due to the introduction of bigger portions and calorie dense and convenience foods.
- *Psychological*: eating for emotional reasons rather than hunger.
- *Behavioural*: poor eating habits, unhealthy and unbalanced food choice.

- *Social*: busy lifestyles leading to increased stress and decreased time spent cooking, availability of fast food which can be cheaper than healthy alternatives, fast food advertising, increased hours watching television.
- *Medical*: diseases such as hypothyroidism and diabetes mellitus can contribute to weight gain.
- *Pharmacological*: examples of drugs that can cause weight gain include corticosteroids (rheumatoid arthritis), tricyclic antidepressants (depression), insulin (type 1 diabetes mellitus).

Obesity is the result of a unique combination of contributing factors where genes interact with environmental and lifestyle factors. However, it is thought that the large increases in obesity observed in modern society are due to changes in diet and particularly physical inactivity (Booth et al., 2000).

Health risks of obesity

The physical and psychological health risks associated with obesity are well documented and are summarised in Box 11.1.

Table 11.1 presents the classification of disease risk based on BMI and waist circumference. Hypertension, high cholesterol levels, type 2 diabetes and coronary heart disease are the most common health consequences associated with obesity (Must et al., 1999). Of particular relevance to physiotherapists is the prevalence of musculoskeletal disorders associated with obesity. Musculoskeletal disorders can cause pain, restricted mobility, decreased physical activity capacity and decreased quality of life. The presence of these disorders can interfere with weight loss

Box 11.1 The health risks associated with obesity.

Physical

- Cardiovascular: coronary heart disease, stroke, hypertension, increased cholesterol levels, increased triglycerides, venous thrombosis
- Metabolic: type 2 diabetes mellitus, insulin resistance, impaired glucose tolerance
- Respiratory: sleep apnoea, breathlessness
- Musculoskeletal: osteoarthritis (knee, hip), gout, low back pain
- Alimentary: gall bladder disease
- Urinary: renal disease, urinary incontinence
- Reproductive: menstrual abnormalities, infertility
- Other: certain cancers, cellulitis

Psychological

- Loss of self-esteem, poor self-image
- Depression
- Prejudice and social stigmatisation
- Decreased quality of life
- Eating disorders

Table 11.1 Classification of disease risk based on body mass index and waist circumference (reproduced from ACSM, 2000, with permission of Lippincott, Williams and Wilkins).

	BMI kg/m^2	Disease risk relative to normal weight and waist circumference	
		Men, < = 102 cm Women, < = 88 cm	Men, > 102 cm Women, > 88 cm
Underweight	< 18.5		
Normal weight	18.5–24.9		
Overweight	25.0–29.9	Increased	High
Obese – Grade I	30.0–34.9	High	Very high
Obese – Grade II	35–39.9	Very high	Very high
Obese – Grade III	> = 40	Extremely high	Extremely high

attempts. Research suggests that there is a positive correlation between obesity and musculoskeletal disorders (Kortt and Baldry, 2002) with back pain and knee pain being the most common musculoskeletal complaints linked with obesity (Jordan et al., 1996; Leboeuf-Yde et al., 1999).

Waist and hip circumference measurement ratios or waist circumference alone can predict increased health risk. In males, waist circumference greater than 102 cm or a WHR (waist to hip ratio) of greater than 0.95 is predictive of increased health risk. In women a waist circumference of greater than 88 cm or a WHR greater than 0.80 predicts increased health risk. The presence of central obesity compared to peripheral obesity increases the risk of insulin resistance, glucose intolerance, type 2 diabetes mellitus, cardiovascular disease, hypertension, certain cancers and increased cholesterol. It is thought that measurement of waist girth may also indicate more strongly the risk of cardiovascular disease than waist/hip ratio.

Skin-fold measurements are used relatively infrequently in adult obesity as they are less reliable than BMI and hip/waist measurements. In some obese patients skin-folds may be too thick to measure accurately. However, they are commonly used measurements in childhood and adolescent obesity.

Treatment of adults with obesity

The current recommendation for achieving weight loss is to attain an initial reduction of 10% body weight over a six-month period, aiming for no more than a 1 to 2 lb (0.45–0.9 kg) weight loss per week (National Heart Lung and Blood Institute (NHLBI), 2000). While this goal may not be consistent with patient expectations it is realistic for patients and thus avoids giving patients the experience of yet another failed weight loss attempt. By losing weight over a long period of time weight maintenance is better achieved and patients can begin to adopt permanent lifestyle changes. A 10% reduction in body weight also results in a significant decrease in obesity related health risks (Pasanisi et al., 2001). After this initial weight loss further weight loss attempts can be made. The main goals of any weight loss programme should be a decrease in body weight and the maintenance of a lower body weight in the long term as recommended by the NHLBI (2000). The very minimum goal should be the prevention of further weight gain.

Successful weight loss results from several interventions, including dietary therapy, physical activity/exercise therapy, psychological therapy, medication and surgery. The amount and timing of each therapy intervention depends on the patient's needs. Combined dietary, physical activity and psychological therapy probably have a more powerful effect on weight loss than individual interventions. The role of the multi-disciplinary team is paramount in successful weight loss programmes, where a range of disciplines can complement each other's efforts. The multidisciplinary team may include doctors, dietitians, psychologists and physiotherapists but this list is not exhaustive and may vary between clinics. The dietitian educates the patient on all aspects of healthy eating. This includes portion control, energy balance, meal structure and timing, and meal planning. Compliance to national healthy eating guidelines is encouraged.

The psychologist provides motivational support and treatment for clinical problems where needed. Psychological input varies from intensive input, for conditions such as binge eating disorders, to less intensive interventions, including stress management training, assertiveness training and communication skills. Two main drugs are currently in use for weight loss. Sibutramine is centrally acting and promotes a feeling of satiety (a feeling of fullness) after eating a meal, by increasing serotonin and adrenaline levels in the brain. Orlistat acts at the periphery and decreases fat absorption in the intestine. Bariatric surgery can be considered when other weight loss attempts have failed or for patients with a BMI > = 40 or BMI > = 35 with coexisting morbidities (Monteforte and Turkelson, 2000). The two most widely used procedures are vertical banded gastroplasty and roux-en-y gastric bypass.

When embarking on a weight management programme the patient should be assessed by all members of the multidisciplinary team. Initially, the patient will be assessed medically, where a history, physical examination and a series of blood tests will be undertaken to see if there is a metabolic cause for their obesity. Depending on the patient's medical history a baseline electrocardiogram (ECG) and/or an exercise test may be performed. Exercise testing has been described in Chapter 6. It may not be realistic or practical to carry out exercise testing on every patient, but it is important that patients are cleared for exercise by the medical team, based on their medical history and examination.

An understanding of medical, dietary and psychological assessment and results thereof is essential as they can have important input to the prescription of exercise, the results achieved and the patient's compliance. For example, a psychological assessment may indicate a person's preference for variety versus routine so an exercise programme should be tailored accordingly.

Physiotherapy management of the adult with obesity

The physical activity assessment is considered below. This is a guide and is not definitive. Patients may be seen by the physiotherapist as part of the multidisciplinary team in the clinic, or they may present to the physiotherapy outpatients with other pathologies, but also be obese. In the latter case, where obesity is not the presenting complaint, it is important to address the problem and try to prevent health complications which will arise due to being obese.

- *How was the patient referred to the service?* Did the patient seek out his or her own referral to the service from their medical practitioner or was it suggested to them? If the latter, were they happy to be referred to the service? This may indicate the patient's motivation to enter a weight loss programme.

- *Previous weight loss attempts with particular emphasis on any exercise involved.* What measures worked/did not work in the past? What was the patient's experience of adding exercise to a weight loss programme in the past? Did they find one type of exercise beneficial?

- *Past medical history and medication.* This can be obtained from the medical chart. It is important to know what coexisting conditions and/or medications may affect weight loss attempts or may affect the patient's ability and safety to exercise. For example, fear of falling due to decreased balance reactions (arthritis, multiple sclerosis, vertigo), previous ischaemic heart disease, diabetes.

- *Musculoskeletal problems.* Are current musculoskeletal problems hindering the patient's ability to exercise, for example, low back pain? Can the patient be given advice to help their condition or do they need a more detailed physiotherapy assessment and course of treatment? Do they need a referral to another service, for example, podiatry. It is vital that the patient is empowered to add exercise to their weight loss attempts. Pain on exercising will not encourage patient compliance and may lead to adverse effects.

- *Past and current physical activity levels.* What activities does the patient currently enjoy or have they enjoyed a particular activity/sport in the past?

- *Barriers/motivators.* What are the barriers that the patient may see as limiting compliance to an exercise programme, for example, time, boredom, self-consciousness? What would encourage the patient to exercise?

- *Is this the right time to embark on this type of programme?* This question need not be asked directly but it is worth getting a sense of other important factors that may be in the patient's life at the moment, for example, changing career, dealing with a family illness, financial worries, etc. It may be better to postpone the patient's entry to the programme for 3–6 months emphasising the need to avoid further weight gain, as a minimum goal.

- *What are the patient's weight loss goals?* Are these realistic? Are they consistent with the weight loss programme's goals?

Based on the information obtained in the assessment a plan is drawn up with the patient. This plan needs to be structured, realistic, safe and tailored to the patient's needs, to ensure optimum compliance and benefit. The ultimate aim of any weight loss programme is to promote permanent lifestyle changes. This will not be achieved if unrealistic goals are prescribed contrary to the patient's needs and lifestyle.

All motivators to exercise should be encouraged, all barriers should be solved, for example, if the patient finds exercise boring try the use of a Walkman. Explore a time that would suit the patient to exercise, for example, morning, lunchtime, straight after work, evening. Is there someone that would join the patient on a walk, etc. Emphasise the commitment involved in a weight loss programme and that it is a high priority.

Exercise prescription

The overall aim of exercise in weight loss programmes is to expend energy to unbalance the energy equation and create an overall calorie deficit. Exercise also provides benefits for the obese patient by reducing health risks associated with obesity, such as hypertension, insulin resistance, hyperlipidaemia, improving body composition and having an impact on the maintenance of weight loss. There have been several reviews of the quantity and quality of exercise necessary for fitness (Pate et al., 1995; AHA, 1996; ACSM, 1998) and the principles of these will be discussed in Chapter 12. While these guidelines may be adequate to promote fitness and attain health improvements, they may not be adequate for weight loss or maintenance of weight loss. This issue was addressed by the ACSM in a recent position stand which justifies the role of exercise in weight loss programmes and discusses strategies for weight loss and prevention of weight regain in adults (ACSM, 2001). The main recommendations are outlined below:

- Progress adults to 200–300 minutes of exercise a week to promote an energy deficit of > 2000 kcal per week. This represents a significant increase from the 150 minutes recommended by the above mentioned guidelines.

- Exercise should be of moderate intensity, that is, 55–69% of maximal heart rate. It is not yet established if there are equal or more significant benefits to exercising more vigorously (> = 70% of maximal heart rate) for less time.

- It appears that undertaking exercise in 10–15 minute bouts several times a day may be as beneficial as one long bout of exercise. This method should be considered for people who dislike long bouts of exercise.

- Lifestyle activity appears to be as effective as structured exercise programmes once it is of a moderate intensity.

- There is no evidence that resistance exercise promotes more weight loss than traditional endurance exercise. However, fat free mass can be maintained or increased with resistance training and as strength improves a more healthy and active lifestyle may be promoted as activities of daily living become easier.

Even if weight loss does not occur within the guidelines provided above it is important to emphasise to the patient the other benefits that are accrued with exercise, including increased health benefits. In a prospective observational study Wei et al. (1999) found that in overweight and obese men low cardiorespiratory fitness (CRF) is as important as type 2 diabetes and other CVD risk factors as a predictor of CVD mortality and all-cause mortality. A recent study by Ross and Katzmarzyk (2003) found that high levels of cardiorespiratory fitness are associated with lower levels of total and abdominal obesity for a given BMI by comparison to those with a low CRF. Therefore exercise can attenuate the health risks attributed to obesity as measured by BMI. It could be argued that the measurement of CRF should be routine in evaluation of these patients in addition to waist circumference.

When prescribing exercise it is important to use FITT principles (Chapter 12) and to agree goals with the patient. Frequency (F), intensity (I), time (T) and type (T) of exercise must be prescribed based on the patient's ability, preferences and medical history. Clinical experience indicates that many obese patients are sedentary and have had negative experience with exercise in the past (for example, self-consciousness, side effects) or feel that they cannot engage in exercise because of their size and/or concurrent medical problems (such as low back pain, breathlessness). Patients must be started slowly, at their own pace, for short periods of time, so that they have a positive experience of exercise and are given realistic goals. Eventually, when the duration and frequency of exercise has increased, the intensity can be increased so that they can start to achieve cardiorespiratory fitness. Patients can use heart rate monitors or the 'rating of perceived exertion' scale to assess their intensity. The type of exercise for many obese patients will be walking. However, any aerobic exercise that uses continuous large muscle groups is appropriate, for example, swimming, rowing, cycling, etc. Exercise can be performed at home (for example, exercise videos, walking), or in a gym/leisure centre. It can be done individually or as part of a group. As with any exercise there are contraindications. Safety and pre-participation screening (Chapter 6 and 12) and constant monitoring and communication with the medical team is essential for safe and successful participation in exercise programmes. Patients must be aware of the warning signs (e.g. chest pain, dizziness) and immediately discontinue exercise and contact their doctor.

Compliance with exercise programmes is always a problem, particularly with obese patients who have been mainly sedentary. Adherence can be improved by many factors, including positive re-enforcement, establishment of a regular routine, variety and enjoyment of programme, encouraging and sensitive staff, use of progress charts and minimisation of injury (ACSM, 2000). In Chapter 13 adherence issues are discussed.

Monitoring/review

It is recommended that patients are seen approximately every four weeks in the first three months of embarking on a weight management programme (NHLBI, 2000). Visits may be more or less frequent depending on clinical judgement. Visits after six months may become less frequent again depending on the needs of the patient.

It is the authors' experience that monthly visits are needed, at least for the first six months, to encourage compliance and to promote lifestyle changes.

Exercise prescription following surgery

There is a scarcity of research available on exercise assessment and prescription for bariatric surgery patients and no established protocols. Patients undergoing bariatric surgery should be assessed in the same way as described previously. Knowing the patient's levels of physical activity and mobility is particularly important, to ascertain their ability to recover from the anaesthetic and to mobilise post-surgery. In the initial six weeks post-surgery normal activities of daily living and physical activity are gradually increased as pain allows. More strenuous physical activity can then be introduced, for example, brisk walking, swimming and stationary bicycle. Any activity that strains the abdominal wall should be introduced slowly and gently due to the risk of incisional hernia (risk of about 10% after open obesity surgery). At three months post-operatively 75% of abdominal muscle strength is regained, but it takes about two years for full recovery. With the emergence of laparoscopic surgery patients leave hospital in 3–4 days and can be mobilised and progressed through physical activity more quickly. The risk of incisional hernia is also eliminated. Surgical and anaesthetic complications are increased in obese patients. Advanced cardiorespiratory disease and heart failure are contraindications to obesity surgery.

Treatment of children with obesity

Increased time spent watching television and video, playing computer games and diminished opportunities for physical activity are contributors to the present epidemic in childhood obesity. Obese children have an increased risk of becoming overweight adults and have a high risk of morbidity and mortality. Obesity that begins early in life can persist into adulthood and increases the risk of obesity related disease later in life. Along with the increase in obesity there is an increase in the incidence of obesity related disease, for example, the incidence in type 2 diabetes in children has risen ten-fold over the last decade. More than 60% of overweight children have at least one additional risk factor for cardiovascular disease, such as raised blood pressure, hyperlipidaemia or hyperinsulinaemia, and more than 25% have two or more risk factors (Freedman et al., 1999).

Intervening in childhood obesity is important due to its associated health risks. However, where this should be done and by whom seems to be debatable. Primary care health providers may be the first to become aware of a problem, but many feel ill equipped to deal comprehensively with this problem (Kristeller and Hoerr, 1997). Obesity prevention and management programmes in children appear to be more successful than those in adults. This may be in part due to it being easier to change behaviours in children than in adults whose habits have been formed over a longer time. New healthier behaviours may then replace the previous behaviours and persist into adulthood (Epstein et al., 1998). While treatment programmes may be expensive it could be argued that the cost of managing the consequences of paediatric obesity, such as hypertension, hyperlipidaemia and diabetes are far higher in both financial and human terms.

Ideally, the overall management of the child with obesity is done by a committed multidisciplinary team, consisting of medical, nursing, physiotherapy, dietetics and psychology personnel. Initial medical assessment may include the exclusion of endocrine disorders and the measurement of anthropometric indices, blood pressure, fasting blood insulin, c peptide and cholesterol. Physiotherapy assessment includes assessment of physical activity levels, exercise tolerance and the presence of any respiratory (for example, asthma) or musculoskeletal problems which may influence exercise prescription. The psychological assessment may include investigation of behaviour problems and internalising and externalising behaviours. An interview with the parents and child may also reveal barriers that may impact on maintaining a healthy lifestyle.

The key message delivered to the child and parents is the importance of a lifestyle approach including healthy eating, daily physical activity and the restriction of sedentary behaviours. Drugs are not approved in children and gastric bypass surgery would only be considered in those with life-threatening complications of obesity (Yanovski, 2001). Occasionally, admission to hospital for caloric restriction may be an option. Frequent visits to a clinic are required (every two weeks to every month), which may be viewed by the parents and child to be disruptive to school, etc. However, acknowledging that obesity is a chronic condition, where rigorous monitoring is important, may help acceptance of these frequent assessments. Time and patience are required by the child, parent and health care providers and small improvements need to be praised. While the child and parents may initially only be encouraged by changes in weight, the importance of other parameters and their beneficial effect on health, such as fitness, waist circumference/body composition, increasing activity levels and blood pressure, need to be highlighted by the health care provider. In children who are growing, maintainence of weight may be the goal, as the child grows in height. The link between obesity and health risks and the fact that obesity is not a 'cosmetic issue' need to be emphasised. Childhood obesity should not be seen as benign, as it is associated with cardiovascular risk factors. Parents may be concerned that restricting food may lead to eating disorders. However, healthy eating based on the food pyramid rather than caloric restriction is advised in children.

The family need to be included in the behaviour changes, such as healthy eating and increasing physical activity levels. The younger child will need to be accompanied by a parent for many of the prescribed activities, such as brisk walking/jogging, because of safety reasons. Family participation in physical activities is the key for successful behaviour change. If time or weather constraints exist then other activities such as skipping or use of home exercise equipment may be a possibility. Sedentary behaviours such as television watching should be limited to 1–2 hours per day, which will impact positively on other family members. Television watching has been associated with body fat in children (Andersen et al., 1998), and reducing time spent sedentary in obese children has been associated with a decrease in body fat (Epstein et al., 2000). When children are watching television they are very still and this time is often associated with snacking, as food advertisements appear.

Physiotherapy management of the child

Physiotherapy management involves assessing exercise tolerance, determining levels of physical activity and prescribing an activity programme. These need to re-evaluated regularly.

Exercise testing

Exercise testing may be performed in many ways and the reader is referred to Chapter 6 for a review of the area. While many children may be familiar with the bleep test (shuttle running test), as a result of having performed it in physical education class in schools, it may be difficult to accommodate in a hospital setting due to environmental constraints. Therefore exercise testing using equipment such as the treadmill or cycle ergometer may be easier in the clinical setting. A protocol such as the Modified Balke Treadmill Protocol can easily be used.

During treadmill testing obese subjects may have a higher cardiac output, oxygen consumption and minute ventilation at a given work rate. Aerobic capacity is reduced when expressed relative to body weight (it can appear to be normal when body weight is accounted for, due to the increased body mass). Exercise tolerance in the obese can be limited by heat intolerance, dyspnoea/hypernoea, movement restrictions, joint pain, muscle weakness or balance problems. In the authors' experience joint pain in the lower limbs is often the reason for terminating the exercise test.

Assessment of activity levels

Activity assessment can be performed by questionnaire and an example of such is the Modifiable Activity Questionnaire for Adolescents. If the child is below 12 years of age this can be completed by the child and accompanying parent (see Chapter 6 for other methods of assessment of physical activity). The reproducibility and validity of the original questionnaire was established by Aaron et al. (1995). Information on the amount of times in the previous two weeks that the child participated in at least 20 minutes of hard and light exercise is sought. Hard exercise is defined as exercise that made the child breathe heavily and their heart beat fast. Light exercise is defined as exercise that does not make the child breathe heavily or their heart beat fast. The number of hours per day that the child spends watching television, videos or playing computer games and the number of competitive activities the child participates in is also recorded. An estimate for energy expended in regular activities each week, such as METs/hr/week is determined by multiplying the hours per week spent at each activity by the metabolic cost of each activity in METs. The modifications to the original questionnaire can include the addition of a question on mode of transport to school and as these children are under nine years of age the question on involvement in competitive activities has been removed. Under the section on 'past year sports regularly played' local or native games can be added.

The physiotherapy assessment should also incorporate the examination of any musculoskeletal or respiratory problems that may need to be considered in exercise prescription. The excess weight put on joints may lead to pain, restricting the child's ability to perform certain activities for prolonged periods. Non-weightbearing activities may need to be included in the exercise programme until the specific joint concerns are alleviated. Asthma is a common respiratory condition. The link between asthma and obesity has been studied and while no causal link has been demonstrated (Chinn, 2003) asthma is considered as a risk factor for obesity in children and adolescents (Gennuso et al., 1998). Physical activity in children with asthma needs to be promoted to prevent obesity. Children with EIA (exercise induced asthma) may need to be instructed in the use of their inhalers prior to exercise so that symptoms do not prevent their activities. Asthma is the most common chronic medical condition that school teachers will encounter and they therefore need to be aware of how exercise induced asthma is managed so children are not excluded from participation in PE.

Exercise prescription

Exercise prescription is done on an individual basis, taking into consideration the types of activities the child enjoys and can do close to home. The guidelines used for children in their teens are:

- Light exercise, such as walking for 30 minutes, accumulated throughout the day every day of the week. Walking to and from school and going for a walk in the evenings would be ways of doing this. The individual does not have to do all the exercise in one session but can break it up into blocks of ten minutes.

- Moderate to vigorous exercise for at least 20 minutes, three times per week. The intensity of this exercise should be about a 5 on the RPE scale. This vigorous exercise could be brisk walking/running/swimming/cycling. The individual could do brisk walking on one day, swimming another day and running another day. Before and after vigorous exercise, light activity for 2–3 minutes to warm up and cool down is advised. In the initial stages of the exercise programme it is recommended to leave a day between vigorous sessions. If home exercise equipment is available it can be suggested that one or two sessions per week could be done this way, which will allow the child to exercise whatever the weather conditions.

- Activity throughout the day is encouraged, as is seeking opportunities for physical activity, such as the use of the stairs instead of a lift/escalator, walking to, or part of the way to, school.

For younger children the recommendation is to accumulate one hour of activity each day of the week and to encourage opportunities for spontaneous play. It is important that the activity chosen is fun for the child, providing excitement and something for the child to look forward to. Even simple programmes such as brisk walking can be made enjoyable by the parent incorporating games such as 'I spy', or counting something. For many, this protected time spent with the parent can provide time for catching up on happenings during the day. In both age groups sedentary behaviours should be restricted.

The fit/fat debate

As the child/adult engages in an exercise programme over many weeks or longer he/she may become disillusioned if their weight does not decrease. The child/adult must be encouraged by other parameters such as a decrease in waist circumference, an increase in fitness or a normalising of blood pressure. The importance of these parameters and their relationship to health benefits needs to be emphasised to parents and child. Regular physical activity decreases many of the health risks associated with overweight or obesity. Individuals who are active and obese have lower morbidity and mortality than normal weight individuals who are sedentary. Inactivity and low cardiorespiratory fitness are as important as overweight and obesity as mortality predictors (Blair and Brodney, 1999). Lee et al. (1999) examined the health consequences of body fatness and cardiovascular fitness in relation to all-cause and cardiovascular disease mortality in men (n = 21 925). Unfit and lean men were at a 2.2 times greater risk of all-cause mortality than fit obese men. Farrell et al. (2002) found cardiorespiratory fitness was a more accurate indicator of all-cause mortality than BMI.

Prevention of obesity

Prevention based activities established within the community and primary care are probably the most obvious way of controlling the epidemic now seen, but how to do this is a more difficult problem. Daily physical activity in schools would go some way towards the prevention of obesity in children, due to the increase in daily energy expenditure, and may also introduce the child to a variety of activities, one or more of which the child may wish to carry on throughout life. Education in schools as regards healthy eating and the health benefits of regular activity should also be considered if education is to prepare the child for life. From a public perspective, increased investment and availability of sporting/leisure facilities would provide opportunities for those on lower incomes. Strategically, aiming programmes at preventing childhood obesity makes sense. Children may be somewhat more flexible than adults in lifestyle habits and therefore behaviour change may be more successful.

Exercise treatment in type 2 diabetes

Physical activity is an important aspect of the management of the patient with type 2 diabetes. In the short term exercise benefits glucose concentrations and in the long term benefits body composition, hypertension, hyperlipidaemia and abnormalities of coagulation/fibrinolysis. Subjects with type 2 diabetes generally demonstrate clustering of multiple cardiovascular risk factors. Increasing physical activity will have a positive influence on many of these parameters. See also Chapter 5.

Exercise improves glycaemic control in type 2 diabetes (Peirce, 1999). Effects of exercise are quickly seen in glucose tolerance and prandial insulin concentration. As well as glycaemic control, physical activity studies also show beneficial effects on lipids and blood pressure. Acute exercise decreases plasma glucose levels and this persists for a number of days. It is probably due to the active muscles' increased insulin sensitivity. Exercise training is associated with improved insulin sensitivity. Mayer-Davis et al. (1998) found that both increased participation in non-vigorous habitual activity as well as overall and vigorous physical activity is associated with significantly higher insulin sensitivity.

Long-term improvements in glycaemic control are probably due to the acute effects of each exercise session and therefore regular exercise is important. In diabetic women increased physical activity, including regular walking, has been found to be associated with reduced risk for cardiovascular events (Hu et al., 2001). The goals of treatment in type 2 diabetes are the prevention and treatment of acute and long-term complications and the management of accompanying disorders such as hypertension and hyperlipidaemia. Modification of hypertension and hyperlipidaemia, through physical activity in these patients, has been shown to reduce mortality from macrovascular disease.

The American College of Sports Medicine's position stand on exercise in type 2 diabetes recommends physical activity, including endurance and resistance training. Beneficial changes in glucose tolerance and insulin sensitivity last for 72 hours after the last exercise session. Therefore regular physical activity is imperative to maintain glucose lowering effects and improved insulin sensitivity. It is recommended that individuals with type 2 diabetes should accumulate a total of 1000 kcal spent in exercise per week. The accompanying chronic conditions of people with type 2 diabetes may make prescription difficult.

Diabetic prevention programmes can be justified on economic grounds as the health consequences of the long-term complications of diabetes will be a huge burden on the health care system. The strong evidence that type 2 diabetes can be prevented raises the question of screening and intervention for those with risk factors.

Exercise treatment in type 1 diabetes

Type 1 diabetes or insulin-dependent diabetes was previously known as juvenile onset diabetes. In type 1 diabetes there is an absolute deficiency of insulin and often other pancreatic hormones. Care is needed to adjust insulin and carbohydrate intake when subjects engage in exercise. For those taking insulin, hypoglycaemia may occur during and after exercise. It can occur during a prolonged exercise session when hepatic glucose production cannot keep up with the use of glucose by the exercising muscles. However, exercise is important for numerous reasons, such as protective cardiovascular effects, optimising bone density and psychological well-being. In children and adolescents who have type 1 diabetes exercise is also important for social reasons. Education for the patient with type 1 diabetes is important to permit safe participation in regular exercise. Unlike subjects with type 2 diabetes exercise in those with type 1 does not improve blood glucose control and therefore subjects treated with insulin can have an imbalance between the plasma insulin level and available plasma glucose. If the plasma insulin level is high, carbohydrate supply may be blocked because hepatic glycogenolysis is blocked due to the high insulin level. In the non-diabetic patient insulin falls shortly after the commencement of exercise but in the type 1 diabetic patient the insulin level depends on the time and dose of the last injection. Therefore the individual needs to plan the timing of strenuous exercise and reduce the insulin dose due to the increased insulin sensitivity in the muscles that occurs.

Hypoglycaemia may occur during exercise or after exercise. It can sometimes be difficult to recognise, as the signs are similar to those normally experienced with strenuous exercise (for example sweating, tachycardia). Hyperglycaemia is a contraindication to exercise and must be corrected by insulin injections to lower blood glucose. Frequent monitoring is recommended for those with hypoglycaemia and those performing exercise of high intensity. Carrying glucose tablets and a diabetic identification bracelet or card is advised. Foot care is essential and correct footwear and skin inspection is essential. In those with neuropathy, alternatives to weight-bearing exercise need to be considered. In those with, or at high risk of, CAD exercise testing to anginal thresholds may need to be performed to avoid ischaemic changes with exercise.

References

Aaron, D.J., Kriska, A.M., Dearwater, S.R., Cauley, J.A., Metz, K.F. and LaPorte, R.E. (1995). Reproducibility and validity of an epidemiologic questionnaire to assess past year physical activity in adolescents. *American Journal of Epidemiology* **142**, 191–201.

American College of Sports Medicine (1998). The recommended quantity and quality of exercise for developing and maintaining cardiorespiratory and muscular fitness, and flexibility in healthy adults. *Medicine and Science in Sports and Exercise* **30** (6), 975–91.

American College of Sports Medicine (2000). *ACSM's Guidelines for Exercise Testing and Prescription*, 6th edn. Lippincott Williams and Wilkins, Philadelphia.

American College of Sports Medicine (2001). Position stand: Appropriate intervention strategies for weight loss and prevention of weight regain for adults. *Medicine and Science in Sports and Exercise* **33** (12), 2145–56.

American Heart Association (1996). Statement on exercise: benefits and recommendations for physical activity programs for all Americans. *Circulation* **94**, 857–62.

Andersen, R.E., Crespo, C.J., Bartlett, S.J., Cheskin, L.J. and Pratt, M. (1998). Relationship of physical activity and television watching with body weight and level of fatness among children. *Journal of American Medical Association* **279**, 938–42.

Blair, S.N. and Brodney, S. (1999). Effects of physical inactivity and obesity on morbidity and mortality: current evidence and research issues. *Medicine and Science in Sports and Exercise* 31, S646–62.

Booth, F.W., Gordon, S.E., Carlson, C.J. and Hamilton, M.T. (2000). Waging war on modern chronic diseases: primary prevention through exercise biology. *Journal of Applied Physiology* 88, 774–87.

Chinn, S. (2003). Obesity and asthma: evidence for and against a causal relationship. *Journal of Asthma* 40, 1–16.

Epstein, L.H., Myers, M.D., Raynor, H.A. and Saelens, B.E. (1998). Treatment of pediatric obesity. *Pediatrics* 101, 554–70.

Epstein, L.H., Paluch, R.A., Gordy, C.C. and Dern, J. (2000). Decreasing sedentary behaviours in treating pediatric obesity. *Archives of Pediatrics and Adolescent Medicine* 154, 220–226.

Farrell, S.W., Braun, L., Barlow, C.E., Cheng, Y.J. and Blair, S.N. (2002). The relation of body mass index, cardiorespiratory fitness, and all-cause mortality in women. *Obesity Research* 10, 417–23.

Freedman, D.S., Dietz, W.H., Srinivasan, S.R. and Berenson, G.S. (1999). The relation of overweight to cardiovascular risk factors among children and adolescents: The Bogalusa Heart Study. *Pediatrics* 103, 1175–82.

Gennuso, J., Epstein, L.H., Paluch, R.A. and Cerny, F. (1998). The relationship between asthma and obesity in urban minority children and adolescents. *Archives of Pediatrics and Adolescent Medicine* 152, 1197–2000.

Hu, F.B., Stampfer, M.J., Solomon, C., Liu, S., Colditz, G.A., Speizer, F.E., Willett, W.C. and Manson, J.E. (2001). Physical activity and risk for cardiovascular events in diabetic women. *Annals Internal Medicine* 134 (2), 96–105.

Jordan, J.M., Luta, G., Renner, J.B., Linder, G.F., Dragomir, A., Hochberg, M.C. and Fryer, J.G. (1996). Self-reported functional status in osteoarthritis of the knee in a rural southern community: the role of socio-economic factors, obesity, and knee pain. *Arthritis Care and Research* 9 (4), 273–8.

Kortt, M. and Baldry, J. (2002). The Association between Musculoskeletal Disorders and Obesity. *Australian Health Review* 25 (16), 207–14.

Kristeller, J. and Hoerr, R. (1997). Physician attitudes toward managing obesity: differences among six speciality groups. *Preventive Medicine* 26, 542–9.

Leboeuf-Yde, C., Kyvik, K.O. and Bruun, N.H. (1999). Low back pain and lifestyle. Part II – Obesity. Information from a population-based sample of 29 424 twin subjects. *Spine* 24 (8), 779–84.

Lee, C.D., Blair, S.N. and Jackson, A.S. (1999). Cardiorespiratory fitness, body composition, and all-cause cardiovascular disease mortality in men. *American Journal of Clinical Nutrition* 69, 373–80.

Mayer-Davis, E.J., D'Agostino, R., Karter, A.J., Haffner, S.M., Rewers, M.J., Saad, M. and Bergman, R.N. (1998). Intensity and amount of physical activity in relation to insulin sensitivity: the Insulin Resistance Atherosclerosis Study. *Journal of American Medical Association* 279 (9), 669–74.

Monteforte, M.J. and Turkelson, C.M. (2000). Bariatric surgery for morbid obesity. *Obesity Surgery* 10 (5), 301–401.

Must, A., Spadona, M.S., Coakley, E.H., Field, A.E., Colditz, G. and Dietz, W.H. (1999). Disease burden associated with overweight and obesity. *Journal of American Medical Association* 282 (16), 1523–29.

National Heart Lung and Blood Institute (2000). *The Practical Guide. Identification, Evaluation, and Treatment of Overweight and Obesity in Adults*. NIH Publication Number 00-4084, Bethesda.

Pasanisi, F., Contaldo, F., de Simone, G. and Mancini, M. (2001). Benefits of sustained moderate weight loss in obesity. *Nutrition Metabolism and Cardiovascular Diseases* 11 (6), 401–6.

Pate, R.P., Pratt, M., Blair, S.N., Haskell, W.L., Macera, C.A., Buchard, C., Buchner, D., Edinger, W., Heath, G.W. and King, A.C. (1995). Physical activity and public health: a recommendation from the centers for disease control and prevention and the American College of Sports Medicine. *Journal of American Medical Association* 273 (5), 402–7.

Peirce, N.S. (1999). Diabetes and exercise. *British Journal of Sports Medicine* 33 (3), 161–72.

Ross, R. and Katzmarzyk, P.T. (2003). Cardiorespiratory fitness is associated with diminished total and abdominal obesity independent of body mass index. *International Journal of Obesity* 27, 204–10.

Wei, M., Kampert, J.B., Barlow, C.E., Nichaman, M.Z., Gibbons, L.W., Paffenbarger, R.S. Jnr. and Blair, S.N. (1999). Relationship between low cardiorespiratory fitness and mortality in normal weight, overweight and obese men. *Journal of American Medical Association* 282 (16), 1547–53.

World Health Organization (2003). *Diet, Nutrition and the Prevention of Chronic Diseases*. Report of a Joint WHO/FAO Expert Consultation. World Health Organization, Geneva (WHO Technical Report Series, No. 916).

Yanovski, J.A. (2001). Pediatric Obesity. *Reviews in Endocrine and Metabolic Disorders* 2, 371–83.

Bibliography

Brown, D. (2003). About Obesity. International Obesity Task Force. Available from http://www.obesite.chaire.ulaval.ca/iotf.htm (Accessed 22 April 2003).

Chipkin, S.R., Klugh, S.A. and Chasan-Taber, L. (2001). Exercise and diabetes. *Cardiology Clinics* 19 (3), 489–505.

International Obesity Task Force (IOTF) (2002). www.iotf.org

McArdle, W.D., Katch, F.I. and Katch, V.L. (2001). *Exercise Physiology. Energy, Nutrition and Human Performance*, 5th edn. Lippincott Williams and Wilkins, Philadelphia.

World Health Organization (2003). Controlling the Obesity Epidemic. Available from http://www.who.int/nut/obs.htm (Accessed 29 June 2003).

Chapter 12

EXERCISE IN TREATMENT OF STROKE AND OTHER NEUROLOGICAL CONDITIONS

Margaret Brownlee and Brian Durward

Key words: aerobic exercise, strength, stroke, Parkinson's disease, multiple sclerosis, spinal cord injury.

Introduction

Muscle strength and cardiorespiratory endurance are recognised as important prerequisites for health and physical function for all individuals. However, conventionally, most of the emphasis in the physical rehabilitation of neurological patients has tended to be given to the management of impairments such as the neurological and biomechanical aspects of muscle tone, and to the re-acquisition of everyday functional skills using neurophysiological (Bobath, 1990; Davies, 1990) or motor learning approaches (Carr and Shepherd, 1992). To date, much less attention has been given to the issues of strength or cardiorespiratory fitness. There is, however, increasing awareness and interest in their relevance and importance to all patients who have a neurological disability.

This chapter will focus on strength and aerobic endurance in relation to cerebrovascular disease (CVD) or stroke, as this is one of the commonest neurological conditions, and furthermore most research has been carried out in this area. Other neurological conditions are also covered, albeit briefly, at the end of the chapter.

Stroke

The World Health Organization definition of a stroke is 'a rapidly developed clinical sign of focal disturbance of cerebral function of presumed vascular origin and of more than 24 hours' duration' (Aho et al., 1980). A stroke is an acute focal neurological deficit resulting from cerebrovascular disease. Lesions such as a stroke, which involve the cortically originating motor system and descending motor pathways, are referred to as upper motor neuron (UMN) lesions. Sensory, cognitive and motor impairments may result, as direct consequences. It is conventional in neuroscience to regard the motor impairments associated with the UMN syndrome, as resulting in both positive and negative features. The positive motor features are exaggerations of normal phenomena and include increased cutaneous and proprioceptive reflexes resulting in spasticity, hyper-reflexia, etc. The negative motor features include weakness, usually referred to as paralysis or paresis, and loss of dexterity (Burke, 1988). The characteristic pattern of weakness is termed hemiplegia or hemiparesis and involves muscles of the arm, leg, trunk, and sometimes face on one side of the body (Fredericks and Saladin, 1996). For patients who survive the cerebrovascular episode leading to stroke, a proportion will recover to some degree (Duncan et al., 1994), and the resulting disability can be classified as 'improving', despite the cause of the stroke. Recovery is related to the site, extent and nature of the lesion, the integrity of the collateral circulation and the pre-morbid status of the patient.

While CVD is not confined to the elderly, its incidence rises with increasing age, and the fact that it is a condition which is primarily associated with older people is significant as there are well documented declines in both strength and aerobic endurance even in the well elderly (Harries et al., 1990; Frontera et al., 1991; Fleg et al., 1995; Rosen et al., 1998). There is, however, evidence that participation in appropriate, regular physical activity (including both aerobic and strengthening exercises) may help to partially reverse or offset these declines. It has been documented that the biological systems of elderly subjects, even those who are frail and very old, retain the ability to adapt to the increasing demands of physical work (Skelton and McLaughlin, 1996; Wood et al., 2001).

It is to be expected that any pre-existing declines in strength and aerobic function will be exacerbated following the onset of CVD, as it results in impaired motor ability, with the consequent further reduction in physical functioning. The issue of maintaining or improving strength and endurance would therefore seem even more pertinent for these individuals.

Strength deficits in stroke patients

Muscle strength may be defined as the ability of a muscle or muscle group to exert force under a given set of conditions. It depends on both neurogenic and myogenic factors, such as the number and type of motor units recruited, the characteristics of motor unit discharge and the properties of muscle itself.

Evidence of strength deficits in stroke patients

For many years the prevailing view in physiotherapy practice was that it was the positive features of the UMN syndrome which were the main cause of stroke patients' movement disorders (Bobath, 1990). It was theorised that the main reason for stroke patients' inability to move was the restraint offered by spastic antagonists to contraction of the agonists, rather than actual weakness in the agonists themselves (Bobath, 1990). This assumption predominated, with little or no experimental confirmation, and in spite of mounting evidence to the contrary (Sahrmann and Norton, 1977; Knutsson and Martensson, 1980).

More recent studies have confirmed the work of earlier researchers, that contrary to the assumptions made by Bobath (1990), actual muscle weakness does exist and is a primary feature of stroke. In a study by Gowland et al. (1992) the electromyographic (EMG) activity of various upper limb muscles in both stroke and control subjects, was investigated during the performance of six tasks. The results showed that there was a significant reduction in agonist muscle activity in subjects who were unable, as compared to those who were able, to complete the tasks. In addition, no evidence was found of abnormally high EMG activity in the antagonist muscles of the stroke subjects. Similar findings were reported in a study by Davies et al. (1996) in which EMG activity and torque were measured in the knee flexors and extensors of stroke and control subjects. It was shown that less torque was generated by the agonist hemiparetic muscles of the stroke subjects, compared to muscles on their contralateral side, and also in comparison to those of the control subjects. In addition, although greater resistance to passive motion was found in the paretic limbs, this was not accompanied by increased EMG activity in the antagonists, thus there was no evidence of spastic antagonist restraint. It was concluded that the source of the increased resistance to motion was of a biomechanical rather than a neural origin.

In summary, muscle weakness is now recognised as a major consequence of stroke and one of the main causes of patients' functional deficits.

Factors contributing to strength deficits in stroke

Many factors may contribute, albeit to different extents, to the reductions in muscle force experienced by patients post-stroke. These include: the direct effects of the neurological lesion, adaptive changes in the musculoskeletal system and age-related changes (Ng and Shepherd, 2000).

Direct effects of the neurological lesion

An upper motor neuron (UMN) lesion such as a stroke, invariably affects the sensorimotor areas of the cerebral cortex and the descending motor pathways. The descending motor tracts exert control over muscle contraction through multiple parallel pathways and any interruption or disruption to them may result in the loss or reduction of descending input to the spinal motor neurons (Gemperline et al., 1995; Kingsley, 1996). The diminished central drive may, in turn, result in loss of motor unit activation and decreased firing rates, which may then be insufficient to cause motor unit discharge at a frequency high enough to generate and sustain a tetanic contraction (Tang and Rymer, 1981; Bourbonnais and Vanden Noven, 1989; Gemperline et al., 1995).

Although morphological changes in hemiparetic muscles are not well understood, some studies have reported that the actual number of functioning motor units is reduced after a stroke. One explanation for this loss is that disruption of the corticospinal tract may result in trans-synaptic degenerative changes, partcularly in type II motor neurons (McComas et al., 1973; Dietz et al., 1986).

There is evidence from various studies that there is a tendency towards selective atrophy of type II (fast twitch) muscle fibres accompanied by a predominance and hypertrophy of type I (slow twitch) fibres (Bourbonnais and Vanden Noven, 1998; Dattola et al., 1993; Toffola et al., 2001).

There is also a suggestion that altered recruitment of motor units may occur (Bourbonnais and Vanden Noven, 1989). In normal circumstances, motor units follow the size principle and are recruited in an orderly manner, with the smaller motor units and muscle fibres (type I) recruited first, and the larger motor units (type II) recruited only at high levels of activation. However, it has been proposed that following a stroke, paretic muscles are unable to develop a high level of force, and therefore type I muscles are predominately recruited and show a more increased contribution to force development than normal, which may in time result in a transformation from type II to type I units (Dattola et al., 1993; Toffola et al., 2001).

Adaptive changes in the musculoskeletal system
In addition to the alterations in muscle structure attributable to altered neural activation, it is likely that muscle atrophy occurs due to reduced activity levels. Histopathological findings from the lower limb muscles of stroke patients have demonstrated that muscle fibre diameter and atrophy had significant correlation coefficients with daily physical activity, but not with the severity of the paralysis, suggesting that disuse is a major mechanism contributing to muscle atrophy subsequent to stroke (Hachisuka et al., 1997).

Relative immobility, imposed as a result of the neurological lesion, may also give rise to other secondary adaptive changes in the musculoskeletal system. A review paper by Singer et al. (2001), documents the changes which occur in the contractile and non-contractile components of muscle, in connective tissue structures and in arthrogenic structures, as a consequence of decreased levels of mobility following acquired brain injury. These include adaptive changes in length, loss of extensibility and increased stiffness or resistance to the passive lengthening of these tissues (Singer et al., 2001). Such mechanical changes in antagonist structures provide passive restraint to agonist muscle contraction during dynamic movement and so contribute to decreased force production or weakness (Ng and Shepherd, 2000).

Age-related changes
The loss of muscle mass (sarcopenia) with increasing age, is well documented (American College of Sports Medicine, 1998). After the age of 70, muscle strength losses are dramatic, with cross-sectional and longitudinal data indicating declines of approximately 15% per decade in the sixth and seventh decade and about 30% thereafter. Although a reduction in fibre size may occur, a decrease in the total number of fibres within muscle is the main cause of sarcopenia. The loss of muscle fibres has been noted to be more marked in type II fibres (ACSM, 1998). The declines in strength associated with ageing have significant consequences for functional capacity.

In summary, the clinical manifestations of strength deficits that have been reported to occur in stroke patients, include an inability to generate normal levels of muscle force or a decrease in the maximum voluntary torque, a slowness in the rate of force development, deficiencies in sustaining force output and a loss of dexterity or ability to make independent movements (Burke, 1988; Bourbonnais and Vanden Noven, 1989; Canning et al., 1999).

Measurement of strength

The quantification of muscle strength should be regarded as a critical aspect of the assessment of stroke patients. It is important to obtain an objective measure of strength in order to monitor changes, identify appropriate treatment methods and assess the effectiveness of therapeutic intervention.

There is abundant literature in relation to strength measurement methods and their validity, accuracy and reliability in non-neurologically impaired individuals. It is not the purpose of this section to provide a comprehensive review of strength testing methods, but rather to consider some of those most commonly used with neurological patients, and to review their reported reliability.

Medical Research Council (MRC) Scale

The MRC Scale is a method that uses manual muscle testing and in which strength is measured using an ordinal scale of 0–5. It is commonly used by physiotherapists for various patient groups. It has also been used in many studies with stroke patients. The reliability of the MRC Scale to measure strength of elbow, wrist, knee and ankle flexors and extensors of stroke patients was assessed by Gregson et al. (2000). The results of this study showed that the inter- and intra-rater agreement for strength measurement was good to very good for all muscle groups tested (Kw = 0.84–0.96, Kw = 0.70–0.96). However, the authors reinforced the need to follow standardised guidelines.

Hand held dynamometry (HHD)

The HHD or myometer may be used to provide a numerical value to quantify muscle force during an isometric contraction. These devices have been used in many research studies involving stroke patients, and have been reported to have good to excellent intra-session reliability (coefficients > 0.80) (Bohannon, 1989, 1992). Excellent inter-session reliability (coefficients > 0.90) has also been reported, mainly for the more affected side (Riddle et al., 1989).

Isokinetic dynamometry

Isokinetic dynamometers have been used to measure both isometric and dynamic muscle strength in numerous studies with stroke patients. In general, there is a limited amount of literature relating to the reliability of this testing method with stroke patients and most of the studies which have been conducted have used muscles of the lower limb. A reliability study of isokinetic knee flexion and extension torque measurements by Tripp and Harris (1991), reported that Pearson Correlation Coefficients and intra-class correlation coefficients (ICCs) were high (0.90) for both involved and uninvolved limbs.

A study by Pohl et al. (2000) examined reliability of knee flexion and extension, and ankle plantar and dorsiflexion. The results confirmed high reliability for both limbs in all measures with the exception of knee flexion in the affected limb, which had ICC values of 0.48 for peak torque and 0.44 for average torque. The reliability of peak and average torque measurements of hip, knee and ankle flexion and extension movements were assessed by Eng et al. (2002a) and were found to be high (ICCs ranged from 0.88–0.99) and similar for both affected and unaffected limbs.

In conclusion, while it is recognised that there is a relative paucity of literature in the use of isokinetic dynamometry with stroke patients, the results of the above studies lend support to the use and further investigation of this testing method with this group.

Distribution of weakness in stroke patients

The paresis or weakness which occurs following a stroke is generally considered to be most severe in the upper and lower limbs contralateral to the brain lesion, in that it presents most obviously as a hemiparesis. However, numerous studies have reported that strength deficits also exist, but to a lesser extent, in the limbs ipsilateral to the brain lesion, those in the so-called normal or unaffected side (Colebatch and Gandevia, 1989; Smutok et al., 1989; Adams et al., 1990; Desrosiers et al., 1996; Andrews and Bohannon, 2000).

In comparison to the limbs, strength impairments in trunk musculature have been given much less attention in research, possibly due to the perceived difficulty in assessing strength in this region. However, several studies have documented that trunk muscle strength is impaired multi-directionally, with muscles involved in forward flexion demonstrating greater deficits than those involved in lateral flexion movements, and with greater impairment being shown in the ability to produce force towards the paretic side compared to the non-paretic side (Bohannon, 1992, 1995; Bohannon et al., 1995). Impairment of the muscles of the neck (Mastaglia et al., 1986), muscles involved in respiration (Annoni et al., 1990) and in mastication (Gruccu et al., 1988) have also been reported.

Such a widespread distribution of muscle weakness should not be unexpected, when it is considered that the descending motor pathways (rubrospinal, reticulospinal and vestibulospinal tracts, in addition to the corticobulbospinal tract) function as an integrated system, and that they are collectively responsible for the innervation of limb and trunk musculature. The involvement of the muscles on the side ipsilateral to the brain lesion, may be explained by the fact that some of the tracts have bilateral projections (Kingsley, 1996; Burke, 1988).

An investigation of weakness in 12 upper limb muscle groups by Colebatch and Gandevia (1989) found that, although the pattern of weakness varied amongst patients, the most affected groups were distal, such as finger and wrist flexors and muscles involved in hand grip, while the least affected were the proximal groups, such as shoulder abductors and adductors. It was also found in this study that elbow flexors were more affected than elbow extensors. The key findings to emerge from a study by Adams et al. (1990), investigating weakness in eight lower limb muscles, were that the proximal muscles of the hip and knee were significantly less affected than the distal muscles of the ankle and hallux. It was also found that there was no significant difference in the extent of weakness between the physiological flexors and extensors. In a similar manner to the upper limb, there was found to be variability amongst patients, with the weakness distribution not conforming to a common pattern.

In contrast, a study by Andrews and Bohannon (2000), examining strength in four muscle groups in each of the upper and lower limbs, found no significant difference in the strength impairments between proximal and distal limb muscles. This study also found no significant difference in the severity of impairments between the upper and lower limbs. It did, however, concur with the findings of Colebatch and Gandevia (1989), by identifying significant differences between elbow flexion and extension strength impairments, with flexion being more impaired.

Work examining the relative strength impairments of seven upper limb muscle groups demonstrated that shoulder abduction was relatively more affected than shoulder extension and that shoulder external rotation was more severely affected than internal rotation (Bohannon and Andrews, 1987).

In summary, although there is some disagreement amongst authors regarding the extent to which different muscle groups in the paretic upper and lower limbs of stroke patients are impaired, there is agreement regarding the generalised strength reduction in stroke patients, the variability amongst patients and the fact that there is bilateral involvement post-stroke. This suggests there is a need to assess strength bilaterally and to be aware that the non-paretic limb does not reflect normal function (Newham and Hsiao, 2001).

Strength training following stroke

If strength training is to be employed as part of a rehabilitation programme for stroke patients, then its use requires to be justified by establishing that no adverse or untoward effects will occur as a consequence of strength training methods, that improvements in strength are possible to achieve within the stroke population and that there is a relation between improved strength and functional ability.

Strength training and spasticity

The strengthening of muscles in individuals who have suffered a stroke, has long been regarded as controversial and inappropriate in certain neuro-rehabilitation approaches (Bobath, 1990; Davies, 1990), in which it is considered that any excessive effort induced by overload training will result in an increase in spasticity and movement abnormalities. These views have not been borne out by the results of several recent studies, which have incorporated resistance or overload training with stroke patients, and which have found no evidence of a resultant increase in neurological tone (Miller and Light, 1997; Sharp and Brouwer, 1997; Brown and Kautz, 1998; Smith et al., 1999; Teixeira-Salmela et al., 1999). Indeed, there is evidence from some studies, that the amplitude of stretch reflex activity is reduced following resistance exercise in the paretic lower limbs (Hsiao and Newham, 1998; Smith et al., 1999). However, a study by Engardt et al. (1995) did report increased EMG activity in antagonist muscles during concentric training with an isokinetic dynamometer, but not with eccentric training. It was reasoned by the authors, that the antagonist restraint was greatest in concentric movements at high velocities due to the velocity dependence of the exaggerated stretch reflexes. Therefore, although the weight of evidence is in support of there being no increase in spasticity with resistance training, the issue concerning velocity of motion is worthy of consideration during both strength training and testing.

Effects of strength training

The following section will review the results of several research trials involving strength training in stroke patients.

A randomised pre- and post-test control group, followed by a single group pre- and post-test design was employed by Teixeira-Salmela et al. (1999), in which 13 stroke patients underwent a ten-week (three days per week) programme of aerobic activities and strengthening of hip and knee flexors and extensors, hip abductors and ankle dorsi and plantarflexors. The strength training protocol was devised using accepted principles of progressive resistance exercise and involved isometric, concentric and eccentric contractions, using body weight and other forms of external resistance. The aerobic component comprised a progressive walking, cycling and stepping regime. Results from this study revealed significant effects for all outcome measures. The total mean peak torque generated by muscle groups of the paretic leg, as measured by isokinetic dynamometry, demonstrated a significant increase of 42.3% (p = 0.000) from baseline values. Walking speed showed a significant improvement of 30.7% (p = 0.004) and timed stair climbing improved by 37.4% (p = 0.000).

A further study by Teixeira-Salmela et al. (2001) evaluated the effects of a ten-week (three days per week) combined aerobic conditioning and lower limb strengthening programme, on gait performance in 13 stroke patients. This work employed a single group pre- and post-test design. The strengthening and aerobic protocols, as described, were the same as those involved in the earlier study by Teixeira-Salmela and associates. Gait was assessed from cinematographic and force plate data and results indicated significant increases in gait speed (37.2% above baseline values) in association with improved ability to generate higher levels of power, and increases in positive work by the ankle plantarflexor and hip flexor and extensor muscles. However, as in the earlier study by Teixeira-Salmela and co-workers (1999), it is not possible to differentiate the specific effects of the strengthening component from those of the task-related aerobic activities.

The study by Engardt et al. (1995) compared the effects of eccentric and concentric training of the paretic leg in two groups, each consisting of ten stroke patients. Training involved generating isokinetic maximal voluntary knee extension motions, through a range of angular velocities, and was performed twice a week for six weeks for each group. Post-training results showed that knee extensor strength had increased in eccentric and concentric actions in both groups ($p < 0.05$). The increases in the eccentric and concentric strength in the paretic leg relative to the non-paretic leg showed statistical significance in the eccentric training group ($p < 0.05$) but were not significant in the concentric training group. The eccentric group demonstrated significant improvement ($p < 0.01$) in symmetry of lower limb weight distribution in the action of standing up from sitting, while the concentric group demonstrated significant increases in walking speed ($p < 0.05$). It was also reported in this study that results of EMG activity indicated that increases in strength were related to enhanced activation of the agonists, in that strength increases were associated with neural factors.

In a non-randomised, self-controlled trial by Sharp and Brouwer (1997), 15 stroke patients took part in a six-week (three days per week) programme of reciprocal knee flexion and extension strengthening of the paretic limb, using an isokinetic dynamometer. The training regime comprised three sets of six to eight repetitions of maximal contractions, at each of three speeds. Results indicated that both hamstrings and quadriceps showed significant gains in strength immediately post-training ($p < 0.05$) at all three speeds of testing. Gait velocity had increased significantly, immediately post-training (by 5.8%) and also at four-week follow-up (by 6.8%) ($p < 0.05$). Although changes were noted for stair climbing and timed get up and go, these values were not significant ($p > 0.37$; $p > 0.91$).

In an investigation by Smith et al. (1999), 14 chronic stroke patients participated in a progressive intensity walking programme on a motorised treadmill, three times per week for 12 weeks. The results demonstrated significant increases in hamstring torque and rate of torque production, as assessed by isokinetic dynamometry in both lower limbs, and a significant reduction in reflexive rate of torque production in the hamstrings of the paretic limbs ($p < 0.027$). The authors hypothesised that although the resultant strength gains could have been due to a reversal of chronic physical deconditioning, it was also likely that the 'forced use' of the paretic limbs may have had an influence in improving spinal motor unit recruitment consistent with central neural reorganisation.

In summary, all of the studies reviewed, reported that strength could be improved in stroke patients and that, depending on the strengthening method employed, there could also be significant functional improvements in selected parameters. However, the limitations of small sample sizes and the lack of randomisation and control in many of the study designs must be recognised. Therefore, in order to further strengthen the evidence in support of this treatment modality, there is a need for larger scale, randomised, controlled studies to be conducted. Nevertheless, since all of the subjects had had their strokes at least six months prior to the investigations, it would have been expected that they would have plateaued with respect to the extent of spontaneous recovery, thus lending support to the strength and functional improvements being due to the experimental interventions.

The studies reviewed in this section, used a variety of different strengthening methods, incorporating isokinetic or isotonic training or repetitive functional activities, different training durations and intensities and different types of muscle contraction, etc. Thus, it must be acknowledged that more research is also required regarding the most beneficial strengthening methods and training regimes, not just for strength increases but also for functional improvement.

Current opinion, based on research evidence, suggests that the amount of force that can be generated within a particular movement context is determined not only by intramuscular factors, but also by the effectiveness of muscle coordination; thus some of the adaptations associated with resistance training may be regarded as motor learning (Carroll et al., 2001). This implies that once a certain level of force generating capacity has been developed by muscles, then that muscle force should be used in the repetitive practice of actual functional tasks, in which the strengthened muscles are being forced to work in a variety of task-specific contexts. Research from studies in both the well elderly and in younger age groups supports this concept of task-specific training for optimal improvement in functional skills (Skelton et al., 1995; Skelton and McLaughlin, 1996; Enoka, 1997).

Cardiorespiratory deficits in stroke

Evidence exists which indicates that the incidence of atherosclerosis, hypertension and coronary heart disease (CHD) are significantly higher in adults with physical disabilities such as stroke (Santiago et al., 1993). Patients with hemiplegia as a result of CVD are disabled by more than just the effect of the stroke; concomitant heart and respiratory disease are common and are clinically significant problems. From the emerging research evidence of the cardiorespiratory deficits associated with stroke it is possible to form two distinctive groupings, co-morbid deficits and resultant deficits.

Co-morbid deficits

The common coexistence of coronary heart disease (CHD) in stroke patients, especially those with ischaemic cerebrovascular accidents, is not surprising because the underlying pathological process of atherosclerosis is the same in both conditions (Gitter et al., 1995). Epidemiological studies indicate that up to 77% of stroke patients have some form of coexisting cardiac disease (Roth, 1993). Heart disease has been shown to be an important independent risk factor for stroke and is the main cause of death of stroke patients who survive acute stroke (Dennis et al., 1993). It is clear, therefore, that stroke rehabilitation should incorporate the goals and principles of cardiac rehabilitation.

Resultant deficits

Lung volume, thoracic movement and pulmonary diffusing capacity are all affected by stroke (Hass et al., 1967; Gitter et al., 1995). Average vital capacity levels have been found to reduce by 88% of normal and the maximal mid-expiratory flow rate is reduced. These deficits are generally attributed to dysfunction in muscles responsible for inspiration and expiration. It is less certain whether the postural alterations associated with stroke also contribute to respiratory deficits. These resultant respiratory deficits affect the ability of patients to perform essential tasks, such as walking, where following stroke the energy costs increase by 1.5 to 2 times compared to normal control subjects (Macko et al., 2001).

Measurement of cardiorespiratory fitness

Exercise stress testing is widely used as a screening method to detect the presence, severity or probable impact of CHD in many different client groups. It is also used to assess patients' functional capacity or ability to tolerate increasing intensities of physical work, and from this information, to prescribe a suitable aerobic fitness programme (ACSM, 2000).

However, exercise stress testing is not routinely used in screening for CHD or as the basis for aerobic exercise prescription in stroke patients. The reasons for this are varied and include concerns about stroke patients' abilities to participate safely and effectively in conventional testing methods using standardised treadmill or cycle ergometers. To circumvent the problem of patients' physical limitations, various researchers have used modified or adapted stress testing methods.

A supine cycle ergometer (Moldover et al., 1984) and a combined arm and leg ergometer (King et al., 1989) have both been used successfully and found to be appropriate for the testing in the disabled stroke population. An upright cycle ergometer (Potempa et al., 1995) and treadmill tests (Macko et al., 1997) have also been used successfully. Functional walking tests such as the six and twelve-minute tests have not proved successful in assessing stroke patients, as physical deficits following stroke are major limitations to distance walked and may have influence on perceived exertion (Eng et al., 2002b).

Safety is of paramount concern during any exercise stress test. It is therefore imperative that guidelines regarding patient screening, exclusion criteria, contraindications, patient monitoring and criteria for test implementation and termination should be consulted and followed (ACSM, 2000). A further point worthy of note to emerge from the studies, was the need to consider the effects of any medication on the patients' physiological responses and exercise capacity.

Aerobic exercise following stroke

While the value of exercise in CHD is now well established, it is only more recently that the potential of aerobic exercise to improve the endurance capacity and minimise the symptoms associated with co-morbid and resultant cardio-vascular deficits in stroke patients has been researched.

Evidence from a number of studies now indicates that chronic stroke subjects may be able to improve their aerobic capacity and physical fitness levels with appropriate training. The inclusion of appropriate aerobic exercise is therefore increasingly being regarded as an important part of a comprehensive rehabilitation programme for stroke. The following section will review the results of several research studies in which stroke survivors have participated in aerobic exercise training.

Effects of aerobic training

The first definitive study which attempted to investigate the effects of intensive exercise for hemiplegic stroke patients was conducted by Potempa et al. (1995). Forty-two subjects were randomly assigned to an exercise training group or to a control group and baseline and post-test measurements were made of maximal oxygen consumption, heart rate, workload, exercise time, resting and sub-maximal blood pressures and sensorimotor function. The exercise programme was delivered three times per week for ten weeks and took the form of adapted cycle ergometer activity for 30 minutes a session (three times per week, for ten weeks). During the initial period of training the intensity was gradually increased and then maintained during the final six weeks of training. The control group received a passive range of movement programme throughout the same period. The results from this study indicated differences between the experimental and control subjects. Only experimental subjects showed significant improvement in maximal oxygen consumption, workload and exercise time. On completion of the study, experimental subjects showed significantly lower systolic blood pressure at sub-maximal workloads during the graded exercise test. This study therefore demonstrated that stroke patients may improve their aerobic capacity and sub-maximal exercise systolic blood pressure response with training.

In response to Potempa's initial study, Macko et al. (2001) investigated the hypothesis that treadmill training will improve peak fitness, while lowering the energy cost of hemiplegic gait in chronic stroke patients. Using an incidental sample, 23 patients with a six-month history of stroke were investigated using a non-controlled repeated measure design. The intervention, which comprised three 40-minute sessions of treadmill exercise delivered weekly for six months, was measured using peak exercise capacity (VO_2peak) and rate of oxygen consumption during sub-maximal effort treadmill walking by means of spirometry. Results from this study revealed that the patients in general increased their VO_2peak and lowered their oxygen demands of sub-maximal effort ambulation. The patients were able to perform the same constant load treadmill task using 20% less of their peak exercise capacity.

The effects of aerobic exercises and lower extremity muscle strengthening were investigated by Teixeira-Salmela et al. (1999). This study was also reviewed in the section on effects of strength training, p. 212. Using a combined programme of physical conditioning and muscle strengthening, the study investigated the effects on reducing impairment in disability in subjects with chronic stroke. A randomised pre-test and post-test control group followed by a single group pre-test and post-test design was adopted. Thirteen community dwelling stroke survivors of at least nine months underwent a ten-week (three days a week) programme, consisting of a warm up, supervised aerobic exercises, lower extremity muscle strengthening based on progressive resistance training, utilising isometric, concentric and eccentric contractions, and a cool down. The outcome measures included peak isokinetic torque of the major muscle groups of the affected lower limb, plantarflexor spasticity, gait speed, rate of stair climbing and measures of activity and health. Significant improvements were measured in all the selected outcome measures for the treatment group ($p < 0.001$). It was notable that the improvement in the outcome measures was not associated with measurable changes of spasticity in either quadriceps or ankle plantarflexors.

The safety and efficacy of graded treadmill training as an aerobic exercise modality in older stroke patients was investigated by Macko et al. (1997). Nine stroke patients who were 50 years of age or older, with mild or moderate hemiparetic gait after ischemic stroke, were enrolled in a six-month programme of low-intensity aerobic exercise using a graded treadmill. Within a repeated measures design, measures of energy expenditure based on steady state oxygen consumption during a standardised sub-maximal effort treadmill walking task were performed before and after training. The six-month low-intensity aerobic exercise training programme consisted of three sessions of 40 minutes each per week or graded treadmill walking at 50% to 60% of heart rate reserve. Upon completion of the six months of exercise training, the patients demonstrated a reduction in energy expenditure during a sub-maximal treadmill walking task. This study again indicates that task orientated aerobic exercise may improve functional mobility as well as the cardiovascular fitness profile in stroke patients.

A study which combined strength, balance and endurance training within a single intervention for individuals with stroke was reported by Duncan et al. (1998). Twenty minimally and moderately impaired stroke patients who were home based and who were 30 to 90 days after stroke onset were randomised to a control group or to an experimental group that received a therapist-supervised, eight-week, three times per week, home-based exercise programme. The home-based exercise programme comprised exercise sessions that lasted for approximately 1.5 hours. Exercise took the form of assisted and resisted proprioceptive neuromuscular facilitation patterns (PNF) or the use of Theraband resisted exercise to the major muscle groups of the upper and lower extremities. In addition, the patients received blocks of balance training, as well as walking or progressive exercise on a bicycle ergometer. The control group received routine care. Outcome measures included ADL indices, measures of health status and functional assessments of balance, gait and hand function. Compared to the control group, the experimental results indicated improvement in terms of general motor function and improved gait and balance. There was no improvement in hand function or activities of daily living. This study is notable in that it demonstrates that a randomised control design, addressing the effects of exercise, can be undertaken within the home setting of stroke patients.

In general, these studies indicate that cardiorespiratory performance could be improved in stroke patients following the delivery of training programmes specific to them. At present, the emerging evidence in support of exercise for cardiorespiratory deficits following stroke is limited. Small sample sizes and the lack of randomised designs incorporating control groups characterise many of the studies in this area. There is a need, therefore, to strengthen the evidence with the adoption of larger, randomised control studies to investigate the stroke population, with a clear indication of sample characteristics. Emerging from existing studies is an indication that training gains plateau at approximately six months. It would be appropriate for future studies to include follow-up measures to identify the long-term benefits of exercise and its effect on cardiorespiratory deficits.

It is clear from the existing studies that a range of methodologies and measurement parameters have been adopted to measure outcomes. There is a need to develop agreed measurement protocols for the stroke population in future studies in an attempt to standardise the outcome measures and enable effective cross-study comparisons.

From existing studies, the emerging evidence would suggest that exercise under controlled conditions has the potential to improve the cardiorespiratory deficits which either occur in premorbid state or as a result of stroke. Further research is required to identify the optimal training strategies that may be used for hospital and home-based exercise intervention programmes.

Exercise in other neurological conditions

This section examines exercise in other neurological conditions and has been added by the editors.

Spinal cord injury

'Tetraplegia or quadriplegia is the impairment or loss of motor and/or sensory function in the cervical region of the spinal cord due to damage of neural elements within the spinal canal. Tetraplegia results in impairment of function in the arms as well as in the trunk, legs and pelvic organs. Paraplegia refers to impairment or loss of motor and/or sensory function in the thoracic, lumbar or sacral segments of the spinal cord. With paraplegia arm function is spared but depending on the level of the injury, the trunk, legs and pelvic organs may be involved.' (Ditunno et al., 1994)

Classification of the lesion is beyond the scope of this text but the reader is referred to Ditunno's reference for this. The clinical effects of the injury depend on the level and the severity of the damage to the spinal cord. Transection of the spinal cord will result in a loss of motor power, loss of sensation, vasomotor control disturbances, bladder and bowel dysfunction and sexual dysfunction. In incomplete lesions some of the nerves may escape injury.

Exercise in the overall treatment of the patient with spinal cord injury will commence early and continue right through rehabilitation and become part of everyday life. Early on in the acute stage passive movements of the paralysed parts will be done by the physiotherapist to maintain range of movement. Active movements of the unaffected areas will begin in an effort to maintain muscle strength. In those with cervical cord lesions no neck exercises are permitted until six weeks post-injury. In those with thoracic or lower lesions resisted arm exercises in supine begin early. Once the fracture has healed mobilisation of the trunk begins gradually. Functional activities such as lifting and moving, moving the paralysed limbs, sitting up and lying down and rolling are then commenced. Transfers are then introduced with the aim of working towards independent transfers.

Sport helps in restoring the patient's strength, balance, coordination and endurance and for other benefits such as interaction with others and for those previously involved in sports it may allow competition in another sport. However, as well as the benefits of socialisation and achievement a certain level of aerobic fitness is necessary to meet the demands of daily life.

Regular exercise in those with spinal cord injury may reduce risk factors for CHD and obesity. Heart disease is among the principal causes of mortality in those with tetraplegia. Due to the nature of the lesion myocardial ischaemia may not be perceived and medical clearance may be necessary prior to commencing an exercise programme. Obesity is likely to occur in this patient group due to the loss of metabolically active tissue and therefore a lower basal energy expenditure.

Upper extremity training will probably be the choice of exercise for those with paraplegia. However, there needs to be consideration of shoulder and upper extremity musculoskeletal problems/overuse injuries. When prescribing exercise the risks of autonomic dysreflexia, areas of skin breakdown, blood pressure responses, osteopenia, and extremes of temperature intolerance need to be considered.

Traumatic brain injury

Traumatic brain injury has been cited as the leading cause of death and lifelong disability in the USA. Such injury is most common in male adolescents and mechanisms of injury include road traffic accidents (RTA), falls and violence (Greenwald et al., 2003). Traumatic brain injury may be classed as primary or secondary, where primary is the damage occurring at the time of impact and secondary being the body's response to the primary injury. The extent of secondary injury can be influenced by medical intervention. The pathology of secondary injury may be divided into intracranial or extracranial insults. Intracranial include hypoxaemia and hypotension and extracranial include various types of haematoma.

The damage to brain tissue following traumatic brain injury (TBI) will in many ways be similar to that following stroke. Thus, there may be focal areas of damage resulting in specific deficits. For this reason much of the rehabilitation will follow the same pathways and the role of exercise may be carried through for a number of pathologies. Thus the previous section, describing exercise in stroke, may be applied with appropriate adaptations in the management of TBI. However, there are a number of special considerations that must be reviewed in the case of TBI. It has already been mentioned that the majority sustaining a TBI are young males. It should be expected that the cardiovascular system should be in better health than that of a subject who sustained a CVA, with the patient demonstrating greater aerobic fitness from the outset. Also, because of the population type, there may be limited existence of other pathologies such as osteoarthritis, which may alter use of exercise. All TBI patients are different and each patient must be considered as an individual.

A number of TBI patients will spend some time in a state of unconsciousness or coma and the role of exercise during this period is invaluable. From necessity, this exercise is passive and is carried out by a physiotherapist. In the acute setting, passive range of movement exercises and stretching will help to maintain joint and soft tissue integrity. Passive trunk rotation may not only help in maintenance of movement but may help normalise tone. As the patient becomes more responsive, bedside exercises, such as balance work with a Bobath ball or active limb exercise, form an important part of rehabilitation (Montgomery, 1995). Stretching continues to form an important part of management, particularly when tone changes alter joint biomechanics.

Maintenance of aerobic capacity following TBI is important. As mentioned previously, many of these patients will have demonstrated good cardiovascular health pre-injury and maintaining these levels may enhance recovery. As has been mentioned many times in this text, aerobic exercise is a core component of prescription. Jackson et al. (2001) investigated the capacity of brain-injured patients to participate in exercise early after injury. They concluded that there was no reason that such a programme should not form an early part of rehabilitation. Further, Gordon et al. (1998), in a retrospective study, found that there were psychological changes when exercise was used in TBI management, with findings suggesting improvement in mood and health status of these patients.

Parkinson's disease

One of the most common lesions of the basal ganglia encountered by physiotherapists is Parkinson's disease. The production of the neurotransmitter dopamine, usually produced in the substantia nigra of the basal ganglia, is reduced in Parkinson's disease, leading to the characteristic symptoms of rigidity, tremor and bradykinesia. Bradykinesia is a disturbance of voluntary movement, which causes a slowness in initiating movement. The severity of the symptoms can vary from stage 1, where there is only unilateral involvement, to stage 5, where the patient is confined to a wheelchair or bed (Hoehn and Yahr, 1967).

There is no treatment that will prevent the onset or effectively delay the progression of Parkinson's disease (Jones and Godwin-Austen, 1998). Physiotherapy is aimed at maintaining optimum function for the patient and will largely depend on the stage and progression of the disease. Exercise in the form of postural correction, flexibility exercises, muscle strengthening and endurance work are all important, especially during the early and middle stages of the disease. Education of the patient about strategies to minimise the effects of the disease on movement are included. Functional activities are also an essential component of treatment.

To maintain aerobic capacity it would seem appropriate to incorporate aerobic-type endurance exercise into the treatment programme. Furthermore, the prevalance of Parkinson's disease increases with increasing age and the mean time of onset is in the seventh decade. Patients therefore may have co-morbitities including cardiovascular disease and respiratory disease. Physical activity has been found to decrease in patients following diagnosis (Fertl et al., 1993). Furthermore, a study by Kuroda et al. (1992) determined that patients with Parkinson's disease who had low levels of activity had a greater risk of dying compared to those with higher levels of activity. The level of activity is related to the severity of disease but activity may be very beneficial.

Reuter et al. (1999) examined the effect of intensive sports activities in patients with Parkinson's disease. Improvements in motor skills were found, along with improvements on the Unified Parkinson's Disease Rating Scale and a basic motor test which measured flexibility, strength and coordination. Bergen et al. (2002) examined the effect of a 16-week aerobic training programme on patients with Parkinson's disease. Only four out of the original eight subjects completed the study. The four subjects, however, demonstrated significantly increased $\dot{V}O_2$peak and improvements in movement initiation time were also found.

The evidence for the beneficial effects of aerobic-type exercise in patients with Parkinson's disease may be limited, but it would appear to be beneficial. Both the studies above were carried out on patients in the earlier stages of the disease. More research is needed to determine the effects of long-term aerobic-type exercise in patients with Parkinson's disease.

Multiple sclerosis

Multiple sclerosis is the most common neurological disease of the young and middle aged adult. It is known as a demyelinating disease, where the myelin sheath of a nerve is destroyed, causing loss of nerve conduction. It is characterised by acute neurological deficit (weakness or sensory disturbance) in one or more limbs, followed by a remission. The pattern may repeat itself over time. Initially the remission may appear complete, but over time, with repeated exacerbations and remissions, a residual deficit will become apparent. As the disease progresses disability will increase and in its most severe form it will cause death within weeks or months of its onset.

The signs and symptoms of multiple sclerosis will depend on the area of the spinal cord or brain affected. The reader is referred to a neurological textbook for a full description. In the limbs, increased tone and weakness are common and tremor may be evident. Symptoms of ataxia and fatigue are also common. Physiotherapy intervention is aimed at preventing contractures, maintaining or increasing range of movement, maintaining weight bearing and postural stability (DeSouza et al., 1998). Manual tasks and walking can become difficult due to the symptoms above. The exercise capacity of a patient may therefore decrease rapidly over time.

For years patients with multiple sclerosis were told to avoid exercise as the symptoms often temporarily worsen on exercising. Aerobic and strengthening programmes can, however, maintain or increase the exercise capacity and prevent disuse atrophy of muscles. Low to moderate intensity exercise is recommended for patients with multiple sclerosis, as high intensity exercise may exacerabate symptoms. A four-week bicycle exercise programme carried out five times per week for 30 minutes was found to increase aerobic threshold, increase health perception and activity levels (Mostert and Kesselring, 2002). Research is needed to determine the appropriate level of exercise for patients with multiple sclerosis.

This chapter provides an insight into the use of strengthening and aerobic exercises in certain neurological conditions. The major proportion of the chapter dealt in depth with stroke. This is due to the fact that it is one of the most common conditions treated by physiotherapists and furthermore most of the research examining the effects of exercise have been carried out in stroke. The use of aerobic exercise in other neurological conditions is relatively new and more research is required to determine the optimium levels for patients with specific neurological conditions.

References

Adams, R.W., Gandevia, S.C. and Skuse, N.F. (1990). The distribution of muscle weakness in upper motor neuron lesions affecting the lower limb. *Brain* 13, 1459–76.

Aho, K., Harmsen, P., Hatano, S., Marquardsen, J., Smirnov, V.E. and Sorasser, T. (1980). *Cerebrovascular Disease in the Community: Results of a WHO Collaborative Study*. Bulletin of the World Health Organization 58 (1), 113–30.

American College of Sports Medicine (1998). Exercise and physical activity for older adults. *Medicine and Science in Sports and Exercise* 30 (6), 992–1008.

American College of Sports Medicine (2000). *ACSM's Guidelines for Exercise Testing and Prescription*, 6th edn. Lippincott Williams and Wilkins, Philadelphia.

Andrews, A.W. and Bohannon, R.W. (2000). Distribution of muscle strength impairments following stroke. *Clinical Rehabilitation* 14, 79–87.

Annoni, J.M., Ackerman, D. and Kesselring, J. (1990). Respiratory function in chronic hemiplegia. *International Disability Studies* 12, 78–80.

Bergen, J.L., Toole, T., Elliott, R.G., Wallace, B., Robinson, K. and Maitland, C.G. (2002). Aerobic exercise intervention improves aerobic capacity and movement initiation in Parkinson's disease patients. *Neuro-rehabilitation* 17 (2), 161–8.

Bobath, B. (1990). *Adult Hemiplegia: Evaluation and Treatment*, 3rd edn. Heinemann, Oxford.

Bohannon, R.W. (1989). Knee extension force measurements are reliable and indicative of walking speed in stroke patients. *International Journal of Rehabilitation Research* 12, 193–4.

Bohannon, R.W. (1992). Lateral trunk flexion strength. Impairment, measurement reliability and implications following brain injury. *International Journal of Rehabilitation Research* 15, 249–51.

Bohannon, R.W. (1995). Recovery and correlates of trunk muscle strength after stroke. *International Journal of Rehabilitation Research* 18, 162–7.

Bohannon, R.W. and Andrews, A.W. (1987). Relative strength of seven upper extremity muscle groups in hemiparetic stroke patients. *Journal of Neurologic Rehabilitation* **1** (4), 161–5.

Bohannon, R.W., Cassidy, D. and Walsh, S. (1995). Trunk muscle strength in impaired multi-directionally after stroke. *Clinical Rehabilitation* **9**, 47–51.

Bourbonnais, D. and Vanden Noven, S. (1989). Weakness in patients with hemiparesis. *American Journal of Occupational Therapy* **43** (5), 313–9.

Brown, D.A. and Kautz, S.A. (1998). Increased workload enhances force output during pedalling exercise in persons with post-stroke hemiplegia. *Stroke* **29**, 598–606.

Burke, D. (1988). Spasticity as an adaptation to pyramidal tract injury. In: *Advances in Neurology, Vol. 47: Functional Recovery in Neurological Disease* (Waxman, S.G. ed.), pp. 401–23. Raven Press, New York.

Canning, C.G., Ada, L. and O'Dwyer, N. (1999). Slowness to develop force contributes to weakness after stroke. *Archives of Physical Medicine and Rehabilitation* **80**, 66 70.

Carr, J.H. and Shepherd, R.B. (1992). *A Motor Relearning Programme for Stroke*, 2nd edn. Butterworth-Heinemann, Oxford.

Carroll, T.J., Riek, S. and Carson, R.G. (2001). Neural adaptations to resistance training. Implications for movement control. *Sports Medicine* **31** (12), 829–40.

Colebatch, J.G. and Gandevia, S.C. (1989). The distribution of muscular weakness in upper motor neuron lesions affecting the arm. *Brain* **112**, 749–63.

Dattola, R., Girlanda, P., Vita, G., Santoro, M., Roberto, M.L., Toscano, A., Venuto, C., Baradello, A. and Messina, C. (1993). Muscle rearrangement in patients with hemi paresis after stroke: an electrophysiological and morphological study. *European Neurology* **33**, 109–14.

Davies, J.M., Mayston, M.J. and Newham, D.J. (1996). Electrical and mechanical output of the knee muscles during isometric and isokinetic activity in stroke and healthy adults. *Disability and Rehabilitation* **18** (2), 83–90.

Davies, P.M. (1990). *Right in the Middle*. Springer-Verlag, Berlin Heidelberg.

Dennis, M.S., Burn, J.P., Sandercock, P.A., Barnford, J.M., Wade, D.T. and Warlow, C.P. (1993). Long-term survival after first ever stroke: the Oxfordshire Community Stroke Project. *Stroke* **25**, 796–800.

DeSouza, L., Bates, D. and Moran, G. (1998). Multiple sclerosis. In: *Neurological Rehabilitation* (Stokes, M. ed.). Elsevier Science, London.

Desrosiers, J., Bourbonnais, D., Bravo, G., Roy, P-M. and Guay, M. (1996). Performance of the 'unaffected' upper extremity of elderly stroke patients. *Stroke* **27**, 1564–70.

Dietz, V., Ketelsen, U.P., Berger, W. and Quintern, J. (1986). Motor unit involvement in spastic paresis: relationship between leg muscle activation and histochemistry. *Journal of Neurological Sciences* **75**, 89–103.

Ditunno, J.F., Young, W., Donovan, W.H. and Creasley, G. (1994). The international standards booklet for neurological and functional classification of spinal cord injuries. *Paraplegia* **32**, 70–80.

Duncan, P.W., Goldstein, L.B., Horner, R.D., Landsman, P.B., Samou, S.P. and Matchar, D.B. (1994). Similar motor recovery of upper and lower extremities after stroke. *Stroke* **25**, 1181–8.

Duncan, P., Richards, L., Wallace, D., Stoker-Yates, J., Pohl, P., Luchies, C., Ogle, A. and Studenski, S. (1998). A randomised, controlled pilot study of a home-based exercise program for individuals with mild and moderate stroke. *Stroke* **29**, 2055–60.

Eng, J.J., Kim, M. and MacIntyre, D.L. (2002a). Reliability of lower extremity strength measures in persons with chronic stroke. *Archives of Physical Medicine and Rehabilitation* 83, 322–8.

Eng, J.J., Chu, K.S., Dawson, A.S., Kim, C.M. and Hepburn, K.E. (2002b). Functional walk tests in individuals with stroke: relation to perceived exertion and myocardial exertion. *Stroke* 33, 756–61.

Engardt, M., Knutsson, E., Jonsson, M. and Sternhag, M. (1995). Dynamic muscle strength training in stroke patients: effects on knee extension torque, electromyographic activity, and motor function. *Archives of Physical Medicine and Rehabilitation* 76, 419–25.

Enoka, R.M. (1997). Neural adaptations with chronic physical activity. *Journal of Biomechanics* 30 (5), 447–55.

Fertl, E., Doppelbauer, A. and Auff, E. (1993). Physical activity and sports in patients suffering from Parkinson's disease in comparison with healthy seniors. *Journal of Neural Transmission* 5 (2), 157–61.

Fleg, J., O'Connor, F., Gerstenblith, G., Becker, L., Clulow, J., Sculman, S. and Lakatta, E. (1995). Impact of age on the cardiovascular response to dynamic upright exercise in healthy men and women. *Journal of Applied Physiology* 78, 890–900.

Fredericks, C.M. and Saladin, L.K. (1996). *Pathophysiology of the Motor Systems: Principles and Clinical Presentations*. F.A. Davis Company, Philadelphia.

Frontera, W.R., Hughes,V.A. and Evans, W.J. (1991). A cross-sectional study of upper and lower extremity muscle strength in 45–78-year-old men and women. *Journal of Applied Physiology* 71, 644–50.

Gemperline, J.J., Allen, S., Walk, D. and Rymer, W.Z. (1995). Characteristics of motor unit discharge in subjects with hemiparesis. *Muscle and Nerve* 18, 1101–14.

Gitter, A. and Haller, E.M. (1995). Cardiac rehabilitation of the patient with stroke. *Physical Medicine and Rehabilitation Clinics of North America* 6 (N2), 297–309.

Gordon, W.A., Sliwinski, M., Echo, J., McLoughlin, M., Sheerer, M.S. and Meil, M. (1998). The benefits of exercise in individuals with traumatic brain injury: a retrospective study. *Journal of Head Trauma and Rehabilitation* 13 (4), 58–67.

Gowland, C., deBruin, H., Basmajian, J.V., Plews, N. and Burcea, I. (1992). Agonist and antagonist activity during voluntary upper-limb movement in patients with stroke. *Physical Therapy* 72 (9), 624–33.

Greenwald, B.D., Burnett, D.M. and Miller, M.A. (2003). Congenital and acquired brain injury.1. Brain injury: epidemiology and pathophysiology. *Archives of Physical Medicine and Rehabilitation* 84, suppl. 1, S3–S7.

Gregson, J.M., Leathley, M.J., Moore, A.P., Smith, T.L., Sharma, A.K. and Watkins, C.L. (2000). Reliability of measurements of muscle tone and muscle power in stroke patients. *Age and Ageing* 29, 223–8.

Gruccu, G., Fornarelli, M. and Manfredi, M. (1988). Impairment of masticatory function in hemiplegia. *Neurology* 38, 301–6.

Hachisuka, K., Umezu, Y. and Ogata, H. (1997). Disuse muscle atrophy of lower limbs in hemiplegic patients. *Archives of Physical Medicine and Rehabilitation* 78, 13–8.

Harries, U.L. and Bassey, E.J. (1990). Torque-velocity relationships for the knee extensors in women in their third and seventh decades. *European Journal of Applied Physiology* 60, 187–90.

Hass, A., Rusk, H.A., Pelosof, H. and Adam, J.R. (1967). Respiratory function in hemiplegic patient. *Archives of Physical Medicine and Rehabilitation* 49, 174–9.

Hoehn, M.M. and Yahr, M.D. (1967). Parkinsonism: onset, progression and mortality. *Neurology* 17, 427–42.

Hsiao, S-F. and Newham, D.J. (1998). Effect of resisted exercises on stretch reflex amplitude in stroke and healthy adults. *Clinical Rehabilitation* 12, 162–3.

Jackson, D., Turner-Stokes, L., Culpan, J., Bateman, A., Scott, O., Powell, J. and Greenwood, R. (2001). Can brain injured patients participate in an aerobic exercise programme during early inpatient rehabilitation? *Clinical Rehabilitation* 15 (5), 535–44.

Jones, D. and Godwin-Austen, R.B. (1998). Parkinson's disease. In: *Neurological Rehabilitation* (Stokes, M. ed.). Elsevier Science, London.

King, M.L., Guarracini, M., Lennihan, L., Freeman, D., Gagas, B., Boston, A., Bates, E. and Nori, S. (1989). Adaptive exercise testing for patients with hemiparesis. *Journal of Cardiopulmonary Rehabilitation* 9, 237–42.

Kingsley, R.E. (1996). *Concise Text of Neuroscience*. Williams and Wilkins, Baltimore, Maryland.

Knutsson, E. and Martensson, A. (1980). Dynamic motor capacity in spastic paresis and its relation to prime mover dysfunction, spastic reflexes and antagonist co activation. *Scandinavian Journal of Rehabilitation Medicine* 12, 93–106.

Kuroda, K., Tatara, K., Takatorige, T. and Shinso, F. (1992). Effect of physical exercise on mortality in patients with Parkinson's disease. *Acta Neurologica Scandinavia* 86 (1), 55–9.

McComas, A.J., Sica, R.E.P., Upton, A.R.M. and Aguilera, N. (1973). Functional changes in motoneurons of hemiparetic patients. *Journal of Neurology, Neurosurgery and Psychiatry* 36, 183–93.

Macko, R.F., Katzel, L.I., Yataco, A., Tretter, L.D., DeSouza, C.A., Dengel, D.R., Smith, G.V. and Silver, K.H. (1997). Low-velocity graded treadmill stress testing in hemiparetic stroke patients. *Stroke* 28, 988–92.

Macko, R.F., Smith, G.V., Dobrovolny, C.L., Sorkin, J.D., Goldberg, A.P. and Silver, K.H. (2001). Treadmill training improves fitness reserve in chronic stroke patients. *Archives of Physical Medicine and Rehabilitation* 82, 879–84.

Mastaglia, F.L., Knezevic, W. and Thompson, P.D. (1986). Weakness of head turning in hemiplegia: a quantitative study. *Journal of Neurology, Neurosurgery and Psychiatry* 49, 195–7.

Miller, G.J.T. and Light, K.E. (1997). Strength training in spastic hemiparesis: should it be avoided? *Neuro-rehabilitation* 9, 17–28.

Moldover, J.R., Daum, M.C. and Downey, J.A. (1984). Cardiac stress testing of hemiparetic patients with a supine bicycle ergometer: preliminary study. *Archives of Physical Medicine and Rehabilitation* 65, 470–3.

Montgomery, J. (1995). *Physical Therapy for Traumatic Brain Injury*. Churchill Livingstone, Edinburgh.

Mostert, S. and Kesselring, J. (2002). Effects of a short-term exercise training program on aerobic fitness, fatigue, health perception and activity levels of subjects with multiple sclerosis. *Multiple Sclerosis* 8 (2), 161–8.

Newham, D.J. and Hsiao, S-F. (2001). Knee muscle isometric strength, voluntary activation and antagonist co-contraction in the first six months after stroke. *Disability and Rehabilitation* 23 (9), 379–86.

Ng, S.S.M. and Shepherd, R.B. (2000). Weakness in patients with stroke: implications for strength training in neuro-rehabilitation. *Physical Therapy Reviews* 5, 227–38.

Pohl, P.S., Startzell, J.K., Duncan, P.W. and Wallace, D. (2000). Reliability of lower extremity isokinetic strength testing in adults with stroke. *Clinical Rehabilitation* 14, 601–7.

Potempa, K., Lopez, M., Braun, L.T., Szidon, J.P., Fogg, L. and Tincknell, T. (1995). Physiological outcomes of aerobic exercise training in hemiparetic stroke patients. *Stroke* 26, 101–5.

Reuter, I., Engelhardt, M., Stecker, K. and Baas, H. (1999). Therapeutic value of exercise training in Parkinson's disease. *Medicine and Science in Sport and Exercise* 31 (11), 1544–9.

Riddle, D.L., Finucane, S.D., Rothstein, J.M. and Walker, M.L. (1989). Intra-session and inter-session reliability of hand-held dynamometer measurements taken on brain damaged patients. *Physical Therapy* 69, 182–9.

Rosen, M.J., Sorkin, J.D., Goldberg, A.P., Hagberg, J.M. and Katzel, L.I. (1998). Predictors of age-associated decline in maximal aerobic capacity: a comparison of four statistical models. *Journal of Applied Physiology* 84, 2163–70.

Roth, E.J. (1993). Heart disease in patients with stroke: incidence, impact and implications for rehabilitation. *Archives of Physical Medicine and Rehabilitation* 75, 75–94.

Sahrmann, S.A. and Norton, B.J. (1977). The relationship of voluntary movement to spasticity in the upper motor neuron syndrome. *Annals of Neurology* 2, 460–5.

Santiago, M.C., Coyle, C.P. and Kinney, W.B. (1993). Aerobic exercise effect on individuals with physical disabilities. *Archives of Physical Medicine and Rehabilitation* 74, 1192–8.

Sharp, S.A. and Brouwer, B.J. (1997). Isokinetic strength training of the hemiparetic knee: effects on function and spasticity. *Archives of Physical Medicine and Rehabilitation* 78, 1231–6.

Singer, B., Dunne, J. and Allison, G. (2001). Reflex and non-reflex elements of hypertonia in triceps surae muscles following acquired brain injury: implications for rehabilitation. *Disability and Rehabilitation* 23 (17), 749–57.

Skelton, D.A. and McLaughlin, A.W. (1996). Training functional ability in old age. *Physiotherapy* 82 (3), 159–67.

Skelton, D.A., Young, A., Greig, C.A. and Malbut, K.E. (1995). Effects of resistance training on strength, power and selected functional abilities of women aged 75 and older. *Journal of American Geriatrics Society* 43, 1081–7.

Smith, G.V., Silver, K.H.C., Goldberg, A.P. and Macko, R.F. (1999). 'Task-oriented' exercise improves hamstring strength and spastic reflexes in chronic stroke patients. *Stroke* 30, 2112–8.

Smutok, M.A., Grafman, J., Salazar, A.M., Sweeney, J.K., Jonas, B.S. and DiRocco, P.J. (1989). Effects of unilateral brain damage on contralateral and ipsilateral upper extremity function in hemiplegia. *Physical Therapy* 69 (3), 195–203.

Tang, A. and Rymer, W.Z. (1981). Abnormal force-EMG relations in paretic limbs of hemiparetic human subjects. *Journal of Neurology, Neurosurgery and Psychiatry* 44, 690–8.

Teixeira-Salmela, L.F., Olney, S.J., Nadeau, S. and Brouwer, B. (1999). Muscle strengthening and physical conditioning to reduce impairment and disability in chronic stroke survivors. *Archives of Physical Medicine and Rehabilitation* 80, 1211–8.

Teixeira-Salmela, L.F., Nadeau, S., McBride, I. and Olney, S.J. (2001). Effects of muscle strengthening and physical conditioning training on temporal, kinematic and kinetic variables during gait in chronic stroke survivors. *Journal of Rehabilitation Medicine* 33, 53–60.

Toffola, E.D., Sparpaglione, D., Pistorio, A. and Buonocore, M. (2001). Myoelectric manifestations of muscle changes in stroke patients. *Archives of Physical Medicine and Rehabilitation* 82, 661–5.

Tripp, E.J. and Harris, S.R. (1991). Test-retest reliability of isokinetic knee extension and flexion torque measurements in persons with spastic hemiparesis. *Physical Therapy* 71 (5), 390–6.

Wood, R.H., Reyes, R., Welsch, M.A., Favoloro-Sabatior, J., Lee, C.M., Johnson, L.G. and Hooper, P.F. (2001). Concurrent cardiovascular and resistance training in healthy older adults. *Medicine and Science in Sports and Exercise* 33 (10), 1751–8.

Bibliography

Eldar, R. and Marinček, Č. (2000). Physical activity for elderly persons with neurological impairment: a review. *Scandinavian Journal of Rehabilitation Medicine* **32**, 99–103.

Jankowski, L.W. and Sullivan, S.J. (1990). Aerobic and neuromuscular training: effect on the capacity, efficiency, and fatigability of patients with traumatic brain injuries. *Archives of Physical Medicine and Rehabilitation* **71**, 500–4.

Potempa, K., Braun, L.T. and Tincknell, Y. (1996). Benefits of aerobic exercise after stroke. *Sports Medicine* **21**, 337–46.

Chapter 13

ADHERENCE TO EXERCISE

John Gormley

Key words: compliance, adherence, patient factors, programme factors.

Introduction

In the preceding chapters the benefits of exercise are documented. The adoption of exercise by an individual is not passive and requires a conscious decision and also necessitates effort. The effort involved is much greater than that involved in other health related activity, for example, taking a pill. In an ideal world if a patient is prescribed a treatment they would adhere rigidly to the prescription. This is, however, not the case, so it is therefore important for professionals involved in the area of exercise prescription to maximise the adherence of individuals. This chapter will therefore explain what is meant by adherence and examine the factors that influence adherence to exercise.

The definition of adherence

The terms adherence and compliance are often used interchangeably but they do not necessarily describe the same thing. Compliance has been defined as the 'extent to which a patient's behaviour coincides with medical or health advice' (Haynes, 1979). The roles are clearly defined, with the health professional issuing the instructions and the patient carrying them out. This definition means that the patient has to do as prescribed, no matter what other factors are present in their lives. The blame for non-compliance lies with the patient, and the health professional administering the advice is absolved of responsibility.

In order to imply a more collaborative relationship between the health professional and the patient the term adherence is more frequently used (Myers and Midence, 1998). Adherence means that the patient is involved in an alliance with the health professional in his or her treatment and is empowered to take responsibility for their own actions. The health professional has therefore a responsibility to enable the patient to adhere to an exercise programme rather than just issue instructions and hope that the patient will comply. In this chapter the term adherence is used extensively as opposed to compliance.

The benefits of exercise to healthy individuals and to those with disease are well documented. It is, nevertheless, apparent that it is extremely difficult to achieve 100% adherence with an exercise programme. This, however, should be the aim and the health professional should enable, as far as reasonably possible, individuals to adhere to their prescribed exercise programme. A high level of adherence will obviously benefit the individual involved, but there are other reasons why achieving high adherence levels are important. In order for most treatment regimes to work the patient must be an active participant, whether it be taking prescribed medication or partaking in exercise. If a doctor prescribes a course of tablets to a patient and the patient does not take the tablets then the treatment administered by the doctor has to be deemed as a failure. The tablets themselves may be very effective but the active participation of the patient is required to enable the intervention to be effective. Exercise, as stated earlier, requires a greater effort on the part of the patient and can only be effective by their active participation. This may be stating the obvious, but one can constantly extol the benefits of exercise to patients; however, unless the patient heeds the advice and adopts the exercise prescription then the treatment will also be a failure. The financial and resource implications for failed treatments are enormous, so it is imperative that adherence rates to exercise prescription are as high as possible and that those working in this area are constantly seeking ways by which adherence to exercise is maximised.

Much of the research in adherence has been conducted in the area of drug therapy. The majority of research in the area of exercise is derived from cardiac rehabilitation programmes and to a lesser extent from primary care schemes operated in the community. While many of the principles that govern adherence to drug therapy are applicable to exercise adherence it is important to remember that the two situations are different. A patient with CHD may well be willing to take their prescribed medication and continue to do so for many years but they may not exercise as prescribed. Indeed, it has been observed in patients with diabetes that there is a high level of adherence to medication yet only 19% engaged in regular exercise (Kravitz et al., 1993).

For many of the diseases discussed in this book exercise is an essential part of treatment. The aim of many programmes is to enable the patient to adopt a new lifestyle which involves regular exercise. In an eight-week phase III cardiac rehabilitation programme, exercise is an essential part. Those attending the programme will derive benefit from exercising for the duration. They will, however, only maintain the beneficial effects if they continue to exercise after the supervised programme is finished. Attendance levels at a supervised programme do not, however, provide information about exercise behaviour beyond the supervised setting (Martin and Dubbert, 1985). The challenge is therefore first to ensure high adherence levels during a period of supervised exercise and second to enable the patient to continue exercising in the long term.

Adherence to exercise is multifaceted, as exercise prescription encompasses frequency, intensity and duration of exercise. It is therefore difficult to determine when an individual becomes a non-adherent. One could exercise at the prescribed duration and frequency of exercise, although not at the prescribed intensity, but is this individual a non-adherent? A similar problem is apparent in adherence to drug therapy, as a patient may take too much or too little medication, not observe the correct interval between doses and not finish the course of medication (Ley and Llewelyn, 1995). The Royal Pharmaceutical Society recommended that terms such as poor or inadequate adherence should be used in drug therapy. The use of these terms in exercise would seem sensible also.

In supervised exercise programmes the measurement of adherence is relatively simple, as attendance is easy to measure. Furthermore, because the individual is supervised, intensity, duration and frequency of exercise can be monitored. Outside the supervised setting determination of adherence is more difficult. Techniques employed include exercise diaries, completed either by a patient or spouse or direct observation. Equipment such as heart rate monitors, pedometers and accelerometers, have also been used. The research examining adherence has concentrated on adherence to supervised exercise with fewer studies examining long-term adherence. The factors that influence adherence to a supervised exercise programme are wide and varied, but knowledge of these factors is essential if one is to maximise adherence. It is important to note that poor adherence in patients may be due to a combination of factors rather than one single factor.

Patient factors

Age

The association between age and adherence to exercise is unclear, with research reporting mixed findings. In 1998 a large study by Evenson et al. found that 42% of those aged 25–49 participated in a cardiac rehabilitation programme compared to 13% of those older than 80 years of age. Oldridge et al. (1992), however, found that attendance rates were higher among older patients than younger age groups. The differences may be due to different effects of age on adoption and maintenance of exercise. Evenson's study was concerned with adoption of exercise, whereas Oldridge's study identified maintenance of exercise. Sallis et al. (1992) found that age predicted adoption of exercise in men but no such trend was obvious for women. This illustrates the point made earlier that a combination of factors influence adherence.

Gender

From studies in cardiac rehabilitation there is a large body of evidence to suggest that: first, women are not referred for treatment as often as men; second, that women when referred are less likely to attend in the first place; and last, that women will have lower adherence rates compared to their male counterparts. There would appear to be more barriers for women attending exercise programmes than men. These can include family/home responsibilities, for example, sick spouse, child care and household duties (Thomas et al., 1996). Radley et al. (1998) found that women had a sense of guilt if they did not resume home duties within 4–6 weeks following a myocardial infarction. The adoption of physical activity in women is increased with strong social support. Lack of social support for women was also identified as a barrier to participation in cardiac rehabilitation programmes (Thomas et al., 1996). Furthermore, in the case of cardiovascular disease, women usually present at an older average age compared to men and are therefore more likely to have more established disease and more co-morbitities.

Socio-economic group

Blue-collar workers have been found to be less adherent to cardiac rehabilitation programmes than those who work in white-collar jobs (Oldridge et al., 1983). Furthermore, those in white-collar jobs reported higher levels of adherence to exercise compared to other socio-economic groups, six months after discharge from a cardiac rehabilitation programme. The likelihood of attending a programme decreases in areas of low deprivation compared to areas of higher deprivation (Lane, 2001). It is important to note that when dealing with socio-economic groups there are numerous confounding factors which can also influence exercise participation, for example, education, nature of work (sedentary versus manual) and ability to take time off to attend an exercise programme.

Fear

There is no doubt that the fear of exercise plays a role in the adoption of exercise and to a lesser extent in the maintenance of an exercise programme. In patients following a myocardial infarction the fear is of a recurrence, for patients with pulmonary disease the fear is breathlessness and in patients with insulin-dependent diabetes mellitus the fear of a reaction to low blood sugar has been cited as a barrier to exercise (Swift et al., 1995). This fear factor can decrease as exercise progresses, and the attendance at a supervised programme helps the patient to overcome their fear. It is more difficult, however, for an individual exercising on their own for the first time. Supervised exercise in the initial stages, along with patient education, are means by which the effect of fear can be negated.

Patient perceptions and beliefs

Self-efficacy is the perception of an individual as to whether they will be able to perform a particular behaviour (Bandura, 1977). Put simply, self-efficacy is the belief of the patient that they will be able to carry out the exercise prescribed. Those with higher self-efficacy scores are more likely to adhere to an exercise programme. Self-efficacy towards exercise is enhanced by constantly engaging in exercise. If a person stops engaging in an exercise programme their levels of self-efficacy towards exercise will decrease. It is unclear, however, whether self-efficacy is a consequence or a determinant of exercise behaviour.

The lack of motivation on the part of a patient can prevent a person commencing an exercise programme and can lead to poor adherence. Professionals should therefore educate and encourage patients prior to commencing an exercise programme and also for the duration of the programme. Patients who believe that their condition is controllable and modifiable through exercise are more likely to adhere to exercise. Participants in cardiac rehabilitation programmes who believe in the benefits of exercise have a lower drop-out rate compared to those who do not have a strong belief. Lack of enjoyment of exercise, unrealistic expectations and the effort involved are other reasons for decreased adherence to exercise.

Social support

Support from family and friends can have a positive effect on the adherence to exercise. Sherbourne et al. (1992) have reported that the quality of social support is a predictor of adherence. One of the most frequent reasons for drop out from cardiac rehabilitation programmes is the lack of spousal support (Andrew et al., 1981). A positive attitude to exercise from a patient's partner has been found to be positively correlated with higher adherence to exercise (Daltroy and Godin, 1989). Many cardiac and pulmonary rehabilitation programmes actively involve the patient's spouse or significant other in all aspects of the rehabilitation programme. As mentioned earlier, the lack of social support in women has been identified as a barrier to exercise in women (Thomas et al., 1996) and therefore women attending exercise programmes may need extra support to enable their participation and adherence.

Programme factors

Personnel

If a patient is referred to an exercise programme by a doctor there is an increased likelihood that adherence will be enhanced. A study by Oldridge (1979) has demonstrated the positive effect of physician referral on adherence to cardiac rehabilitation programmes. Another individual who has a positive effect on exercise adherence is the exercise leader. Indeed, it one of the most important factors in increased adherence. Research has indicated that exercise leaders who are of a similar age to participants are preferred (Lee, 1993). A friendly atmosphere fostered by the leader, coupled with positive reinforcement aimed at improving participants self-efficacy, both enhance adherence.

Education

Education of the patient has been an integral part of many exercise based rehabilitation programmes as the patient takes such an active part in their own treatment. Educating the patient about their condition and how exercise can help them allows the patient to develop an understanding of his/her condition, which enables them to develop self-efficacy and adherence (Mahler et al., 1999). The information provided to any patient should be easily understood and based on the patient's background level of knowledge. It is important that patient information is not all given at one session but spread out over a period of time. This approach allows the patient time to assimilate the information (Sluijs, 1991). Education provision to the patient can have a detrimental effect if the patient receives different or contradictory information from the different professions involved in his/her treatment (Nordin, 1995). It is therefore imperative that all professionals involved in patient education provide similar information and avoid contradiction of one another.

Individualised attention

Every person is different and patients with similar pathologies all require and react positively to individual attention. The attitude to exercise, the expectations of exercise, the level of social support and ability to exercise will all differ in patients. It is therefore important that each patient receives an individual programme that takes into account his/her individual preferences, abilities and attitudes. An individualised programme based on realistic expectations will enhance adherence (Jones et al., 1998). Activities and exercise that the patient favours can be encouraged and the variety of exercise is important to prevent boredom.

Group dynamics

In order to achieve benefit from exercise it is important that patients have an individualised programme. It would therefore appear a contradiction to suggest that adherence is enhanced by working in a group. The evidence would, however, point to the positive effects on adherence of group work. Exercising in a group has been shown to have a positive relationship with adherence (Carron et al., 1996). The use of group work has long been recognised by physiotherapists as an important method of treatment. Group work involving patients with similar pathologies was used extensively 15–20 years ago, but has become less common in recent years. The 'knee class' or 'shoulder class' involved a group of patients exercising together supervised by a physiotherapist. Cardiac and pulmonary rehabilitation programmes also use a group approach for exercising. Two things are important to point out. First, it is necessary to have patients who have similar levels of fitness or abilities exercising together. If a person finds the programme too hard or too easy then this will have negative effects on their adherence to the programme. Second, individualised prescription is not incompatible with group work. Patients in a cardiac rehabilitation programme can all work to their individualised prescription, yet they can derive the benefits of the exercise and be more likely to adhere to the programme by working in a group.

Logistics of a programme

In the last 10–15 years health professionals have started to recognise the problems patients experience in adhering to treatment. An exercise programme should therefore be organised, as far as reasonably possible, to suit the patient rather than the health professional. Issues such as timing of sessions, location of centre, etc. have an impact on adherence to exercise programmes. Andrew et al. (1981) determined that factors such as inconvenient location of centre, parking difficulties and difficulty in attending on time, all negatively impacted on adherence to a cardiac rehabilitation programme. It may not always be necessary to conduct an exercise programme in the hospital or clinic environment. Local halls and leisure centres can provide an environment for exercise programmes. They also have the added advantage for those working, especially in rural areas, that the programme can be held in close proximity to the patients.

The timing of programmes can present major problems for patients. Job requirements and family responsibilities are just two areas that can impact on an individual attending a programme during normal working hours. A more flexible attitude on the part of the physiotherapist and other professionals with regard to the timing of programmes can enable individuals to attend, where previously they would have been unable.

The aim of many supervised exercise programmes is to enable an individual to modify their lifestyle and incorporate exercise into their daily lives where previously it may have been absent. Individuals may be able to attend organised exercise programmes but then face difficulties when the period of supervision of exercise is completed. The importance of an individualised programme that is tailored to the individual's needs is imperative at this stage. The prescribed programme has to incorporate the individual's preferences as to the mode of exercise and also allow him/her to incorporate the prescription as much as possible into their daily lives, for example, walking or cycling to work rather than taking the car.

The exercise prescription

Exercise is prescribed to individuals in terms of frequency, intensity and duration of exercise. The mode or modes of exercise are often suggested rather than prescribed. The adherence to exercise can be influenced by these elements of prescription and each one is discussed individually below.

Frequency

The frequency of exercise is usually described in terms of number of times per week. The frequency should be sufficient for the individual to achieve a beneficial effect, but also not be so frequent that it decreases adherence. The results of studies examining the relationship of frequency to adherence differ depending on the subjects involved. A study by Dressendorfer et al. (1995) found high adherence levels in patients post-myocardial infarction, whether they attended for one, two or three sessions per week. In healthy subjects King et al. (1995) found that frequencies of five times per week of low intensity exercise for 30 minutes reduced adherence compared to 40 minutes of high intensity exercise three times per week. Higher injury rates have been associated with increased frequency of exercise (Pollock et al., 1977), which could have a detrimental effect on adherence. It is important to note that the increased adherence in this study may have been due to the altered intensities or duration of exercise. There is evidence to suggest that with overweight women adherence was enhanced when subjects exercised for shorter periods but more frequently (Jakicic et al., 1995). The optimium frequency of exercise to ensure maximum adherence is unclear and more research is required.

Duration

For many people 'lack of time' is frequently cited as a reason for not adhering to an exercise programme (Dishman et al., 1985; Sluijs et al., 1993). The duration of exercise, as with frequency, should be of sufficient length of time to obtain benefit but not too long to affect adherence. Adherence to exercise decreases when the duration increases (Milesis et al., 1976). Furthermore, as with increased frequency, an increase in duration of exercise can result in an increase in injuries (Pollock et al., 1977). The incorporation of exercise into the daily routine can overcome some of the problems. Also, accumulating three bouts of exercise of ten minutes duration over the course of the day rather than one bout of thirty minutes may be more feasible for individuals. There is, however, a lack of research to determine whether the health benefits are similar from the two forms of exercise prescription (Hardman, 2001).

Intensity

In prescribing exercise for health gain one must remember that high intensities are often not required to elicit a health gain. Evidence suggests that subjects are more adherent to a low intensity exercise programme, compared to high intensity. In a study of patients with coronary heart disease adherence was significantly higher ($p < 0.05$) with low intensity exercise (50% $\dot{V}O_2max$) compared to high intensity exercise (85% $\dot{V}O_2max$) (Lee et al., 1996). Lower intensities of exercise may allow the individual to incorporate exercise into their daily routine and also provide more enjoyment for the individual.

Behavioural change

In many of the conditions described in this book exercise has beneficial health enhancing effects. The benefits of exercise are quickly diminished if an exercise programme is ceased. In prescribing exercise one is attempting to bring about a lifelong, lifestyle change in the individual. The interaction of motivation to change and the behavioural change required have been classified into five stages by Marcus et al. (1992) based on the work of Prochaska and DiClemente (1983):

(1) Pre-contemplation
(2) Contemplation
(3) Preparation
(4) Action
(5) Maintenance

Pre-contemplation

An individual at this stage does not intend to change his/her behaviour. This could be at the initial assessment of a patient with coronary heart disease or obesity. The patient lacks the knowledge or has not been made aware of the need to change, for example, starting exercise. It is therefore important at this stage for the health professional to present information to the patient about the need to change and also instil confidence in the patient about their ability to change. Booklets and educational material can be used and the involvement of spouse or family can help in moving the individual to the next stage (ACSM, 2000).

Contemplation

At this stage the individual is thinking about changing, but has, as yet, not done anything about this. The individual has now realised the need to change but needs help. An examination of potential barriers to exercise can be helpful, as can defining with the individual the potential benefits of exercising and the hazards of continuing with their present lifestyle.

Preparation

In the preparation stage the individual has decided to change and may even have adopted some changes. For example, they may have started some exercise but are, as yet, not carrying out the full prescription. (ACSM, 2000). It is important for the health professional to be positive about the changes already made and devise short-term objectives with the individual to enable him/her to reach the desired level of change. The process of helping someone to move from exercising one day per week to most days of the week may require time and numerous interventions on the part of the health professional.

Action

The individual is meeting the exercise prescription at this stage, but has not, as yet, maintained the programme for a sufficiently long period of time. Positive reinforcement and encouragement are important. The individual may experience boredom or find the exercise monotonous, so changes to the mode of exercise may be helpful. Incorporation of exercise into their daily routine may also enable maintenance.

Maintenance

This is the objective of many exercise prescriptions. If an individual has maintained the exercise programme for at least six months then exercise can be thought to be habitual. Interventions by the health professional can still be beneficial to prevent a return to a sedentary lifestyle.

The adoption and maintenance of an exercise programme requires an individual to change their lifestyle. This chapter has focused on the factors that prevent an individual from adhering to a programme. For the health professional an awareness of these factors is important. Furthermore, an awareness of how these factors can impact on the individual is essential. The stages of change described above enable the health professional to identify the phase that the individual is at and to adapt their intervention to move the individual to the next phase. If, through an intervention, an individual moves from pre-contemplation to contemplation then this in itself is an achievement. It is seldom that one can move an individual from the pre-contemplation to action immediately.

References

American College of Sports Medicine (2000). *Guidelines for Exercise Testing and Prescription*, 6th edn. Lippincott Williams and Wilkins, Baltimore.

Andrew G.M., Oldridge, N.B., Parker, J.O., Cunningham, D.A., Rechnitzer P.A., Jones, N.L., Buck, C., Kavanagh, T., Shephard, R.J., Sutton, J.R. and McDonald, W. (1981). Reasons for drop out from exercise programs in post-coronary patients. *Medicine and Science in Sports and Exercise* 13, 164–8.

Bandura, A. (1977). Self-efficacy: toward a unifying theory of behavioral change. *Psychological Reviews* 84 (2) March, 191–215.

Carron, A.V., Hausenblas, H.A. and Mack, D. (1996). Social influence and exercise: a meta-analysis. *Journal of Sport and Exercise Psychology* 18 (1), March, 1–16.

Daltroy, L.H. and Godin, G. (1989). The influence of spousal approval and patient perception of spousal approval on cardiac patient participation in exercise programs. *Journal of Cardiopulmonary Rehabilitation* 9, 363–7.

Dishman, R.K., Sallis, J.F. and Orenstein, D.R. (1985). The determinants of physical activity and exercise. *Public Health Reports* 100 (2), March–April, 158–71.

Dressendorfer, R.H., Franklin, B.A., Cameron, J.L., Trahan, K.J., Gordon, S. and Timmis, G.C. (1995). Exercise training frequency in early post-infarction cardiac rehabilitation. Influence on aerobic conditioning. *Journal of Cardiopulmonary Rehabilitation* 15 (4), July–Aug., 269–76.

Evenson, K.R., Rosamond, W.D. and Luepker, R.V. (1998). Predictors of outpatient cardiac rehabilitation utilisation: the Minnesota Heart Surgery Registry. *Journal of Cardiopulmonary Rehabilitation* 18 (3), May–June, 192–8.

Haynes, R.B. (1979). Introduction. In: *Compliance in Health Care* (Haynes, R.B., Taylor, D.W. and Sackelt, D.L. (eds). John Hopkins University Press, Baltimore.

Jakicic, J.M., Wing, R.R., Butler, B.A. and Robertson, R.J. (1995). Prescribing exercise in multiple short bouts versus one continuous bout: effects on adherence cardiorespiratory fitness, and weight loss in overweight women. *International Journal Obesity and Related Metabolic Disorders* 19 (12), Dec., 893–901.

Jones, F., Harris, P. and McGee, L. (1998). Adherence to prescribed exercise. In: *Adherence to Treatment in Medical Conditions* (Myers L. and Midence, K. eds), pp. 343–62. Harwood Academic Press, UK.

King, A.C., Haskell, W.L., Young, D.R., Oka, R.K. and Stefanick, M.L. (1995). Long-term effects of varying intensities and formats of physical activity on participation rates, fitness and lipoproteins in men and women aged 50–65 years. *Circulation* **91** (10), 15 May, 2596–604.

Kravitz, R.L., Hays, R.D., Sherbourne, C.D., DiMatteo, M.R., Rogers, W.H., Ordway, L. and Greenfield, S. (1993). Recall of recommendations and adherence to advice among patients with chronic medical conditions. *Archives of Internal Medicine* **153** (16), 23 Aug., 1869–78.

Lane, D., Carroll, D., Ring, C., Beevers, D.G. and Lip, G.Y. (2001). Predictors of attendance at cardiac rehabilitation after myocardial infarction. *Journal of Psychosomatic Research* **51** (3), Sept., 497–501.

Lee, C. (1993). Attitudes, knowledge, and stages of change: a survey of exercise patterns in older Australian women. *Health Psychology* **12** (6), Nov., 476–80.

Lee, J.Y., Jensen, B.E., Oberman, A., Fletcher, G.F., Fletcher, B.J. and Raczynski, J.M. (1996). Adherence in the training levels comparison trial. *Medicine and Science in Sports and Exercise* **28** (1), Jan., 47–52.

Ley, P. and Llewelyn, S. (1995). Improving patients understanding recall, satisfaction and compliance. In: *Health Psychology: Processes and Applications* (Broome, A. and Llewelyn, S., eds), 2nd edn. pp. 75–98. Chapman and Hall, London.

Mahler, H.I., Kulik, J.A. and Tarazi, R.Y. (1999). Effects of videotape information intervention at discharge on diet and exercise compliance after coronary bypass surgery. *Journal of Cardiopulmonary Rehabilitation* **19** (3), (May–June), 170–7.

Marcus, B.H., Selby, V.C., Niaura, R.S. and Rossi, J.S. (1992). Self-efficacy and the stages of exercise behavior change. *Research Quarterly in Exercise and Sport* **63** (1), March, 60–6.

Martin, J.E. and Dubbert, P.M. (1985). Adherence to exercise. *Exercise and Sports Science Reviews* **13**, 137–67.

Milesis, C.A., Pollock, M.L., Bah, M.D., Ayres, J.J., Ward, A. and Linnerud, A.C. (1976). Effects of different durations of physical training on cardiorespiratory function, body composition, and serum lipids. *Research Quarterly* **47** (4), Dec., 716–25.

Myers, L.B. and Midence K. (1998). Concepts and Issues in Adherence. In: *Adherence to Treatment in Medical Conditions* (Myers, L.B. and Midence, K. eds). Harwood Academic Publishers, UK.

Nordin, M. (1995). Back pain: lessons from patient education. *Patient Education and Counselling* **26** (1–3), Sept., 67–70.

Oldridge, N.B. (1979). Compliance of post-myocardial infarction patients to exercise programs. *Medicine and Science in Sports* **11** (4), Winter, 373–5.

Oldridge, N.B., Donner, A.P., Buck, C.W., Jones, N.L., Andrew, G.M., Parker, J.O., Cunningham, D.A., Kavanagh, T., Rechnitzer, P.A. and Sutton, J.R. (1983). Predictors of drop out from cardiac exercise rehabilitation. Ontario Exercise-Heart Collaborative Study. *American Journal of Cardiology* **51** (1), Jan., 70–4.

Oldridge, N.B., Ragowski, B. and Gottlieb, M. (1992). Use of outpatient cardiac rehabilitation services: factors associated with attendance. *Journal of Cardiopulmonary Rehabilitation* **12** (1), Jan.–Feb., 25–31.

Pollock, M.L., Gettman, L.R., Milesis, C.A., Bah, M.D., Durstine, L. and Johnson, R.B. (1977). Effects of frequency and duration of training on attrition and incidence of injury. *Medicine and Science in Sports* **9** (1), Spring, 31–6.

Prochaska, J.O. and DiClemente, C.C. (1983). Stages and process of self-change of smoking: toward an integrative model of change. *Journal of Consulting and Clinical Psychology* **51**, 390–395.

Radley, A., Grove, A. and Thurston, H. (1998). Problems of women compared with those of men following myocardial infarction. *Coronary Health Care* **2** (4), 14–7.

Sallis, J.F., Hovell, M.F. and Hofstetter, C.R. (1992). Predictors of adoption and maintenance of vigorous physical activity in men and women. *Preventative Medicine* **21** (2), March, 237–51.

Sherbourne, C.D., Hays, R.D., Ordway, L., DiMatteo, M.R. and Kravitz, R.L. (1992). Antecedents of adherence to medical recommendations: results from the Medical Outcomes Study. *Journal of Behavioural Medicine* **15** (5), Oct., 447–68.

Sluijs, E.M. (1991). Patient education in physiotherapy: towards a planned approach. *Physiotherapy* **77**, 503–8.

Sluijs, E.M., Kok, G.J. and Van der Zee, J. (1993). Correlates of exercise compliance in physical therapy. *Physical Therapy* **73** (11), Nov., 771–82.

Swift, C.S., Armstrong, J.E., Beerman, K.A., Campbell, R.K. and Pond-Smith, D. (1995). Attitudes and beliefs about exercise among persons with non-insulin-dependent diabetes. *Diabetes Education* **21** (6), Nov.–Dec., 533–40.

Thomas, R.J., Miller, N.H., Lamendola, C., Berra, K., Hedback, B., Durstine, J.L. and Haskell, W. (1996). National survey on gender differences in cardiac rehabilitation programs. Patient characteristics and enrollment patterns. *Journal of Cardiopulmonary Rehabilitation* **16** (6), Nov.–Dec., 402–12.

Bibliography

Bailey, W.C., Richards, J.M. Jr, Brooks, C.M., Soong, S.J., Windsor, R.A. and Manzella, B.A. (1990). A randomised trial to improve self-management practices of adults with asthma. *Archives of Internal Medicine* **150** (8), Aug., 1664–8.

Hardman, A.E. (2001). Physical activity and health: current issues and research needs. *International Journal of Epidemiology* **30** (5), Oct., 1193–7.

Royal Pharmaceutical Society of Great Britain, Merck Sharp & Dohme (1997). *From Compliance to Concordance: Achieving Shared Goals in Medicine Taking*. Hoddesdon, London.

Chapter 14

PROMOTING PHYSICAL ACTIVITY: BUILDING SUSTAINABLE INTERVENTIONS

Lindsey Dugdill and Rebecca Graham

Key words: physical activity promotion, primary care based exercise promotion.

Introduction

Physical activity has been defined as 'any bodily movement produced by skeletal muscles that results in energy expenditure' (Caspersen et al., 1985) and as defined here, it encompasses all activities from sport and exercise-based activities, leisure activities, activities of daily living (such as washing, stair climbing), occupation-ally related activity (such as commuting to work by bicycle or foot) and specific prescribed interventions (such as exercise referral programmes).

Health is a multidisciplinary and contested concept, which encompasses psychological, physiological and spiritual domains and states of both positive and negative well-being. It is now accepted that complex states of health can exist co-terminally rather than on a wellness-illness continuum only. As Downie and Macnaughton (2001) state: 'In whatever guise it appears, health is regarded as a value, for it frequently appears in lists alongside other values, as in phrases such as "healthy, wealthy and wise".' In contemporary models, the health of the indi-vidual is seen to be influenced by the broader sociocultural context or environment (for example, Dahlgren and Whitehead, 1991). Health promotion has emerged as an increasingly important academic and professional multidiscipline 'encompass-ing health education, lifestyle and preventative approaches alongside environ-mental, legal, policy and fiscal measures designed to advance health' (Scriven and Orme, 2001). As such it embraces the notion that health is influenced by a range of factors at every level of the 'system', from the biosphere down to the cellular level. This holistic stance is discussed in the section on socio-ecological models (p. 243).

Traditionally, health and physical activity research has focused on the natural science paradigm (for example, physiological change of individuals) rather than social science paradigm (for example, psychosocial factors, such as social support).

Consequently, the importance of exploring the role of family and the sociocultural environment has received less attention until recently (Stokols, 1992). However, these are now being recognised as factors of extreme importance in physical activity promotion. Physical activity research has clearly established the link between inactivity and poor health status in populations, but we are a long way from understanding how to design, develop and implement physical activity interventions that are effective in sustaining behaviour change as the quote from McKay et al. (2003) illustrates:

> '. . . the evidence for the health benefits of physical activity is firmly established, but people remain inactive . . . research must focus on discovering (a) precise exercise prescriptions (to make exercise more palatable) and (b) methods of delivering exercise more cost effectively (so that it is accessible and sustainable).'

Consequently, this chapter aims to explore the rationale for physical activity promotion, the difficulties of trying to reverse the trend towards increasingly sedentary lifestyles in the UK through behaviour change and proposes strategies for physical activity promotion. Two case studies of physical activity interventions being developed and evaluated on Merseyside, for adults, are discussed.

Rationale for the promotion of physically active lifestyles

Physical inactivity is becoming an issue of extreme public health concern to all health professionals and agencies within the UK, across Europe and other Western industrialised countries. There is considerable evidence to indicate that individuals who are more physically active across the lifespan suffer from reduced morbidity and mortality from a wide range of diseases (US Department of Health and Human Services, 1996). Despite such convincing evidence, physical activity levels in the UK population remain low; approximately three fifths of men and three quarters of women are not active at the recommended levels to achieve any health benefits (DoH, 2000a). Also, growing levels of childhood obesity (Bundred et al., 2001), diabetes and depression can all be linked to sedentary behaviour (Sallis and Owen, 1999) and are causing concern for health care and other professionals in the UK. Decreasing levels of sport participation in schools (Sport England, 2003) has been identified as one key factor leading to physical inactivity in childhood. The importance of physical activity as a risk factor for coronary heart disease is increasingly being recognised throughout Europe (HEPA Guidelines, 2000). Physical activity is cited as a key intervention in the National Service Framework for CHD (DoH, 2000b) and should be considered as a potential intervention for many other health problems.

Strategies for changing physical activity behaviour

Enabling sustained health-related behaviour change is acknowledged to be one of the most difficult and complex challenges facing health professionals today, especially amongst communities which suffer from social deprivation, lack of opportunities and facilities. Behaviour change must take place at a societal level, as well as an individual level, if real health gains are to be seen at a population level and long-term patterns of 'healthy' behaviour established. Also, structural change within communities (for example, policy development) must mitigate for the promotion of individual change. It is now an imperative of the National Service Framework for CHD (DoH, 2000b) that all local authority areas must develop and implement physical activity strategies. Ireland (2001) stated that:

> '. . . local authorities are actively involved in promoting physical activity in different ways. There is still little evidence to determine the most effective form of intervention, and this must generally be determined by local partnerships agreeing local objectives through a process of consultation. Whether the intervention is through GP referral schemes . . . physical activity strategies, or cycling and walking forums, it is important wherever possible, to measure its impact.'

Hence, interventions provided must be needs led and reflect the community agenda for successful uptake and maintenance to be achieved: in essence the community must be the main driving force behind the change processes sought (Popay and Williams, 1994). Health professionals and academics can act as enablers of this process by working with community members to design the intervention and research processes. Previous health-related behaviour research has often failed to reflect the complexity of context within which behaviours are carried out and the interrelationships between behaviours and other factors.

It is important that physical activity, as a behavioural pattern, is established when children are young, and then maintained by support from the family and community settings (Sallis and Owen, 1999). Much is known about the barriers to physical activity participation within individuals; however, little research has focused on the family as a unit and 'driver' of behavioural change. Also, the development of appropriate risk-taking behaviours (smoking, drinking, drug-taking) in young adults may be influenced if positive psychological constructs (self-esteem and self efficacy) are developed at an early age. A longitudinal study of smoking behaviour in Liverpool (Porcellato et al., 1999) has shown the complexity of children's perspectives towards health behaviour at ages as young as five. If children are forming multifaceted perspectives about health from this young age then they are ideally placed to be educated about physical activity at this time. Thus, appropriate intervention with family groups could be a major influence on future health-related behaviour, such as physical activity and societal attitude.

Promoting physical activity in different settings

In the UK, increasing interest in using a 'settings-based' approach to health promotion developed throughout the 1990s. Settings include workplaces, schools, primary health care and other community settings. This approach was strengthened when

Saving Lives: Our Healthier Nation (DoH, 1999) was published, as this overtly recognised such settings as important structures for reaching and involving the general population in health interventions (Dooris and Thompson, 2001). There are many positive reasons for using a settings-based approach when attempting to promote physical activity:

- It allows individual behaviour and lifestyle to be related to the psycho-social-cultural environment.
- It moves practice from an individual to an organisational or community approach.
- It has its foundation in management science and organisational development.
- It uses existing cultural structures for implementation rather than setting up new structures.
- Any intervention is developed in conjunction with the relevant population and is delivered in a familiar environment (more likely to be sustained and successful).
- It provides a venue and captive population for ongoing intervention.
- It targets existing funding structures.
- It allows intervention at individual, organisational, community and policy levels.
- The diffusion and/or transferability of programmes is possible, and facilitated by organisational networks.
- Communication networks are already in operation.

Therefore, settings provide ready-made organisational structures through which interventions can be developed. Despite all the positive reasons for working at this level there are some potential drawbacks with a settings-based approach, which are worth mentioning. For example, settings may have gatekeepers who are difficult to circumvent or get on board (for example, senior management); marginal groups may be missed out (for example, if physical activity interventions target the workplace then all home workers may be missed); and people may feel disempowered or coerced by the action. Of the two case studies discussed in the latter stages of this chapter, one was targeted at the workplace setting and was implemented in the community (Liverpool Corporate Cup) and the second was targeted at the primary care setting and was implemented in a leisure/community setting (EXCEL – exercise referral intervention).

Socio-ecological models for physical activity promotion

Sallis and Owen (1999) have championed the importance of the concept of socio-ecological models in understanding physical activity behaviour. Socio-ecological models are holistic, multi-level models that endeavour to understand behaviour at a variety of levels from the individual, intra-personal, community/organisation up to policy level. All levels of the system are considered to be influential on physical activity behaviour.

Sallis and Owen (1999) explain that such models are vital in understanding physical activity settings (as discussed above):

'. . . few studies have directly applied ecological models to understanding or intervening on physical activity. A key concept that we believe is helpful in understanding the potential impact of social and physical environmental influences is "behaviour settings". Behaviour settings are especially critical in understanding physical activity, because activities are done in specific places. Some places have characteristics that make it easy for people to be active, and some places make it hard to be active.'

Such models have moved the agenda for physical activity promotion away from a focus on individual behaviour change alone (which has had limited success) to a broader focus on the environmental structures and policies it is necessary to have in place to help mitigate change. Stokols (1992) articulated the importance of using a social ecological approach to health promotion, in that it helped to represent the true complexity and transactions that occurred in people's lifestyles. Manipulating the environment to enhance health opportunities (for example, providing safe cycle lanes) might be much more effective than trying to persuade people to change behaviour in an unsupportive environment.

A European perspective on physical activity promotion: HEPA – Health Enhancing Physical Activity

The main structure for promoting physical activity across the European region is the European Network for the promotion of Health Enhancing Physical Activity (the HEPA network). It is one of seven European Commission health promotion networks and has been responsible for initiating the development of physical activity promotion policy across the EC. One recent, significant document produced from the HEPA network was the *Guidelines for HEPA Promotion Programmes* (2000), which offer principles of good practice for physical activity promotion. The guidelines were developed from a multidisciplinary panel of expert practitioners from across the EC.

The guidelines set out a practical framework to help policy makers, health professionals and other relevant personnel develop, implement and evaluate physical activity interventions. In summary, the guidelines include the following stages:

- *Stage 1: Preparing a HEPA Programme.* The key components of programme preparation include identifying potential stakeholders, identifying relevant evidence to justify the programme and the use of evidence to develop the political justification, support and funding for the programme.
- *Stage 2: Developing a HEPA Programme.* The components for development include: exploration of the roles of health and sport related bodies responsible for physical activity promotion; recruiting stakeholder groups; identifying pilot project work; conducting a good practice audit (to locate models of good practice); and assigning the programme a clear name and identity.
- *Stage 3: Designing a HEPA Programme.* Design components include the involvement of stakeholder views in programme design, development of a

programme strategy, aims, objectives and indicators (including key health promotion messages).

- *Stage 4: Implementing a HEPA Programme.* Components at this stage include developing the organisational structure for the programme, establishing participant ownership of the programme, development of the promotional networks involved and monitoring of take-up rate for interventions (poor response may be seen in certain population groups for instance).
- *Stage 5: Evaluating a HEPA Programme.* Evaluation components include making a commitment to evaluation, designing an evaluation framework for the programme using existing auditing systems and creating new, independent evaluation mechanisms where required.

These guidelines illustrate that in order to develop a rigorous, effective, well-structured physical activity intervention, health professionals need to work in partnership with other professional groups, for example, sport development, transportation. The planning and design process is complex and involvement of participants, through consultation mechanisms, will take time to set up properly. The following section focuses on two applied research case studies which have explored the impact and effectiveness of two different physical activity interventions implemented within Merseyside, UK.

Research case study 1: evaluation of the Liverpool Corporate Cup

Rationale for the corporate series

The Corporate Series is a programme of 5 kilometre, team-based running events staged at various locations around the north west region of the UK, targeting employees to participate. The adult, working population is an extremely important population to target with physical activity interventions, due to the sedentary nature of most occupations today. Also, it is estimated that UK adults spend approximately 60% of their waking hours at work and have the longest working hours/week in the European Union. This makes the workplace a priority setting for the promotion of health enhancing physical activity. There is an increasing evidence base which links the physical activity behaviour of workers to increased effectiveness and productivity in the workplace (Kaman, 1995). From an 'ecological' perspective, workplace interventions should target the organisation itself, not just the employees, and attempt to create a 'corporate culture' that is supportive of physical activity. This is precisely what the Corporate Series set out to achieve when it was launched in 1995.

Development of the corporate series

The Corporate Series is a unique intervention within the UK. Although many running events are staged, and they target currently inactive people, none directly aim to promote sustained behavioural change. The NW Corporate Series was developed by Robin Ireland, Director of Healthstart (an events management organisation in Merseyside), who experienced a YMCA Corporate Cup in New Orleans in the 1980s. Ireland returned to the UK and instigated the first run in Crewe, followed in 1990 by the Liverpool Corporate Cup, which successfully recruits several thousand runners every year. By 2002, runs had taken place in Birkenhead, Blackburn, Chester, Chorley, Crewe, Knowsley, Liverpool, Macclesfield, Manchester, Oldham, Preston, Southport, St Helens and Warrington. Currently, the Series attracts over 8000 runners/walkers each year, representing 2000 teams from a range of occupational settings, including the NHS.

Developing the evidence base: the research design

A recent evaluation (Evans, 2002) of the NHS North West Corporate Series has confirmed that the Corporate Series successfully promotes physical activity, encourages previously inactive women to run, can sustain participation over time and offers an excellent support mechanism for health enhancing physical activity. The evaluation sought to answer the vital question: 'Do running events lead to sustainable health gain and behaviour change?' The research focused on the 5 km team event held annually in the city centre of Liverpool, UK: the Liverpool Corporate Cup (LCC). The LCC primarily aims to recruit teams of participants from the workplace setting and is the biggest event within the Corporate Series. It is organised by Liverpool City Council and Healthstart (on behalf of the local primary care trusts) and annually attracts more than 2500 participants.

Lifestyle events are frequently used in the UK to raise health awareness within communities, but there is little evidence to support their effectiveness, especially with running events. As mentioned earlier, increasingly, the use of ecological models in the promotion of physical activity has been advocated (Sallis and Owen, 1999). Such models incorporate action aimed at multiple levels of change from the level of the individual, through to organisational and policy development. Most evaluation studies focus measurement at the level of individual behaviour change and fail to assess changes at a higher level of the system. Consequently, the wider benefits of physical activity interventions are often not understood. This research project used a unique ecological evaluation design, incorporating quantitative and qualitative studies, to measure the effectiveness of the event from personal, interpersonal, organisational, community, environmental and policy perspectives (Evans, 2002). Participant and stakeholder views were actively sought through a series of focus groups, interviews and specially constructed questionnaires.

Research findings

The evaluation study established that:

- 52% of runners had previously participated in the LCC
- 38% took part for enjoyment

- 18% joined in to team build with colleagues
- 12% participated for health and fitness reasons
- 46% said they took part in additional physical activity in order to train for the event

Also, very importantly, it was clear that behavioural change had been established in many partipants, as 96% believed that the Corporate Series helped previously inactive people to become more active and 76% could identify someone who had become more active as a result of taking part. Women runners, in particular, seemed to benefit from the team-based approach as they gained support from family, friends and work colleagues.

Focus group statements clearly illustrated the increase in self-confidence and self efficacy in female runners: 'I always thought I would never run, ever. When I started I used to feel embarrassed but I don't care now. We do more than just the Corporate Cup events now' and:

'. . . no, I don't think we'd have gone on to do the running that we've done.'

'The interest we now have in running has taken us further . . . after the Corporate Cup we did the women's 10 K (Liverpool Women's 10 K) and then . . . a half marathon and in 1997 a full marathon.'

In conclusion, this evaluation showed that the Liverpool Corporate Cup was successful in attracting, and sustaining, running behaviour in previously inactive adults, particularly women. Interestingly improving health was not a strong motivator for people taking part (only 12% cited this as a reason for participation): fun, enjoyment and the social aspects were much more important reasons for participation.

Research case study 2: evaluation of an adult exercise referral scheme, EXCEL, Sefton, Merseyside

Rationale for primary care based exercise promotion

The concept of promoting physical activity within the primary care setting: exercise referral, is a growing phenomenon in the UK. Primary care has a key role to play in helping people achieve lifestyle change, with 78% of the UK population visiting their GP each year and the GP being considered as a credible source of advice (Calnan and Johnson, 1983). Research conducted in 1994 identified that there were 200 exercise referral schemes in operation in the UK (Fox et al., 1997) and now there are approximately 600. However, the expansion of such schemes has not been paralleled with an evidence base to support their effectiveness (Riddoch et al., 1998).

This statement is corroborated by Hillsdon and Thorogood (1996) who suggested that the effectiveness of strategies that promote physical activity uptake remains largely unknown. Promotion of physical activity within the primary care setting is no exception, despite numerous studies that have attempted to examine the role and potential of exercise referral schemes as a means of physical activity promotion in the least active segment of the population (Biddle et al., 1994; Ayres and Pocock, 1995; Lord and Green, 1995; Stevens et al., 1998; Taylor et al., 1998; Harland et al., 1999; Tai et al., 1999; Smith et al., 2000; Hillsdon et al., 2002).

EXCEL – Excel to Health exercise referral intervention

This study evaluated a fully operational exercise referral scheme (Excel to Health) located in Sefton, Merseyside. The primary aim of EXCEL is to reduce the incidence of coronary heart disease (CHD) in the population, by promoting physical activity in sedentary individuals suffering from at least one CHD risk factor. CHD accounts for 21% of deaths before the age of 75 in England. This prevalence rate is mirrored in Sefton with 21.2% of the population suffering from CHD before 75 years, in 1999 (Sefton Health Authority, 2001). EXCEL operates according to the most common model of exercise referral (as described by the *National Quality Assurance Framework for Exercise Referral Systems*, DoH, 2001) whereby a GP or practice nurse refers patients to a leisure centre or gym for a supervised exercise programme. A 14-week programme of physical activity is provided during which three health assessments take place; before starting the programme, midway through the programme (seven weeks) and at the end point of the programme (14 weeks).

Research design

Research in the literature, to date, has focused on experimental methods that have predominantly examined the outcomes of referral schemes, often to the neglect of processes (Riddoch et al., 1998). The effectiveness of experimental research, such as randomised controlled trials (RCT), as a means to evaluate health promoting activity has been questioned for a number of reasons (Riddoch et al., 1998; DoH, 2001).

- It is not always ethical to assign participants to a control group as this is denying them access to a necessary service.
- Randomised controlled trials do not examine the real exercise referral process in its entirety, for example limitations are placed on the ability to study the effect of practitioner advice as subjects are often recruited via postal letters (Puska, 2001).
- The ability to examine the broader, more complex factors that relate to programme success are inhibited by the strict, highly controlled nature of the RCT.
- Experimental methods can give us an indication as to the outcomes of an intervention, but give very limited information as to why the outcome has occurred (Puska, 2001).

More recently it has been suggested that 'a case study approach to evaluation may be as rewarding as a randomised controlled trial approach' (Riddoch et al., 1998), but few exercise referral studies using alternative evaluation techniques have been carried out to date in the UK. Consequently, a triangulation of data collection techniques were used in this study, combining qualitative methods (semi-structured interviews) with quantitative techniques (closed format questionnaires, physiological tests), to enhance validity of the data and strengthen the study design (Patton, 1990).

Some of the research questions asked are illustrated below:

- What are the demographic and physiological characteristics of individuals who attend an exercise referral scheme having been referred by their medical professional and who subsequently complete the intervention?
- Are there any significant differences in physiological parameters recorded at baseline and upon completion of the intervention?
- What are the outcomes of an operational exercise referral scheme (both intended and unintended)?
- What are the factors within the implementation environment, treatment and intervening mechanism domain that mediate attainment of programme outcomes?

Research findings

Between March 2001 and February 2002, of the total number of the 667 clients referred to EXCEL:

- 43% attended the initial assessment only (n = 287)
- 15% attended both the initial and seven-week assessment (n = 100)
- 42% (n = 280) attended the initial, seven-week and 14-week assessments and were considered to be 'adherers' to the programmes

Consequently, adherence to the programme, during 2001–2002, was only 42%, but this rate of adherence is considerably more successful than many other types of community based, physical activity intervention. It is important that exercise referral schemes examine the characteristics of attendees and non-attendees so that potential modifications can be made to the programme in order to prevent this relatively high drop-out rate.

Referral is more prevalent in older clients, with the age category 46–60 years of age being the most prevalent. This is consistent with population statistics for Sefton Borough (Sefton Health Authority, 2001).

The most popular reason for referral was for being overweight (Figure 14.1), 39% (n = 262). When examined in conjunction with adherence data for the 14-week intervention (Table 14.1) overweight individuals had a lower than average adherence rate at 39%. This is an important finding, especially with the growing levels of obesity amongst socially deprived groups within the population.

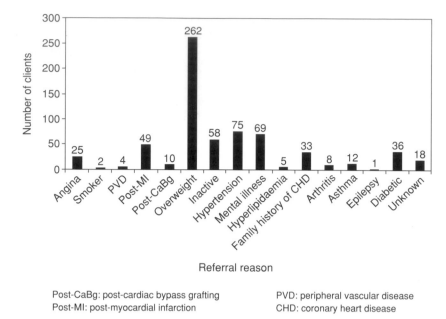

Post-CaBg: post-cardiac bypass grafting   PVD: peripheral vascular disease
Post-MI: post-myocardial infarction   CHD: coronary heart disease

Figure 14.1 Distribution of referrals according to primary referral reason.

Patients referred with myocardial infarction had one of the highest adherence rates, 61% (n = 49), possibly due to the fact that these individuals had taken part in a structured, tertiary-based, cardiac rehabilitation programme prior to attending the exercise referral scheme and had learned the necessary skills to sustain physical activity behaviour. The issue of varying adherence rates for different pathologies suggests that different mechanisms may be affecting the individuals in terms of exercise behaviour change.

Only mean diastolic blood pressure reduced significantly post-intervention ($p < 0.05$). The 14-week programme of exercise is probably too short, and practiced at too low a level of intensity, to change other physiological parameters significantly (Table 14.2). However, continued adherence after the end of the referral programme should lead to gradual improvements in these factors. Measurement of physiological parameters alone during an exercise referral audit can result in some of the other psychological benefits being missed, so it is recommended that any evaluation study should measure a *range* of relevant variables (for example, self-esteem, self efficacy, sustained physical activity behaviour).

The proportion of females referred 62% (n = 416) was greater than males 38% (n = 251), but the proportion of males completing the scheme (49%) was greater than females (37%). The higher proportion of females at the initial stages of the research is consistent with findings of other studies, for example Stevens et al. (1998) reported that initially 60% of subjects referred were women, and may be reflective of the higher presentation rate of women at their GP practice.

Adherence was found to increase with age. This may be due to the fact that younger individuals take part in physical activity for different reasons from those of the

Table 14.1 Primary referral reason (according to pathology) and subsequent adherence.

Referral reason	Total number referred	Percentage of those adhering to the 14-week programme
Angina	25	52%
Smoker	2	50%
PVD	4	75%
Post-MI	49	61%
Post-coronary artery bypass grafting	10	10%
Overweight	262	39%
Inactive	58	34%
Hypertension	75	43%
Mental illness	69	33%
Hyperlipidaemia	5	40%
Family history	33	33%
Arthritis	8	50%
Asthma	12	58%
Epilepsy	1	0%
Diabetic	36	55%
Unknown	18	0%

Table 14.2 Change in physiological parameters throughout the 14-week intervention period (n = 667).

Physiological parameters	Initial assessment	7 week assessment	14 week assessment
Weight (kg)	86.5	84.3	84.8
Body mass index (BMI)	31.5	30.9	30.9
Systolic BP (mmHg)	135.9	134.1	134.8
Diastolic BP (mmHg)	81.1	80.0	79.8
Heart rate (beats/min)	71.7	70.2	69.8

older population; thus, younger individuals may be more interested in issues of image whereas the older population may be more interested in taking part in physical activity for the purposes of health gain. Also, it could simply be due to an issue of time; older, retired individuals may have more time to commit to structured physical activity than younger counterparts.

GPs' views and opinions on the EXCEL programme

A postal questionnaire (2002) yielded a response rate of 26% (n = 38). In terms of the self-reported barriers that prevented GPs referring to the scheme: 20% of GPs cited lack of time to complete paperwork (exercise referral forms).

'I have found the referral process and forms a barrier to using a service that I otherwise really believe in.'

Table 14.3 GP ranking of health promotion services that are most utilised in Sefton.

	Smoking cessation	Dietary advice	Physical activity
1st	**67%**	10%	21%
2nd	8%	**48%**	21%
3rd	12%	21%	**35%**

Of the other reasons put forward, 20% cited time as a barrier, 6% cited lack of knowledge on their behalf, 15% thought that they lacked knowledge of the processes and aims of the EXCEL scheme, 12% were unsure as to the effectiveness of EXCEL in achieving behaviour change and 21% felt that patients did not take advice.

'Please, please, please sort out the referral process. This is a good scheme which is irritatingly difficult to access.'

In addition to the criteria stated on the questionnaire other issues included medico-legal implications for the GP and the process of referral.

'Lack of resolution as to who is clinically responsible if patient has a myocardial infarction etc, whilst attending the scheme. As a referral implies that I am still responsible.'

Of the GPs responding to the questionnaire, 31% (n = 15) indicated that they did not refer any patients to the scheme, whilst the remaining 69% indicated that they referred 1–3 patients to the scheme each week.

Table 14.3 shows how GPs in Sefton used the referral service. Smoking cessation was the most popular referral service for Sefton GPs. The most common reasons given for this were:

- Evidence of benefit: *'Cessation of smoking is so important for all aspects of health and we know we have an effect. Not evidence for other two as much.'*
- Efficiency of service and medico-legal responsibility: *'The protocols and clinical accountability are clear for dietician and smoking cessation'* and *'Smoking is an efficient service, diet, month long wait – demotivates. Exercise, medical recommendation is a medico-legal case waiting to happen.'*

In terms of the impact of the scheme only 25% (n = 12) of GPs thought that patients would adhere for the 14-week intervention period, and only 15% of GPs thought clients could sustain this behaviour in the long term. However, despite these seemingly disappointing opinions, 75% (n = 36) of GPs felt that EXCEL should become a mainstream funded service.

Summary of main findings

- Adherence was variable across age, gender and referral reason:
  — Older clients were more likely to adhere.

—   More females were referred, but, more males completed the scheme.
—   Clients who were overweight, hypertensive and suffered from depression
    had the highest rates of referral.

● Diastolic blood pressure was the only physiological parameter to show significant change pre- and post-intervention, and a focus on physiological change
  alone could lead to other benefits being missed.

● GPs had a wide range of views about the effectiveness of exercise referral. This
  suggests that data from the scheme should routinely be fed back to GPs (and
  other stakeholders) so as to enhance the learning about the referral process and
  its impacts.

● The main barriers preventing GPs referring to the scheme were concerns regarding medico-legal responsibility (in the case that a patient suffers a heart attack
  or similar event whilst exercising) and lack of knowledge about the operation
  of the scheme and its effectiveness.

Conclusions

Promoting physical activity is a complex activity that requires the input of many
professional groups to achieve success. Individual behaviour change models have
been unsuccessful in halting the trend towards sedentary behaviour in the UK.
Consequently, health promotion professionals now advocate the use of socio-
ecological models that reinforce behaviour change at every level of the system, from
health promoting policy (such as physical activity strategies), through supportive
environments and settings for behaviour change (such as workplaces that encourage physical activity), to the development of specific programmes and interventions
that target population groups that are most in need of physical activity involvement (such as exercise referral). More evaluation studies are needed to measure
the effectiveness of physical activity promotion at each of these levels of delivery
so that health practitioners can become more informed about the processes
involved and the successful components of a physical activity intervention.

Acknowledgements

The authors would like to thank Lee Evans and Robin Ireland for their involvement in the evaluation of the Liverpool Corporate Cup, and all the participants
who took part in the research case studies.

References

Ayres, R. and Pocock, E. (1995). Exercise on prescription. *British Journal of General
Practice* 46, 325–6.

Biddle, S., Fox, K. and Edmunds, L. (1994). *Physical Activity Promotion in Primary Health Care in England – Final Research Report for Health Education Authority*. Health Education Authority, London.

Bundred, P., Kitchiner, D. and Buchan, I. (2001). Prevalence of overweight and obese children between 1989 and 1998: population based series of cross-sectional studies. *British Medical Journal* **322**, 326–8.

Calnan, M.W. and Johnson, B.M. (1983). Influencing health behaviour: how significant is the general practitioner? *Health Education Journal* **42**, 39–45.

Caspersen, C.J., Powell, K.E. and Christenson, G.M. (1985). Physical activity, exercise and physical fitness: Definition and distinctions for health-related research. *Public Health Reports* **100**, 126–31.

Dahlgren, G. and Whitehead, M. (1991). Tackling inequalities: a review of policy initiatives. In: *Tackling Inequalities in Health: An Agenda for Action* (Benzeval, M., Judge, K. and Whitehead, M. eds). King's Fund Institute, London.

Department of Health (1999). *Saving Lives: Our Healthier Nation*. The Stationery Office, London.

Department of Health (2000a). *Health Survey for England*. The Stationery Office, London.

Department of Health (2000b). *National Service Framework: Coronary Heart Disease*. Department of Health, London.

Department of Health (2001). *Exercise Referral Systems: A National Quality Assurance Framework*. London, Department of Health.

Dooris, M. and Thompson, J. (2001). Ch. 14: Health promoting universities: an overview. In: *Health Promotion: Professional Perspectives* (Scriven, A. and Orme, J. eds). Palgrave, Hampshire.

Downie, R. and Macnaughton, J. (2001). Ch. 2: Images of health. In: *Working for Health, Open University* (Heller, T., Muston, R., Sidell, M. and Lloyd, C. eds). Sage, London.

Evans, L.J. (2002). 'Evaluating the effectiveness of corporate running events in the north west region'. M.Phil. thesis, Liverpool John Moores University, Liverpool.

Fox, K., Biddle, S., Edmunds, L., Bowler, I. and Killoran, A. (1997). Physical activity promotion through primary health care in England. *British Journal of General Practice* **47**, 367–9.

Harland, J., White, M., Drinkwater, C., Chinn, D., Farr, L. and Howel, D. (1999). The Newcastle exercise project: a randomised controlled trial to promote physical activity in primary care. *British Medical Journal* **319**, 828–32.

HEPA Guidelines (2000). *European Network for Health Enhancing Physical Activity*. British Heart Foundation, European Commission, Oxford University, Oxford.

Hillsdon, M. and Thorogood, M. (1996). A systematic review of physical activity promotion strategies. *British Journal of Sports Medicine* **30**, 84–9.

Hillsdon, M., Thorogood, M., White, I. and Foster, D. (2002). Advising people to take more exercise is ineffective: a randomised controlled trial of physical activity promotion in primary care. *International Journal of Epidemiology* **31**, 808–15.

Ireland, R. (2001). Ch. 10: Promoting physical activity with local authorities. In: *Health Promotion: Professional Perspectives* (Scriven, A. and Orme, J. eds). Palgrave, Hampshire.

Kaman, R.L. (1995). *Worksite Health Promotion Economics*. Human Kinetics, Leeds.

Lord, J.C. and Green, F. (1995). Exercise on prescription: does it work? *Health Education Journal* **54**, 453–64.

McKay, H.A., Macdonald, H., Reed, K.E. and Khan, K.M. (2003). Exercise interventions for health: time to focus on dimensions, delivery and dollars. *British Journal of Sports Medicine* **37**, 98–9.

Patton, M.Q. (1990). *Qualitative Evaluation and Research Methods*. Sage, London.

Popay, J. and Williams, G. (1994). *Researching the People's Health*. London, Routledge.

Porcellato, L., Dugdill, L., Springett, J. and Sanderson, F. (1999). Primary schoolchildren's perceptions of smoking: implications for health education. *Health Education Research* **14**(1), 71–83.

Puska, P. (2001). Commentary: physical activity promotion in primary care. *International Journal of Epidemiology* **30**, 815–6.

Riddoch, C., Puig-Ribera, A. and Cooper, A. (1998). *Effectiveness of Physical Activity Promotion Schemes in Primary Care: A Review*. Health Education Authority, London.

Sallis, J.F. and Owen, N. (1999). *Physical Activity and Behavioural Medicine*. Sage, London.

Scriven, A. and Orme, J. (2001). *Health Promotion: Professional Perspectives*. Palgrave, Hampshire.

Sefton Health Authority (2001). *Sefton's Health: The Annual Report of the Director of Public Health*. Sefton Health Authority, Sefton.

Smith, B.J., Bauman, A.E., Bull, F.C., Booth, M.L. and Harris, M.F. (2000). Promoting physical activity in general practice: a controlled trial of written advice and information materials. *British Journal of Sports Medicine* **34**, 262–7.

Sport England (2003). *Young People and Sport in England: Trends in Participation 1994–2002*. Sport England, London.

Stevens, W., Hillsdon, M., Thorogood, M. and McArdle, D. (1998). Cost-effectiveness of a primary care based physical activity intervention in 45–74 year-old men and women: a randomised controlled trial. *British Journal of Sports Medicine* **32**, 236–41.

Stokols, D. (1992). Establishing and maintaining healthy environments: towards a social ecology of health promotion. *American Psychologist* **47**(1), 6–22.

Tai, S., Gould, M., Smith, P. and Iliffe, S. (1999). Promoting physical activity in general practice: should prescribed exercise be free? *Journal of the Royal Society of Medicine* **92**, 65–7.

Taylor, A., Doust, J. and Webborn, N. (1998). Randomised controlled trial to examine the effects of a GP exercise referral programme in Hailsham, East Sussex, on modifiable coronary heart disease risk factors. *Journal of Epidemiology and Community Health* **52**, 595–601.

United States Department of Health and Human Services (1996). *Physical Activity and Health: A Report of the Surgeon General*. US Department of Health and Human Services, Centers for Disease Control and Prevention, National Center for Chronic Disease Prevention and Promotion, Atlanta.

INDEX